T0177729

Precision Medicine and Distributive Justice

Precision Medicine and Distributive Justice

Wicked Problems for Democratic Deliberation

LEONARD M. FLECK

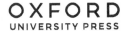

OXFORD
UNIVERSITY PRESS

Oxford University Press is a department of the University of Oxford. It furthers
the University's objective of excellence in research, scholarship, and education
by publishing worldwide. Oxford is a registered trade mark of Oxford University
Press in the UK and certain other countries.

Published in the United States of America by Oxford University Press
198 Madison Avenue, New York, NY 10016, United States of America.

Library of Congress Cataloging-in-Publication Data
Names: Fleck, Leonard M., author.
Title: Precision medicine and distributive justice : wicked problems for
democratic deliberation / Leonard M. Fleck, Ph.D.
Description: New York, NY : Oxford University Press, [2022] | Includes bibliographical references.
Identifiers: LCCN 2022025824 (print) | LCCN 2022025825 (ebook) |
ISBN 9780197647721 (hardcover) | ISBN 9780197647745 (epub)
Subjects: LCSH: Medical care, Cost of—Moral and ethical aspects—United States. |
Personalized medicine—Costs—United States. |
Health care rationing—Moral and ethical aspects—United States. |
Public health—Moral and ethical aspects—United States. |
Personalized medicine—Moral and ethical aspects—United States. |
Health services accessibility—United States. | Right to health—United States. |
Health care reform—United States. | Social justice—United States.
Classification: LCC RA410.53 .F63 2022 (print) | LCC RA410.53 (ebook) |
DDC 338.4/33621—dc23/eng/20220615
LC record available at https://lccn.loc.gov/2022025824
LC ebook record available at https://lccn.loc.gov/2022025825

DOI: 10.1093/oso/9780197647721.001.0001

This material is not intended to be, and should not be considered, a substitute for medical or other
professional advice. Treatment for the conditions described in this material is highly dependent on the
individual circumstances. And, while this material is designed to offer accurate information with respect
to the subject matter covered and to be current as of the time it was written, research and knowledge about
medical and health issues is constantly evolving and dose schedules for medications are being revised
continually, with new side effects recognized and accounted for regularly. Readers must therefore always
check the product information and clinical procedures with the most up-to-date published product
information and data sheets provided by the manufacturers and the most recent codes of conduct and
safety regulation. The publisher and the authors make no representations or warranties to readers, express
or implied, as to the accuracy or completeness of this material. Without limiting the foregoing, the
publisher and the authors make no representations or warranties as to the accuracy or efficacy of the drug
dosages mentioned in the material. The authors and the publisher do not accept, and expressly disclaim,
any responsibility for any liability, loss, or risk that may be claimed or incurred as a consequence of the use
and/or application of any of the contents of this material.

1 3 5 7 9 8 6 4 2

Printed by Integrated Books International, United States of America

To Jean: My partner
In life
In love
In labor

Contents

Contents

Acknowledgements

This book began during a sabbatical at the Brocher Foundation outside Geneva Switzerland. I am grateful for the hospitality of the Foundation during those five months as well as my fellow bioethics researchers with whom we shared many good meals and even more productive conversations.

I need to offer a special word of thanks to Mitchell Pawlak, MD, who was my undergraduate professorial assistant for four years at Michigan State University from 2011-2015. He introduced me to the wealth of literature emerging regarding precision medicine. He proved to be an outstanding intellectual companion for this journey. He earned his medical degree at the University of Buffalo and is now completing his residency training.

I am grateful to Michigan State University and the College of Human Medicine for the time needed to complete the research and writing for this book. I am especially grateful to my physician colleagues who endured my persistent questioning regarding many of the details regarding precision medicine and oncology.

Most of the work in this volume has been presented at numerous bioethics conferences, such as the American Society for Bioethics and Humanities, the Paris Retreats sponsored by Cambridge University Press, the European Society for the Philosophy of Medicine and Health Care, the International Society for Priorities in health, and the biomarker conferences sponsored by the University of Bergen. I am most appreciative for the comments and discussion proffered by my bioethics and health policy colleagues at those conferences, especially Dr. Thomasine Kushner for multiple invitations to the Paris Retreats.

Finally, I thank Springer publishers for permission to use large portions of an essay I did: "Precision Health and Ethical Ambiguity: How Much Cancer Can We Afford to Prevent?" in *Precision Oncology and Cancer Biomarkers: Issues at Stake and Matters of Concern*, edited by Anne Bremer and Roger Strand (Springer, early 2022), chapter 13. This material is now part of Chapter 8 in this volume.

Leonard M. Fleck, Ph.D. May 2, 2022

A Provocative Prologue

I think I can safely assume that anyone reading this book has some significant familiarity with precision medicine, targeted cancer therapies, and immunotherapies. What you likely understand is that precision medicine in the context of oncology is about using various pharmacologic agents to disrupt the further spread of a metastatic cancer at the molecular level. Two dominant messages have been part of that medical reporting. The first is that these interventions are described with a range of scientific and medical superlatives, such as "breakthrough," "game changer," "revolutionary," "transformative," "lifesaving," and so on (Feller, 2015; Abola and Prasad, 2016). Likewise, medical centers have not been shy in their use of superlative language. The University of Chicago Medical Center (2018) had as its website banner "Supercharging Your Blood Cells to Defeat Cancer" (as opposed to "Doing Our Best to Buy You a Little More Time on Earth with Your Cancer").

The second message is that these targeted cancer therapies and immunotherapies are extraordinarily expensive by any standard. By late 2020 approximately 150 of these cancer therapies had received Food and Drug Administration approval as well as approval for coverage by Medicare. Virtually all of them have a cost of $100,000 or more for a course of treatment (or a year of treatment) with front-end costs of $475,000 for a form of immunotherapy that uses chimeric antigen receptor T cells. These drugs are generally used with metastatic cancer, a terminal illness. Given these costs and given the hyperbolic language used to characterize the effectiveness of these drugs, one would expect that these patients are gaining extra years of life of reasonable quality. In fact, however, the clear majority of these patients who have access to these drugs will gain no more than extra weeks or extra months of life (Walker, 2018; Szabo, 2018), when compared to current available cancer therapies. A small number of patients might gain an extra year or two. A very small number of patients, often referred to as "super-responders," will gain several extra years of life.

This book is about ethics and health policy. More specifically, I intend to address what I refer to as the "just caring" problem in the context of precision medicine. The just caring problem is best captured in this question: What does it mean to be a "just" and "caring" society when we have only limited resources to meet virtually unlimited health care needs? The term "limited resources" refers to the money we are willing to spend as taxpayers or insurance premium payers to purchase health care services. The term "unlimited health care needs" refers to the fact that what we judge to be health needs (as opposed to mere desires that do not represent medical necessity) has been rapidly expanding since the early 1970s as emerging medical technologies effectively create new needs. Cardiac bypass surgery, organ transplantations, intensive care unit (ICU) care, kidney dialysis, and, of course, these targeted cancer therapies are all illustrative of this point. The word "need," as a term with ethical connotations, is quite apt, given that patients with the relevant disease process who are denied access to these technologies will suffer severe, irreversible health consequences, such as premature death. A "caring" society, with an abundance of all these therapeutic technologies, could hardly continue to think of itself as caring if it permitted hundreds of thousands of patients with these needs to be denied access to these technologies. For the most part (not completely), the United States has tried to be a caring and compassionate society seeking to meet all these health needs for those with the relevant medical problems.[1] Why then do we need to address the just caring problem?

The primary implication of the just caring problem (limited resources, unlimited needs) is that there are limits to our ability to meet all medically legitimate health care needs. Health care spending is crowding out other important social needs that require funding from social budgets (governmental and non-governmental). To provide a quick statistical picture, in 1960 in the United States we spent a total of $26 billion on health care, 5.2% of gross domestic product (GDP) at the time, roughly $240 billion in 2020 inflation-adjusted dollars. In 2020 in the United States, we spent $4.0 trillion on health care, or 17.9% of our present GDP (Keehan et al., 2020). On this trend line, projections to 2027 put aggregate US health spending at $5.96 trillion, or

---

[1] This sentence fairly represents the efforts of the not-for-profit portions of our health care system. However, more than 40% of the US health care system operates in the for-profit mode. This is true for 25% of our hospitals, the large majority of long-term care facilities and assisted-living facilities, home care agencies, hospice programs, occupational therapy offices, physical therapy offices, medical equipment makers, private insurance companies, and, of course, pharmaceutical companies. For a trenchant assessment of what this means for patients needing care, see Rosenthal (2017), *An American Sickness: How Healthcare Became Big Business and How You Can Take It Back.* See also Brill (2015), *America's Bitter Pill: Money, Politics, Backroom Deals, and the Fight to Fix Our Broken Healthcare System.*

20% of projected GDP (Sisko et al., 2019). There is nothing intrinsically un-ethical about spending all that money on health care.

Despite all that spending on health care, we must also take note of the fact that in 2020 we still had over 30 million individuals without any health in-surance and, hence, no access or only uncertain, marginal access to needed health care. In addition, another 40 million Americans had very inadequate health insurance with very high deductibles or co-payment requirements such that they were forced to deny themselves and their family members costly needed care because they were unable to pay for that care.[2] These indi-viduals had relatively inexpensive health insurance because that was all they could afford, or that was all their employers were willing to pay for as a ben-efit of employment. As aggregate health costs have increased steadily since the late 1980s, more and more employers have either ceased offering health insurance as a benefit, required employees to pay a larger share of the an-nual premium, or provided only skimpy health insurance (high deductibles, narrow provider networks). You might be inclined to think this is just an awkward and unfortunate economic problem for families that find them-selves in this situation. However, some research shows that as many as 45,000 Americans die prematurely each year because of a lack of health insurance that would otherwise pay for the effective health care that would have saved their lives (Wilper et al., 2009; Woolhandler and Himmelstein, 2017). A sta-tistic such as this makes it more difficult to characterize the American health care system as "caring," unless we attach an asterisk to that term.

As noted already, the just caring problem implies limits regarding access to needed health care. "Limits" means that not everyone can get everything that has any therapeutic value for meeting health care needs. This is often referred to as the problem of health care rationing or health care priority-setting. This is what generates the ethical problem of distributive health care justice. Some philosophers and policy analysts will assert that we live in a capitalistic society, which implies that you have a "right" only to those goods and services you are able to pay for, including health care. This is a very harsh view if you were to put such a view into practice. It would mean we would turn away from hospital emergency rooms individuals who could not pay

---

[2] Papanicolas et al. (2018) write: "The United States spends more per capita on health care than any other nation, substantially outpacing even other very high-income countries. However, despite its higher spending, the United States performs poorly in areas such as health care coverage and health outcomes. Higher spending without commensurate improved health outcomes at the population level has been a strong impetus for health care reform in the United States" (at 1024).

for the lifesaving care they needed immediately. In effect, we would direct such patients to reserved space in the hospital parking lot where they could die without interfering with hospital routine. This is unthinkable for anyone with a microgram of ethical sensitivity for a conscience. However, the exact opposite is equally unthinkable.

Imagine a patient with end-stage metastatic cancer who will die within the next two weeks. Imagine that we have a very rare drug that cost $1 million and that would give that individual one extra week of life. Are we, citizens of a society that aspires to be just and caring, ethically obligated, as a matter of justice, to provide that drug to that individual at social expense? I doubt that any of my readers would believe we were ethically obligated to do that. That thought experiment demonstrates that we do respect the need for limits regarding health care spending, even when that spending is technically connected to saving/prolonging a life. If we had to offer an ethical justification for concluding that it was ethically acceptable (not unjust) to deny that patient that extra week of life that was going to cost $1 million, we might say that that was too little medical good at much too high a price. We might also wonder whether there was anything "ethically special" about that patient. They were in the end stages of their cancer. We might consider that their terminal status generated some sort of special claim on health care resources. However, more than 610,000 Americans die every year of some form of cancer. If our hypothetical patient were not absolutely, uniquely special, then moral logic would seem to require that we be prepared to spend comparable extravagant sums for every cancer patient who would desire some gain in life expectancy *or some chance of gain.*

In my original thought experiment, I made it clear that it was certain this patient would gain that extra week of life for $1 million. Consider some alternative thought experiments. Would a just and caring society be ethically obligated as a matter of justice to provide a patient with a cancer drug that cost $1 million but was certain to give that patient six extra months of life of acceptable quality? I suspect I will lose some readers on that scenario, that you would think that six months is significant but that a mere week is not ethically significant. Consider another scenario. In this next scenario, we have a cancer drug that costs $1 million, and it promises a 10% chance of six extra months of life. That six extra months is still ethically significant, but now only 1 of every 10 patients would realize that benefit, which would mean that the real aggregated cost of achieving that outcome would be $10 million. Of course, it is easy to imagine that each of those patients would see *their cost* *to society as being only $1 million.* What is a just and caring society ethically obligated to do in this latter scenario?

Consider another scenario, one that might be called a thought experiment but that reflects a situation in the real world. Patients with cystic fibrosis have a limited life expectancy, roughly 30–40 years on average. They have cystic fibrosis because of a genetic deficiency (Phe508del) that results in a failure of their body to produce a key protein necessary for proper lung functioning. Today (in 2021) there are at least three drugs that can at least partially correct for that deficiency. Ivacaftor is the generic name of one of those drugs; lumacaftor and tezacaftor are the other two (Holguin, 2018). This is part of precision medicine. Each of these drugs costs $300,000 per year, but each might add 10–20 years to the life expectancy of these patients.[3] Unlike targeted cancer drugs given to patients in the later stages of cancer, these drugs would be taken early on. If a patient lived with one of these drugs for 30 years (at current prices), the aggregated cost over those years would be $9 million. Is a just and caring society ethically obligated, as a matter of justice, to make certain that eligible patients had secure access to these drugs, whether or not those families had the financial ability to pay for these drugs? Keep in mind that these are all patients in the early stages of life.

It should be noted that for a cystic fibrosis patient to gain 10 extra years of life, they would have to have been taking the drug for 30 years. That means that the actual cost of each year of life gained would be $900,000.[4] Would you, the reader, still argue that a just and caring society was ethically obligated to provide this drug at social expense to these patients? Next, I ask you to compare this situation to that of a patient with metastatic cancer who needs $150,000 worth of some targeted cancer therapy to gain two extra months of life. If we agree to provide this drug to this patient (and all others like this patient), then we are saying (from an economist's perspective) that we are

---

[3] No one knows at this time whether this drug, or some combination of these three cystic fibrosis drugs, will yield one or two extra years of life for these patients. It could be a decade or longer before we would have a correct answer to this question. This raises a problem of health care justice. These drugs have some beneficial effect right now, but long-term gains in life expectancy might still be marginal. Would a just and caring society be justified in providing the drug only to patients in a clinical trial for some number of years until a definitive answer is achieved? If the drug proved successful, the ethical cost of that strategy would be the preventable deaths of other cystic fibrosis patients outside that trial. On the other hand, if these drugs were provided to all cystic fibrosis patients beginning immediately and if it turned that out overall gains in life expectancy were marginal, billions of dollars would have been wasted that could otherwise have been used for other life-prolonging interventions. This is one example of what we later identify as a "wicked problem."

[4] The Institute for Clinical and Economic Review (2018) has done formal economic analysis and concluded that the cost per life-year gained would be $1.2 million to $1.5 million.

willing to spend $600,000 for an extra year of life. This is what economists refer to as the "incremental cost-effectiveness" of that drug. The question I pose to you, my reader, is this: If we are willing to spend $900,000 for each *extra* year of life for a cystic fibrosis patient, are we ethically obligated, as a matter of ethical consistency, to purchase those extra months of life for our cancer patients, given that those years are less expensive? The just caring problem is about limits. Who should decide what those limits ought to be? Is this for Congress to decide? Is this for your state legislature to decide? Is this for each insurance company to decide? Is this for an employer to decide? Should this be decided by an individual's personal ability to pay? These are additional examples of "wicked problems." Let us go back to our scenarios.

What sort of ethically relevant considerations would you believe are relevant to answering our questions? We have limited resources. We must do some priority-setting. Should we give higher priority to our cystic fibrosis patients or to our patients with late-stage cancers? We might start with the recognition that both sorts of patients are faced with a terminal prognosis. However, our cystic fibrosis patients have many more years of life at stake than our cancer patients, who generally have extra months of life to gain rather than extra years. Moreover, our cystic fibrosis patients will always be much younger (have had less opportunity to live a life) compared to the clear majority of late-stage cancer patients. Should these two considerations be ethically decisive in not awarding priority to our cancer patients?

Alternatively, should the fact that death is imminent for our metastatic cancer patients be decisive in giving them ethical priority for our limited resources, given that we have no alternative therapeutic interventions? Does our sense of compassion require this? Often, we judge to be morally relevant for priority-setting purposes giving priority to those who are "medically worse off." Are our cancer patients correctly judged to be more medically worse off than our cystic fibrosis patients? What are the criteria for making comparative judgments regarding who is medically worse off? Is that a judgment that should be made at a point in time? Alternatively, should we consider a whole lifetime for comparative purposes? Should it be ethically relevant that the actual cost (real dollars expended) for any one cancer patient (maybe $200,000) is so much less than what we would expend for a cystic fibrosis patient (maybe $9 million over 30 years)? Alternatively, from the perspective of public budgets and real aggregated dollars expended annually, there are about 30,000 Americans alive with cystic fibrosis today (potential recipients of ivacaftor or tezacaftor) compared to more than 600,000 patients who will die of metastatic cancer this year (potential recipients of a targeted cancer therapy). To put this in numerical terms, if all those cystic fibrosis patients received ivacaftor or tezacaftor, the aggregated cost would be $9 billion annually, compared to $60 billion annually if all those metastatic cancer patients received a targeted cancer drug. Should these economic numbers tip the balance toward priority for cystic fibrosis patients? Still more "wicked problems" for consideration.

I am sure some clinicians might be reading these prefatory comments. I can imagine their thinking with considerable frustration, "These are just the worst sort of philosophic examples. We are ethically obligated to provide the life-prolonging drugs that are available to all these patients. Granted, we must reduce the overall costs for health care in our society. We should do that by getting rid of wasteful and low-value uses of health care resources. We should be doing far fewer diagnostic CT and MRI scans." In 2015 in the United States, we did 80 million computed tomography (CT) scans and about 32 million magnetic resonance imaging (MRI) scans (Papanicolas et al., 2018). Many of these would be judged to be of questionable value, both medically and economically. I agree that this is a reasonable response. However, I also need to point out that it is more difficult in actual clinical practice to identify "low-value" care. Very few diagnostic or therapeutic interventions represent low-value care in all the clinical circumstances where they might be employed. The classic example of low-value care is the patient with a severe tension headache who wants a CT or MRI scan to rule out brain cancer. The likelihood that that patient would have both a very stressful life and brain cancer is very remote. Still, some very small number of patients will have both stressful lives and brain cancer. That cancer will now be missed, with potentially tragic consequences as a result. Is that outcome ethically problematic?

In that connection, consider a 56-year-old patient with metastatic lung cancer who can be given a targeted cancer drug at a cost of $75,000 that will *most likely* yield an extra month of life, though there would be a very small chance that they *might be* a very strong responder and gain two extra years of life. Does that drug represent "low-value" care? Again, the clear majority of patients in this circumstance would only get a very marginal benefit at a very high cost. At present, we have no way of identifying before the fact which individuals might turn out to be very strong responders. If we deny the drug to that whole cohort of patients because we (societal decision makers with limited resources for unlimited health needs) judge that use of resources to be of low value, should we conclude that any premature loss of life, ethically speaking, should be considered tragic and unfortunate, not unjust? Should we think of this as being in the same category of low-value care as our patient with a stressful life and brain cancer? The wickedness is spreading.

Perhaps you are tempted to make a distinction. Perhaps you find it ethically troubling (unjust and uncaring) that we would deny metastatic cancer patients a drug that might yield some life-prolonging benefit for them. If so, then we need to ask whether metastatic cancer patients with an imminent terminal prognosis are in any sense "ethically special." That is, do they deserve more in the way of life-prolonging resources, as a matter of justice, than, say, patients with various forms of late-stage heart disease or non-cancerous late-stage lung or liver disease? I cannot think of any ethically relevant considerations that would justify an affirmative answer to that question. Cancer seems to be more dreaded as a disease process than almost any other disease process (Mukherjee, 2012). However, that social or psychological fact has virtually no ethical weight. It does not make cancer an "ethically special" disease for which a disproportionate share of life-prolonging resources would be justified.

It seems obvious that if we (societal decision makers with limited resources) were to provide unlimited sums of money to provide late-stage cancer patients with any therapeutic intervention, no matter how small the life-prolonging gain, and if we offered nothing comparable to patients with other late-stage terminal prognoses, those other patients could rightly complain that they were treated unjustly. Perhaps this ethical challenge could be resolved through being more inclusive. Should we endorse a social policy that would guarantee to all individuals with a late-stage chronic degenerative condition any intervention that would offer any degree of benefit (postponing death) at whatever cost? This proposal certainly has the appearance of generous and inclusive compassion. However, would such social compassion also be just, all things considered (such as non-terminal health care needs)? In addition, would such social compassion be economically reasonable, given limited monetary resources?

Inclusive compassion is ethically desirable. However, what do we imagine are the boundaries of that inclusiveness? Are we including all patients with a chronic degenerative condition and a terminal prognosis, perhaps because such patients would be regarded as being among the medically least well off, and therefore deserving of more health care resources? However, what are the boundaries for having a "terminal prognosis"? Patients diagnosed with end-stage renal disease have a terminal prognosis, though they can survive for an indefinite number of years with access to renal dialysis. Patients with rheumatoid arthritis also have a terminal prognosis, as well as patients with multiple sclerosis or congestive heart failure or chronic obstructive pulmonary disease or amyotrophic lateral sclerosis, and the list goes on and on. No doubt, all these patients have serious health needs that often require costly medical interventions to slow disease progression and forestall for as long as possible reaching the terminal phase of the disease.

We might conclude that this way of thinking about all these patients is "too inclusive" because they are not "terminal enough." That is, they are not imminently terminal, which is what would elicit that strong compassionate response. Consequently, we can embrace the hospice (bureaucratic) sense of being terminal, meaning a predicted life expectancy of less than six months. That puts some "reasonable" boundaries around that cohort of patients who would have presumptively just claims to unlimited health care resources that might yield any gain at all in life prolongation no matter what the cost. However, we again need to recall that we are faced with resource limits. We must ask ourselves: Are we committed to the view that this category of patients should be thought of as our highest-priority cohort of patients so far as health care justice is concerned? If we are committed to that view, then one practical implication is that we might have many fewer resources to provide those patients in earlier stages of those chronic degenerative conditions. That would mean that many of these patients would progress more quickly to the strictly terminal phases of their disease process, where they would then garner loads of social compassion. They would also garner unlimited access to life-prolonging medical resources, though those resources would generally yield a lot less in the way of medical benefit compared to having those resources securely provided at an earlier stage in their disease process. The ethical wickedness is getting thicker and more pervasive as we consider the implications of precision medicine.

From a purely rational, prudentially self-interested point of view, it makes the most sense to invest limited life-prolonging health care resources in the earlier stages of a disease process, where they would do more health good at a lower cost per unit of health gained. Nevertheless, if we were to reallocate resources away from patients in the very late stages of a terminal illness to earlier stages of that illness, that would still have some awkward social consequences. More specifically, physicians would have to face patients in these very late stages and say something like this, "I know you have read about drugs that we used to provide to patients like you in the very late stages of an illness. Occasionally, those drugs yielded a significant gain in life expectancy, though for the clear majority of patients the gains were only a few months. It was decided [a deliberately impersonal 'it'] then that it made more sense to spend that money earlier in the disease process where we believed it would do more good. Likely, you have been a beneficiary of that policy change. Consequently, neither Medicare nor your insurance plan are willing to pay for the drugs we used to use this late in the disease process. You need to consider hospice." Many patients would not graciously accept this conclusion. They would not have heard from that physician that the therapeutic interventions no longer covered did little good and caused excessive pointless suffering for patients. On the contrary, they would have heard that some patients (maybe only a small minority) might have gained an extra year of life. Those were the patients, they would believe, who were fighters. These patients would see themselves as fighters who at least deserved a chance to gain an extra year of life. They would expect their doctors to be strong advocates for them, not lackeys for some insurance company.

Maybe this scenario is too dramatic; maybe it is not dramatic enough. Maybe this scenario is just unrealistic. Any such policy proposal in our world would instantly elicit the rhetoric of "death panels," condemning patients to a premature death for the sake of saving money. The moral imperative that would seem to drive this sort of commitment might be stated this way: "We should never deny individuals access to effective life-prolonging therapies, no matter what the cost, most especially when those individuals have no other life-prolonging alternatives and are faced with death in the relatively near-term future." This imperative has a compelling compassionate ring to it. Perhaps we ought to embrace this imperative. Before doing that, however, maybe we ought to consider another perspective.

We need to realize we are only saving brief extensions of lives with a small number of exceptions. More desirable would be embracing a prevention strategy. For example, several recent news accounts have called attention to "liquid biopsies" able to detect circulating cancer cells in the blood for eight common cancers (Kaiser, 2018). These tests are intended for use when there is a suspicion of cancer in an early stage. However, the presence of such circulating cancer cells would not necessarily mean either that a cancer had established itself somewhere or that it was certain to establish itself somewhere relatively soon (Cha, 2015). A company called Grail is seeking to identify such "homeless" circulating cancer cells with a test that costs $300. We will pass over the obvious risk of overdiagnosis associated with this technology (Mukherjee, 2018). We will assume instead that this technology could indeed identify some number of either very-early-stage cancer patients or future possible cancer patients whose lives might have otherwise ended prematurely with a deadly metastatic cancer. At present, no empirical evidence exists that these tests could prevent 10% or 20% or 50% of future possible metastatic cancer deaths. We pass over this concern as well.[5]

The health care justice question is whether a just and caring society would be ethically obligated to underwrite the cost of this test through Medicare, Medicaid, or mandates on private insurance companies. If so, there would be 200 million anxious adult Americans who would be eligible for this screening test four times per year at an annual cost of $1200, or an aggregated annual cost of about $240 billion for this test alone (not any of the follow-up cancer care that might be required). If we thought this was a poor use of social resources, we might appease our consciences with the thought that none of these individuals is imminently dying. Hence, neither medical nor moral urgency would require social funding for this test. We might hypothesize, for the sake of argument, that 20,000 lives might be saved annually from a premature death from cancer, but these might be dismissed as just "statistical lives"—no names, no faces, unlike actual patients with metastatic cancer. Hence, those 20,000 "lives" really do not have any moral weight. Do you, the reader, agree with that conclusion?

How should we think about that potential $240 billion in annual costs for that test? That surely seems as if it would create a huge distortion in any just or reasonable allocation of health care resources. Further, two-thirds of those 200 million potential users of the test would never develop cancer for their entire life. Of course, we have no idea who the other third is who will develop some form of cancer, most of whom are now treated and cured in relatively early stages. This last sentence is not entirely accurate. Several million of those individuals could be members of so-called cancer families. They would be at elevated risk of developing cancer, perhaps somewhat earlier in life. Those are the individuals, it might be argued, that a just and caring society should provide with these liquid biopsy tests at social cost (not

---

[5] More recently (2021), Grail has introduced a yet more sophisticated version of a liquid biopsy that can detect more than 50 types of circulating cancer cells at a cost of $ 950. In theory, every adult American (200 million+) could have such a test every year. Do the math!! Would that be a good buy with public resources?

personal cost). I imagine that many of my readers would endorse this conclusion. However, complexities abound in what seems like a simple and clear
commitment.

How does one identify an eligible "cancer family"? We might say that if
an individual has three or more first-degree relatives diagnosed with cancer,
that will identify a cancer family. Does it matter (for just resource allocation
purposes) that none of those three relatives died of their cancer, that they
were all successfully treated (without need for any costly liquid biopsy)?
What if one of them did in fact die of their cancer at age 65? What if all three
relatives died of their cancer at ages 74, 78, and 82? After all, cancer is largely
a disease of the elderly. None of these individuals would have died prematurely, at least relative to average life expectancy. Should we then conclude
that a current 30-year-old in such a family would not have a just claim to have
a liquid biopsy covered at social expense?

Some cancers have very definite links to specific DNA mutations (e.g.,
Lynch syndrome or breast cancer linked to mutations in BRCA1). Most
cancers, however, are linked either to DNA damage caused by a very broad
range of environmental factors or else to complex causal relationships among
multiple genes that might result in a lifetime risk of cancer of 2% or 10%
or 20% and so on. Soon, we might be able to do whole genome sequencing
of an individual at an early age and provide a small percentage range of the
lifetime risk of some cancer for that individual. What number would be
sufficient, such that a just and caring society would be ethically obligated
to provide an individual with that liquid biopsy test four times per year at
social cost? This question does not have an obvious answer. Relative to the
resource needs of cystic fibrosis patients, should the cancer risk percentage
be set somewhat high so that fewer resources are devoted to liquid biopsies,
thereby making more resources available for cystic fibrosis patients *with an
actual disease process established*? Likewise, relative to the resource needs
of patients with metastatic cancer, should the cancer risk percentage be set
somewhat high so that fewer resources are devoted to liquid biopsies, thereby
making more resources available for those patients in the advanced stages of
a life-threatening cancer? This is what is known in the literature (Callahan,
1990) as the "ragged edge" problem. How are we, citizens in a just and caring
society, supposed to determine where a justice-relevant line should be drawn
when nature does not provide us with a bright objective basis for such a line?
Wickedness is ubiquitous.

Now you understand why this is a "provocative preface." Precision medicine may have many of the virtues associated with the term "precision." Nevertheless, precision medicine is also the source of considerable ethical ambiguity. In Chapter 1, I provide a sketch of what precision medicine is in practice. Among other things, it is important to understand the complexity and wiliness of cancer, which generates the problem of cancer drug resistance. Despite the accuracy of these targeted cancer therapies, metastatic cancers survive and advance toward their deadly goal. These biological facts, in conjunction with the extraordinarily high cost of these targeted therapies, create more challenging ethical problems, most especially about health care justice. If we had unlimited resources for meeting all health care needs, no problem of health care justice would exist. However, that is contrary to fact. Moreover, no single conception of health care justice can respond adequately to the ethical complexity associated with the medical complexity of cancer and its treatment. This is directly related to the "ragged edge" problem. Consequently, I argue, the most we can hope to achieve in this regard is "rough justice," outcomes that can garner reasonable agreement through respectful democratic deliberation.

I provide several personal stories of patients who have benefited from precision cancer medicine in Chapter 1. Those stories are ethically important. If we, as a society, must address the just caring problem, if we must make rationing and priority-setting decisions because we cannot afford to do everything for everyone that might yield any degree of medical benefit, then the ultimate consequences will fall upon individual patients and the physicians charged with caring responsibly and compassionately for those patients. Recall that in 2020 we spent $4.0 trillion on health care in the United States. Somewhere between 70% and 80% of those dollars are effectively spent by physicians who are authorized to establish a diagnosis, recommend a treatment plan, prescribe drugs, approve home health care, and so on. That means in practice that policy efforts to control health care costs will focus considerable attention on managing the behavior of physicians. From an ethical perspective, it is one thing to incentivize physicians to be more parsimonious in ordering diagnostic tests. Withholding what metastatic cancer patients perceive to be very expensive life-prolonging targeted therapies, however, would appear to be considerably more ethically problematic. A recent headline from *Stat News* (Ross, 2018) says it all: "A New Cancer Care Dilemma: Patients Want Immunotherapy Even When Evidence Is Lacking."

In Chapter 2, I review the medical literature in more detail regarding several of the more common metastatic cancers and cutting-edge therapeutic interventions aimed at addressing those cancers. Despite the medical precision of these targeted therapies, only a minority of patients achieve any substantial benefit, as measured by progression-free survival or overall survival. From an economic perspective, none of these drugs reflect reasonable cost-effectiveness. From an ethical perspective, do these economic facts have any relevance for addressing the problems of health care justice? Alternatively, should the fact that these patients have a terminal prognosis and no alternative therapeutic interventions be ethically decisive, no matter what the economic cost? Earlier, however, we saw that virtually no one would endorse spending $1 million to provide a cancer patient with an extra week of life. That suggests that cost matters. How should we decide how and when cost should matter so far as the just allocation of health care resources is concerned?

Chapter 3 introduces the notion of "wicked problems." Very briefly, the core element of a wicked problem is that every proposed solution seems to be as problematic as the problem that was supposed to be solved. I will argue that the problems of health care justice generated by precision cancer medicine are of the wicked variety. To give just a brief illustration, precision medicine, just like the rest of medicine, is peppered with diagnostic, prognostic, and therapeutic uncertainty, much of it related to the molecular complexity of metastatic cancer and its ability to mutate around these targeted therapies. On top of that, these drugs are extremely expensive and yield only marginal gains in life expectancy for the clear majority of patients who receive them. However, a small number of patients gain more than a year of life, sometimes several years, though we generally do not know who those super-responders might be. However, research is being pursued to identify biomarkers that would yield that information. What then, ethically speaking?

Could we justify not "wasting" resources on patients we knew before the fact would be only marginal responders? That might be a reasonable response from the perspective of a utilitarian conception of health care justice. How does that square with either a moderate or a strict egalitarian conception of health care justice? Should it matter, for resource allocation purposes, that some cancers are clearly a result of "bad health choices" individuals might have made, as a luck egalitarian would emphasize? Alternatively, should the morally decisive consideration be, for resource allocation purposes, that all these individuals with metastatic cancers are facing death soon, as prioritarians would emphasize? These individuals are among the medically "least well off." Should we conclude instead that these individuals are "beyond the domain of justice," that social compassion might warrant providing these targeted therapies at social expense? In other words, in the strict sense, metastatic cancer patients would not be treated unjustly if these drugs were not provided.

We think of compassion, a charitable response, as something freely given. Individuals are not open to moral criticism for donating to heart disease rather than cancer. Is the same true when we are talking about governmental resources? Sufficientarians are committed to the view that we owe everyone in our society access to a decent or adequate or sufficient level of health care as a matter of justice. No one has a just claim to health care beyond a sufficiency threshold. How should we, citizens in a just and caring society, decide where that threshold lies? Further, how medically or ethically appropriate can a single threshold be, given the heterogeneity and complexity of many health problems, not to mention the uncertainty of an effective therapeutic intervention? Finally, the need for complex and contentious social judgments in all these matters seems to disappear if we adopt a libertarian view and agree that no one has a just claim to any health care they might need if they are unable to pay for that health care. That would seem to result in a greatly attenuated social sense of both justice and compassion. If there are no atheists in foxholes, it is likely also true there are no middle-class libertarians with metastatic cancer in ICUs graciously accepting their fate once their funds are exhausted. Hence, the conclusion of Chapter 4 is that our conceptions of health care justice are too abstract to address the complexities of clinical practice and social policy in relation to cancer and precision medicine, not to mention respect for reasonable pluralism in a liberal society. Ultimately, what we need (I argue) is a Rawlsian understanding of *public justice* or *political justice*, analogous to his notion of political liberalism (i.e., a non-comprehensive conception of health care justice).

In Chapter 5 we turn to the role of rational democratic deliberation in addressing the wicked problems generated by precision medicine. Readers familiar with my work will know that I have a distinctive account of rational democratic deliberation which I elaborated and defended in an earlier volume (Fleck, 2009). I summarize that view in this chapter and start to provide an account of how that deliberative process might yield a more just response to the ethical ambiguity associated with precision medicine. An awkward balancing act is needed. On the one hand, if I were able to offer clear and compelling accounts how all these wicked problems could be addressed so as to yield more just outcomes regarding access to these targeted therapies, the deliberative process would be otiose. Philosophic wisdom and analytic acuity would have triumphed without the divisiveness and conflict and messiness of the deliberative process. On the other hand, if I offered as a magical incantation "rational democratic deliberation," as if this well-described process would surely yield outcomes that were "just enough," this would certainly leave readers deeply dissatisfied. Consequently, in many places, I have tried to develop plausible arguments and analyses that could be embraced through a democratic deliberative process as being "just enough" without implying that that was the only resolution that would satisfy the requirements of reasonableness, reflective equilibrium, and an overlapping consensus. This is essentially what I am trying to accomplish in Chapter 6.

Chapter 7 introduces the notion of social beneficence, obligatory and non-obligatory. My starting point for this discussion is the sufficientarian conception of health care justice, such as that offered by Segall (2010). We start with the question of what belongs in a basic or decent or adequate package of health care benefits that ought to be guaranteed to everyone in our society as a matter of health care justice. Are all of these marginally beneficial, extraordinarily expensive cancer therapies included? An affirmative answer is not obvious. If all these precision therapies are outside that universal benefit package, are they then beyond justice and dependent upon individual ability to pay for those therapies? That does not seem like a satisfactory prospect either for a society that wishes to see itself as just and caring. The space I want to create and defend is the space of social beneficence, sometimes ethically obligatory, sometimes not. The task of this chapter is to defend the creation of that space.

Chapter 8 addresses a recent challenge generated by a cancer researcher in her book, *The First Cell* (Raza, 2019). She argues that we have wasted enormous resources in trying to prolong the lives of individuals with late-stage metastatic cancer. She rejects as wasteful and ethically problematic most of precision medicine. She argues instead that we ought to apply all those resources to defeating cancer when it is first initiated. This would require taking full advantage of the emerging technologies associated with liquid biopsies. This has a certain attractiveness to it, but it also generates some very politically and ethically challenging prospects. In particular, if taken seriously, it would force us to confront directly as a society the challenge of sacrificing hundreds of thousands of identified lives (metastatic cancer patients within a year of dying) in order to save statistical lives that do not yet have an established cancer.

One final point. The US health care system is a libertarian haven and a den of health care wickedness made all the more visible and tragic by the emergence of precision medicine. The enormous fragmentation of health care financing in the United States is an insuperable obstacle to achieving a more just health care system because the wicked problems I address in this volume are truly unsolvable in that context. To have a reasonable chance of achieving even a "roughly just" health care system with some control over all these wicked problems, we need something much closer to the single-payer system of Canada or the highly coordinated and centralized pluralistic system of Germany. Wickedness is not intrinsic to precision medicine, but it is highly infectious for precision medicine in a profit-centered medical world.

1

Precision Medicine

An Introduction to Its Ethical Ambiguity

1.1. Precision Medicine: A Patient Story

And that's why we're here today. Because something called precision medicine—in some cases, people call it personalized medicine—gives us one of the greatest opportunities for new medical breakthroughs that we have ever seen. Doctors have always recognized that every patient is unique, and doctors have always tried to tailor their treatments as best they can to individuals. You can match a blood transfusion to a blood type. That was an important discovery. What if matching a cancer cure to our genetic code was just as easy, just as standard?[1]

Dr. Randy Hillard, formerly a psychiatrist at Michigan State University, is a perfect illustration of the hopes expressed by President Obama in the passage above. In 2010, Dr. Hillard was diagnosed with Stage IV stomach cancer. He was given a year to live. However, his gastric cancer had a somewhat distinctive genetic feature. It was HER2-positive (Millman, 2015), which is a distinguishing feature of breast cancer that afflicts about 20% of women with breast cancer. HER2-positive breast cancer is treated with a "targeted therapy" drug called trastuzumab (Herceptin˚). Trastuzumab cannot be properly described as curing anyone of their advanced breast cancer, but for many women it has yielded significant gains in life expectancy. Dr. Hillard has been given this drug at three-week intervals for the past 11 years. The medical literature describes him as a "super-responder." This is an amazing result. It clearly

---

[1] "Remarks by the President on Precision Medicine" (Jan. 30, 2015). Accessed April 24, 2016. https://www.whitehouse.gov/the-press-office/2015/01/30/remarks-president-precision-medicine

Precision Medicine and Distributive Justice. Leonard M. Fleck, Oxford University Press. © Oxford University Press 2022.
DOI: 10.1093/oso/9780197647721.003.0001

exemplifies the best hopes associated with "precision" or "personalized" medicine.[2]

What exactly does "precision" or "personalized" medicine mean? What preceded precision medicine? The most common response to that last question has been "one-size-fits-all" medicine. If someone has very high blood pressure, a beta-blocker will be given. That someone can be anyone with very high blood pressure. ACE inhibitors can also be given for the same purpose. Bacterial infections will be treated with antibiotics. There are many antibiotics. The more common ones usually work for most people. Often enough, however, they fail. Then it takes a bit of guesswork, empirical trial and error, to find the antibiotic that will achieve the desired therapeutic effect without undesirable side effects. The treatment of various cancers with various chemotherapeutic agents will typically have such on-target and off-target effects. The Precision Medicine Initiative is intended to minimize those random non-therapeutic effects. The National Research Council: Committee on a Framework for Development of a New Taxonomy of Disease (2011) defines precision medicine this way:

> Precision medicine refers to the tailoring of medical treatment to the individual characteristics of each patient. It does not literally mean the creation of drugs or medical devices that are unique to a patient, but rather the ability to classify individuals into subpopulations that differ in their susceptibility to a particular disease, in the biology and/or prognosis of those diseases they may develop, or in their response to a specific treatment. Preventive or therapeutic interventions can then be concentrated on those who will benefit, sparing expense and side effects for those who will not.[3]

Much of the research that comes under the rubric of precision medicine has been driven by the completion of the Human Genome Research Project (1993–2003). To give some quick examples, the cytochrome P-450 family and its polymorphisms determine to some extent whether someone is a normal,

---

[2] The story of Randy Hillard has garnered considerable positive media attention for precision medicine. Those stories would not suggest that precision medicine might itself generate medical, economic, political, or ethical problems requiring careful thought and research.

[3] This passage is from National Research Council: Committee on a Framework for Development of a New Taxonomy of Disease. 2011. *Toward Precision Medicine: Building a Knowledge Network for Biomedical Research and a New Taxonomy of Disease.* Appendix E, 125. As the title suggests, this research group recognizes that rethinking prevailing taxonomies of disease will be a necessary first step toward discovering more effective and less harmful therapeutic interventions.

fast, or slow metabolizer of various drugs (Mega et al., 2009). The standard drug dosage will work fine for individuals who are normal metabolizers. However, if someone is a slow metabolizer, a normal dose of that drug will accumulate in that individual with potentially toxic effects. Hence, the dosage will need to be adjusted accordingly. Alternatively, if someone is a fast metabolizer, the drug will fall short of achieving the expected therapeutic result because it is metabolized too quickly. Again, the dosage will need adjusting.

Here are other examples of what precision medicine is about. (1) Patients who are candidates for simvastatin therapy (high levels of low-density lipoprotein, so-called bad cholesterol) and who have a variant of SLCO1B1 are at increased risk of myopathy (SEARCH Collaborative Group et al., 2008). If those same patients have two copies of the SLCO1B1 variant, they have a 20-fold increased risk of myopathy. (2) Patients who are HIV+ are at risk of a hypersensitive reaction if they have the HLA-B*5701 allele and are given the drug abacavir (Mallal et al., 2008). That represents about 5.6% of this patient population. Genetic screening for this allele can prevent this potentially fatal reaction. The take-home message from these examples is that precision medicine prevents serious and costly harms to patients. However, precision medicine is also about achieving more positive therapeutic effects, as the next examples illustrate.

The average life span today of a person with cystic fibrosis is 37 years. Cystic fibrosis is the result of a gene mutation that produces a defective version of the CFTR protein. About 4%–5% of cystic fibrosis patients have a variant of that mutation known as G551D. Those patients can now receive a drug, ivacaftor (Kalydeco®), which partially corrects the results of that mutation (Ramsey et al., 2011). The hope is that this drug may allow these patients to achieve something closer to a normal life expectancy. This is perfectly illustrative of what precision medicine is supposed to be. However, the cost of that drug is $300,000 per year, and patients would need to take this drug for the rest of their lives.[4]

---

[4] Lifetime costs for patients with cystic fibrosis will typically exceed $1 million, given the multiple hospitalizations required for disease exacerbation. Those are costs (and patient suffering) that will be reduced with ivacaftor. Still, at current prices 30-year survival would be achieved at a cost of $9 million per patient. More problematic would be the annual and lifetime costs of the cohort of 15,000 with the Phe508del mutation for the drug combination Orkambi. The annual costs would be $4.2 billion and 30-year lifetime costs $126 billion. Ferkol and Quinton (2015) ask the right question in the title of their essay, "Precision Medicine: At What Price?" They ask that as an economic and ethical question.

There is also some good news for cystic fibrosis patients with the most common genetic variation, what has been known as F508del but now is known as the Phe508del CFTR mutation. Approximately 45% of cystic fibrosis patients have this mutation. They can now take a drug combination, lumacaftor–ivacaftor (Orkambi˚), that ameliorates the effects of their cystic fibrosis but not nearly to the dramatic degree for those patients with the G551D mutation (Wainwright et al., 2015). The annual cost of that drug combination is $279,000. The cited research did show reduced hospitalizations for these patients, but it is unknown whether that will include a substantial gain in life expectancy. The take-home message is that money is saved, and patients are spared the risk of harm by only giving these drugs to patients who are known to be likely to benefit before the fact. One could hardly have any ethical qualms about that outcome.

Here is another example of the positive outcomes of precision medicine. In 2001 imatinib (Gleevec˚) was featured as the cover story for *Time* magazine (Lemonick and Park, 2001). Imatinib was hailed as a "magic bullet" in the arsenal against cancer. Imatinib is a tyrosine kinase inhibitor (TKI). It targeted what is known as the BCR-ABL "fusion gene" that was responsible for overproducing a molecule known as tyrosine kinase that encouraged white blood cells to grow incessantly and multiply. That process resulted in chronic myeloid leukemia (CML) (Querido, 2012). Approximately 80% of patients achieve complete remission (not a cure, just effective disease suppression) with imatinib. Approximately 70% of them gain substantially more than 10 extra years of life, which would seem to justify being featured on the cover of *Time* magazine. Still, many of these patients will develop *resistance* to imatinib (discussed later, see Section 1.2), which will require their being switched to another TKI.

Thompson et al. (2015, at 1448) write: "Identification of specific BCR-ABL1 mutations is critical to subsequent TKI choice. Patients with a T315I mutation are resistant to all TKIs except ponatinib. Patients with the F317L mutation are resistant to dasatinib but responsive to nilotinib. Y253H, E255K/V, and F359V/C mutations are resistant to nilotinib but sensitive to dasatinib." I use this passage to illustrate the increasing precision of precision medicine, which is clearly related to our ability to employ extraordinarily refined genetic testing. Such precision does have a price, and it is not cheap. In 2015, the annual cost of imatinib was $106,000 (Knox, 2015). The 10-year cost would be more than $1 million.[5] Speculation exists regarding

---

[5] Imatinib went off-patent in 2016 at a cost of $140,000 per year. However, the early generic versions were priced at about $72,000 for a one-year supply. The second-generation TKIs are priced

the question of whether patients might be taken off imatinib safely after some number of years with no evidence of recurrence (Bansal and Radich, 2016). That would obviously save money. However, no one knows how risky that might be for patients.[6]

Genetic heterogeneity develops in tumors, sometimes in reaction to the cancer therapies themselves, sometimes for intrinsic biological reasons (such as epigenetic alterations or molecular changes in the tumor's micro-environment). In either case, this tumor heterogeneity will characterize the vast majority of these patients with metastatic disease. Corless et al. (2011, at 873) write: "Additional studies using more sensitive assays have identified secondary mutations in more than 80% of drug-resistant GIST lesions. More sobering is that there is considerable heterogeneity of resistance across different lesions, and even within different areas of the same lesion." This heterogeneity affects the efficacy of salvage TKI therapy because there are now a number of genetically distinct mutations, both within individual lesions and among these lesions. The practical implication of this heterogeneity is that no particular TKI will result in the systemic eradication of a specific cancer. This has cost consequences and ethical consequences as far as distributive justice is concerned. Keep in mind that these patients have a terminal illness. None of these drugs can alter that fact. Some of these drugs might offer a gain of additional months of life, typically at a cost of $10,000 per month or more, just for the drug. Often, considerable uncertainty will exist regarding which TKI might be most medically appropriate, given that multiple drivers of the cancer might be active in different lesions. How many of these drugs might a patient have a just claim to try at social expense, given uncertain and limited efficacy as well as high cost?

---

at about $150,000 per year. Why is this important? "Meanwhile, the prices of Sprycel [dasatinib] and Tasigna [nilotinib] continued to increase after generic imatinib became available, the researchers found. Sekeres explains that patients with chronic-phase CML need tailored treatment for their disease, which can mean that a newly diagnosed patient found to have intermediate- or high-risk disease begins therapy with one of the higher-cost TKIs" (Azvolinsky, 2020).

[6] One biological reason behind this problem pertains to the cancer "stem cell hypothesis." These stem cells, in the language of cancer biologists, are not "addicted" to BCR-ABL kinase activity. Winger and Shah (2015, at 409) write: "These and other data led many to believe imatinib kills dividing CML cells but cannot penetrate the quiescent CML stem cell pool, which theoretically needs to be eradicated to effect cure." The problem of cancer stem cells is not unique to CML. The effective treatment of many other cancers may be affected by this same problem.

1.2. Precision Medicine: What Is It?

The term "precision medicine" has really emerged in the context of cancer treatment and research. An enormous amount of molecular research has been focused on cancer, aimed primarily at understanding how cancers begin and evolve. Ultimately, the goal is to find drugs that can interrupt the evolution of a cancer and destroy those cells as well. To allow the reader to better appreciate the ethics issues discussed later in this volume, allow me to offer a sketch of this research over the past couple of decades.

Cancer typically develops "from a single cell that, as it divides into a clonal population, accumulates function-altering mutations in the genes that control cell growth, survival, and differentiation" (Schoenberger and Cohen, 2017). Among those mutations are loss-of-function mutations in DNA-repair proteins. What that means is that we ordinarily have proteins in our cells that "correct" these mutations that occur during cell division. When those repair proteins are disabled, these mutated cells can begin to multiply themselves uncontrollably. The result is a cancer.

If those repair proteins are disabled, then the daughter cells can gradually accumulate more and more mutations as the cancer evolves. Quite literally, thousands of mutations can develop in those cells. Those mutations are described by cancer researchers as either "driver" mutations or "passenger" mutations. Only a small percentage of those mutations are of the driver variety. Nevertheless, those are the mutations that are critical to the evolution and dissemination of that cancer. In the medical literature, this is referred to as the problem of cancer "heterogeneity." This heterogeneity is one of the primary reasons why cancer is so difficult to treat, especially after it has metastasized.

I have already introduced the term "targeted therapies." That phrase refers to drugs that "target" one or another of these "driver" mutations. For example, in the case of lung adenocarcinoma, the mutated driver of the cancer will be KRAS 25% of the time, EGFR 15% of the time, ALK 8% of the time, BRAF 5% of the time, NRAS 1% of the time, and still other drivers (many unknown) 33% of the time (Garraway, 2013). The clinical implications can be illustrated in the following way. If the primary driver of a tumor is a mutated (rearranged) ALK (anaplastic lymphoma kinase) gene, the first drug given will be crizotinib, which is an ALK inhibitor. The drug is designed to hit that target. Success means that the relevant tumors stop growing, which is referred to as "progression-free survival." This is tumor control, not complete tumor destruction. That growth cessation may be sustained for a period of several months, maybe somewhat longer for the strong responders. Some patients may barely respond to the drug, even though it is the correct drug for that target. Researchers at present have no idea why that drug failed in those patients.

Failure often occurs because the cancer continues to evolve genetically. This phenomenon is described as cancer drug "resistance." A number of biological explanations are available for the resistance. One of them is that the targeted cancer drug itself, say, crizotinib, precipitates additional mutations in the ALK gene. When this occurs, and cancer progression is medically detectable, another targeted therapy will be given, such as ceritinib or alectinib. These targeted therapies have proven effective against most of the acquired mutations in ALK. However, after some limited period of time, resistance will develop, and progression will occur. Then brigatinib can be used (Honey, 2017). In the pipeline is lorlatinib, which has received expedited review by the US Food and Drug Administration (FDA), in part because it has been successful in reducing ALK-related brain metastases (Shaw et al., 2017). Again, in spite of this succession of drugs, all of which "work" to some degree for some period of time for some portion of that patient population, the cancer will progress and will prove fatal.

Earlier I referred to the *primary* driver of a cancer, which clearly implies the existence of *secondary* drivers. Consequently, what often happens is that one of these targeted therapies is successful in controlling a primary driver of a cancer, which then results in a secondary driver becoming the new primary driver. This is analogous to what medical researchers have seen in connection with the evolution of HIV in AIDS patients. HIV mutates in response to the drugs that are given. To achieve control of HIV today, three- and four-drug combinations are used with these patients, and the combinations are altered if there is evidence of disease progression. The clinical implication of this strategy for cancer control is that a different targeted therapy will be needed to manage this new driver. If mutated BRAF becomes the new driver of the cancer, then a BRAF inhibitor will be needed. The BRAF variant that researchers have identified as being most significant for control of the cancer is the V600E variant. Dabrafenib and trametenib are the two drugs used in combination to achieve the desired control. Only 1%–2% of lung cancer tumors harbor the V600E mutation. However, given the nature of cancer, it should be obvious that completely destroying the other 98%–99% of lung cancer cells without that mutation would not result in a cure for that cancer.

The reader might imagine that if researchers can just find a good match between a targeted therapy and a specific driver mutation, some significant therapeutic benefit will ensue. However, that will be true only about 30% of the time. Imatinib and its success as a targeted therapy may have generated excessive optimism. Imatinib is a therapeutic outlier. As noted already, acquired resistance occurs when a drug, such as erlotinib, provokes a response from a different driver mutation in that cancer, which undercuts the effectiveness of that drug. Alternatively, compensatory signaling pathways may leave the effectiveness of that drug intact but instead provide the cancer with the biochemical means to continue to progress, thereby defeating the therapeutic potential of one of these targeted therapies (Van Allen et al., 2014). Yet another reason for the defeat of these targeted cancer drugs is the presence of cancer stem cells. Just like normal stem cells in our bodies that serve as a source of biological renewal in our bodies, cancer stem cells serve as a source of biological renewal for various cancers. These cancer stem cells are largely *undifferentiated*, which means they "look different" from the cancer cells that have genetic features that make them a target for drugs such as erlotinib. Consequently, they evade destruction. At present (2021), no drugs are available that can target these cancer stem cells without also destroying normal stem cells (Batlle and Clevers, 2017).

The other main strategy that has emerged over the past few years for attacking cancer is immunotherapy. Ordinarily, our immune system is good at recognizing cancer cells spontaneously generated in our bodies as "not me" and destroying those cells. Still, some cancer cells use their "immune checkpoints" to block the immune system from attacking the cancer. "Immune checkpoints are specialized proteins that act as brakes on the immune system, ensuring that immune defenses are engaged only when they are needed and for as long as they are needed" (Burstein et al., 2017, at 1346). Immune checkpoints are normal and necessary parts of our cellular machinery. They prevent the immune system from becoming overactive, which can result in either excessive inflammation or autoimmune disease.

Over the past few years, a number of drugs have been developed, collectively known as "checkpoint inhibitors." They "take the brakes off" those cancer cells so that the immune system can destroy that cancer. The drugs to which I am referring include nivolumab (Opdivo˚), ipilimumab (Yervoy˚), pembrolizumab (Keytruda˚), and atezolizumab (Tecentriq˚). Again, these drugs are used to treat *metastatic* cancer. None of these drugs can promise a cure.[7] At present, these drugs are used to treat melanoma, lung and renal cancers, and Hodgkin lymphoma (though their use is rapidly expanding to other cancers). Broadly speaking, they have had somewhat more success than the targeted therapies discussed earlier with respect to disease-free progression. However, that success has been mostly marginal, mostly for 30%–40% of patients treated.

The targets of these checkpoint inhibitors are PD-1 and PD-L1 receptors, the first of which is on T cells, and the second of which is on cancer cells. These are the receptors that put the brakes on the immune system. The obvious questions to raise are why less than half the patients treated have a positive response to these drugs, and why is it that the response is of only limited duration for virtually everyone. The short answer is that resistance mechanisms are at work again (Zaretsky et al., 2016; Bifulco and Urba, 2016). We could simply accept this as a regrettable outcome, except that the cost of these drugs for such marginal outcomes raises issues of health care justice.

The cost of the combination of atezolizumab and bevacizumab for renal cancer is about $195,000 per year. Since the median gain until progression was three months, the incremental cost-effectiveness of that combination would be almost $800,000. This is an extraordinarily high relative price for that median gain of three months. One way of addressing this problem is to find biomarkers that would identify individuals who were much more likely to gain greater clinical benefit from access to these checkpoint inhibitors. One such biomarker is PD-L1 expression. Patients with metastatic non-small cell lung cancer, for example, with >50% PD-L1 expression who are treated with pembrolizumab will have a median gain in life expectancy of 14.9 months compared to 8.2 months with current chemotherapy (Reck et al., 2016). Unfortunately, this is not some neat cutoff such that patients with 30% PD-L1 expression can be told they will not benefit from pembrolizumab and must settle for standard chemotherapy instead. The clinical reality is that they *might* still have some marginal gain in life expectancy, and they might very much desire to have that chance. However, Temel et al. (2018, at 1654) write: "Although checkpoint inhibitors can be effective in patients with

---

[7] I am reporting here what every reputable medical journal will confirm. However, I did see a TV commercial from the Dana-Farber Cancer Institute titled "Change the World," which focused on these PD-1 and PD-L1 immunotherapies. In that commercial three individuals say "PD-L1 saved my life." This would create a gross misimpression in the mind of any TV viewer that these drugs "cured their metastatic cancer" (and would likely cure your metastatic cancer as well). https://www.youtube.com/watch?v=ZRKKAmTniGQ (Accessed 3/14/2021).

low or no PDL-1 expression, the majority of those without this biomarker will not benefit from these therapies" (see also Carbone et al., 2017). The ethical issue is whether patients with a predicted low probability of benefit would still have a just claim to "that chance." Would they have been treated unjustly if they were denied that chance, given some range of uncertainty regarding the clinical outcome? Buyx et al. (2011), for example, want to defend the justness of minimum effectiveness thresholds for socially funded access to these very expensive cancer drugs. They would set that threshold at a three-month gain in life expectancy. This is a fairly low bar. However, they undermine that low bar when they add that if there are "a few patients who might respond very well" despite a very low median of effectiveness, then "cutting the treatment would deprive these patients of substantial benefits." This is not an ethically acceptable outcome for them. The problem is that very few drugs that offer some marginal benefit will not have a few patients at the long tail of the curve.

I want to call attention to one more novel cancer therapy certain to generate problems of health care justice. This is CAR-T cell therapy (chimeric antigen receptor),[8] which is very much *personal* precision medicine. T cells are removed from a patient and genetically modified to respond to certain targets (CD19+ B cells) expressed on a patient's cancer cells. Those modified T cells (now millions after three weeks) are reinfused into the patient. These cells then secrete a number of programmed substances, including inflammatory cytokines that ultimately destroy the cancer cells. This is an extraordinarily complex process. Three forms of CAR-T cell therapy had FDA approval in early 2021, tisagenlecleucel (Kymriah°) for acute lymphoblastic leukemia and axicabtagene ciloleucel (Yescarta°) and lisocabtagene maraleucel for large B-cell lymphoma. In all cases therapy involves just a single infusion. The cost of tisagenlecleucel is about $475,000, while the cost of axicabtagene is $373,000. However, this is only the beginning of the cost problem.

Roughly half the patients who receive CAR-T cell therapy experience a "cytokine release syndrome," which involves an extraordinarily high fever, hypotension, a risk of multi-organ failure, confusion, lethargy, stroke-like symptoms, and coma, all of which require prolonged intensive care unit care (Bach et al., 2017). There have also been deaths. Bach et al. add, "CAR-T

---

[8] CAR-T cell therapies are actually one version of what is more broadly described as "adoptive cell transfer" therapies (National Cancer Institute, 2017).

therapies are effective at killing any cell, normal or cancerous, that expresses the target, so damage to normal cells and tissues and long-term and likely permanent toxic effects can be considerable" (2017, at 1861). Bach et al.'s ultimate conclusion is that the cost per patient for tisagenlecleucel is actually closer to $1 million, on average, when all the relevant medical costs are taken into account.[9] It is noted that response rates are around 80%, but 25% of those patients will have recurrence of their cancer within six months. One-year survival for those patients is 70%–80%. Some number of these patients have survived for several years. However, no one can justifiably claim that any of these patients has been cured of their cancer. Further, 46% of the patients who responded initially to this therapy had disease relapse at one year (Prasad, 2018). This looks like another instance of cancer therapy resistance. What should we conclude as far as the problem of health care justice is concerned? Is a just and caring society with limited resources to meet unlimited health care needs obligated as a matter of justice to provide a million dollars' worth of health care to purchase this extra year of life for these patients? In answering this question, does it matter that the intended primary beneficiaries of tisagenlecleucel are the 600 children with ALL (acute lymphocytic leukemia) each year in the United States who have failed primary therapy for their ALL?

One final point regarding this particular version of immunotherapy: It is described by its advocates as a "living drug" (McGinley and Johnson, 2017). Just as our immune system "learns" to recognize over the course of our lives many disease-causing invaders of our bodies, which it then "knows" need to be destroyed, so in this case the immune system is biochemically engineered by medical researchers to have the same ongoing therapeutic efficacy with regard to specific cancers. This is not an external drug that needs to be given repeatedly. One infusion of these altered T cells "teaches" the immune system how to attack some specific cancer, in much the same way that a vaccine would work. Lim and June (2017) write: "Living cells are radically different from inanimate platforms, such as small molecules or antibodies, in that cells are capable of intelligent sensing and response behaviors" (at 724). Further, Sharma et al. (2017) add: "A hallmark of immunotherapy is the durability of

---

[9] Bach et al.'s conclusion regarding costs is further documented in a *Wall Street Journal* article (Rockoff, 2018). The enormous uncertainty associated with the overall cost of providing this therapy has made many hospitals reluctant to take on these patients because insurers, including the Medicare program, have been uncertain about how to pay for these therapies in the most cost-effective way possible.

responses, most likely due to the memory of the adaptive immune system, which translates into long-term survival for a subset of patients" (at 707).[10]

1.3. Precision Medicine and the "Just Caring" Problem

We return to the story of Randy Hillard. It must be noted that most of the other patients with that same advanced gastric cancer and the same "genetic signature" as Dr. Hillard who were given trastuzumab achieved much smaller gains in life expectancy, roughly a median gain in life expectancy of 10 months (Shitara et al., 2013; Boku, 2014). One obvious follow-up question would be: What *really* set apart Dr. Hillard's HER2-positive gastric cancer from that of all those others who seemed to be genetically similar? Why was his cancer so dramatically responsive to trastuzumab? Was his tumor *really responsive to the drug,* as opposed to having an intrinsic biological feature that has yielded prolonged survival? Further, there are always individuals at the far end of a survival curve (Prasad and Vandross, 2015; Zimmerman and Peters, 2019). This last question is one for medical research, not ethical analysis. However, it does have considerable potential ethical relevance.

The cost of Dr. Hillard's therapy has been about $17,000 for each three-week transfusion. He estimates that his care has cost a bit over $1.7 million as of early 2021. His personal costs have been somewhat above $100,000, the rest having been covered by insurance. For that, he has enjoyed more than 11 extra years of very good quality of life. One of the clear goals of the Precision Medicine Initiative is to make this same outcome a reality for every patient with advanced or metastatic cancer. The hope is that metastatic cancer will become a chronic well-managed medical problem, like AIDS, rather than a fatal medical condition. Probably no one would deny that this represents a noble goal. Is that goal affordable? Approximately 610,000 individuals die of cancer each year in the United States (though this number will increase dramatically over the next two decades because of the post–World War II "baby boom" generation). If there were targeted therapies for their cancers that were

---

[10] Though immunotherapy has been associated with an increased proportion of durable responses for more patients than is generally true with targeted therapies, evidence has emerged of late that immunotherapy may also precipitate rapid progression of a cancer. According to one study, 9% of a subset of patients with non-small cell lung cancer had precisely this outcome in response to PD-1/PD-L1 inhibitors (Powers, 2017). Precision medicine might not always be as precise as we might hope. See also Champiat et al. (2017). This latter study saw the risk of hyperprogression as more of a potential problem in elderly cancer patients treated with these inhibitors.

as effective as trastuzumab for Dr. Hillard, the aggregated cost of such therapeutic success at Year 6 and every year thereafter would be $600 billion.[11] That kind of expenditure is simply not economically feasible. Nor would that represent a just allocation of limited health care resources, given all the other life-threatening non-cancer medical needs. The domain of health care needs has rapidly expanded over the last five decades along with the health care expenditures that have supported that expansion. To be more precise, in the United States in 2020 we spent about $4.0 trillion on health care, or approximately 18.0% of our gross domestic product (GDP) then (Keehan et al., 2020). Projections to 2028 in the United States put expenditures at $6.2 trillion, or approximately 19.6% of projected GDP. Projections to 2030 put health care expenditures then at $6.75 trillion (Poisal et al., 2022).

The practical import of this largely uncontrolled expenditure growth has been increasing business and political pressure to limit the growth of health care costs, at least to business enterprises, state government, or the federal government. This has had two major consequences, both with substantial ethical import. First, physicians are generally seen as being responsible for about 70%–80% of health care expenditures ($2.8 trillion in 2019). This is because they alone have the legal and professional authority to order surgery for a patient, prescription drugs, home health care, some form of rehabilitative care, some costly diagnostic test, and so on. Hence, hospitals and insurers have devised various rules and incentive schemes aimed at eliciting from physicians more restrained use of health care resources. Often, the behavior elicited is described as "minimizing the wasteful use of resources," the implication being that nothing of ethical concern is at stake. Frequently enough that description is disingenuous because the intervention withheld might represent at least marginally beneficial care, though from the payer's perspective it might be regarded as not being cost-effective. Such withholdings of care are more properly described as being instances of health care rationing.[12] This is a matter of ethical concern because physicians are

[11] To explain the derivation of that number, if there are 610,000 patients who die of cancer annually, and we are successful in prolonging their lives for six years, that equals $610 billion. In Year 1 that cost is "only" $100 billion. In Year 2, it is $200 billion (because there is a second cohort). In Year 3, it is $300 billion, until Year 6 and beyond, for each of which the cost would be $600 billion. Recall that roughly 70% of CML patients treated with imatinib survive for 10 years or more.

[12] What is properly described as health care rationing? Peter Ubel (2000) carefully addresses this definitional issue in a chapter titled "The Politics of Defining Health Care Rationing" (pp. 11–30). That title is perfectly apt. Defining rationing is deeply politically tainted. Neither government nor businesses wish to be accused of imposing or endorsing health care rationing decisions at the expense of their workers or citizens, though both do. It is typically accomplished "invisibly," in ways that are hidden from those most affected. This can be accomplished through either linguistic

then placed in the ethically awkward position of being expected to be loyal advocates of the best interests of their patients as well as prudent stewards of corporate or governmental resources. Patients, of course, are typically unaware of the fact that their physician may really be a double agent at times.

Second, to control escalating health care costs, employers and insurers are also shifting more health care costs to consumers, typically invoking the rhetoric of motivating "health care consumers" to make smart choices because they "have more skin in the game." The mechanism for accomplishing this might be requiring employees to pay 30% or more of the cost of their health insurance premium. Alternatively, employers might require their employees to purchase a high-deductible plan, one in which they would be responsible for the first $5,000 each year for their own care and $10,000 each year for their family care. The ethically problematic aspect of this approach to cost control is that employees in highly paid managerial roles will likely not stint on needed care for themselves or their families while lower-wage workers will often deny themselves health care that is needed and effective but excessively costly *to them*. This will be regarded by many as an unethical disparity in access to needed care. It is also accurately described as self-imposed rationing, which is to say that employers and insurers can distance themselves from any accusation that they have *imposed* rationing on their workers. Again, I would regard that as disingenuous at best.[13]

Many insurance contracts also include steep co-pay requirements for things such as specialty drugs. Those co-pays can be 30% or higher.[14] Most of the targeted cancer therapies alluded to above have prices of $100,000 or more for a course of treatment. Workers in the lower 60% of the income spectrum would rarely be able to afford $30,000 as their portion of that cost. If most of these drugs yield only extra weeks or extra months of life

legerdemain (i.e., the language of parsimonious care) or bureaucratic obscurantism, such as Medicare DRGs (Diagnosis-Related Groupings). I critically assess appeals to the language of parsimonious care (Fleck, 2016a), and in an earlier essay I demonstrated that DRGs represent a form of invisible rationing (Fleck, 1987). See also Fleck (1990).

[13] Our first-year medical students have as an assignment recalling a patient, acquaintance, or family member who was denied access to needed health care because of insurance issues, along with the consequences of that denial. These are terribly painful essays to read. Fewer than half these stories are about patients who have no health insurance for a variety of reasons. The other half are patients with health insurance and high deductibles or co-pays that result in their rationing their own care, such as cutting their insulin in half or simply avoiding getting timely attention to an emerging medical problem, often with disastrous consequences.

[14] Medicare offers a clear chart of how drug formularies work. See https://www.bcbsm.com/medicare/help/understanding-plans/pharmacy-prescription-drugs/tiers.html (accessed June 18, 2020).

for someone with metastatic cancer, then maybe they really are not worth it. That would seem to diminish ethical concern. Maybe it is not *so unjust* that these workers cannot afford access to these drugs. However, we must also note that for those in the upper tiers of the income spectrum who can afford such co-pays for these drugs the insurance company is paying the other 70% of that cost. Who contributes to that other 70%? The ethically problematic response is that all those workers in the lower economic tiers would have contributed their "fair share," though they will not be able to derive a corresponding fair share of any benefit. In other words, the economically less well off are providing a substantial subsidy to those who are much better off. How should a just and caring society respond to this state of affairs?

One response to that last question would be that there should be no financial barriers to having access to these drugs. This certainly seems like a decent and generous policy choice. However, the obvious critical comment coming from any of a number of patients with end-stage heart disease, end-stage lung disease, end-stage liver disease, or any number of other chronic degenerative conditions is: What is so morally special about cancer that patients with cancer would have unlimited socially subsidized access to any beneficial cancer treatment, no matter what the cost, while individuals with other life-threatening, or quality of life–diminishing, health problems would be at the mercy of insurance markets, employer budgets, or personal ability to pay? No doubt, cancer is widely feared, in part because it is common, in part because its effects, both the disease and the therapy, are so destructive of the lives of individuals. Still, these considerations are not ethically weighty enough to justify "special access" to these costly targeted therapies for cancer while denying comparable socially subsidized access to other costly therapies for other life-threatening illnesses.

The obvious way to remedy this apparent injustice is to provide comparable socially subsidized financial coverage for at least all life-threatening illnesses. However, that would ignore the chief implication of the "just caring" problem: We have only limited resources for meeting unlimited health care needs. That is, we cannot avoid the problem of health care rationing. Some health care needs will not be met.

It is one thing for a physician to have to say to a patient, "I am sorry, but there is nothing more we can do to forestall your dying." But it is quite another for a physician to have to say to a patient, "I am sorry, but you have no ability to pay for the left ventricular assist device [LVAD] that would otherwise provide you with three extra years of life with your heart failure. You likely have only a six-month life expectancy. I realize that the federal government is paying $100,000 for a targeted cancer treatment that will give your neighbor six extra months of life, but you do not have cancer." If the physician added as further explanation that society has only limited resources to meet virtually unlimited health care needs, and hence that rationing decisions were inescapable, it should not come as a surprise that a patient in these circumstances would feel that not funding an LVAD was neither fair nor just. Further, our heart failure patient could reasonably complain that he was paying taxes to provide this costly cancer care to someone who was not paying taxes to subsidize his access to the costly cardiac care he needed to prolong his life.

1.4. Precision Medicine: Another Case, More Ethics Issues

We return for a moment to the case of Dr. Hillard. His care has cost a bit more than $1.7 million, but it has gotten him 11 high-quality extra years of life (and that is continuing). Can anyone argue that this outcome is fundamentally unjust or ethically wrongheaded? No one with an ounce of compassion could argue that he simply should have been allowed to die of his cancer, even though there was this extraordinarily effective treatment available to him. In case it matters, he is (as of 2021) 68 years old.

Then there is the story of Evan Johnson, as reported in the *Wall Street Journal* (Winslow, 2016). Mr. Johnson was a 23-year-old senior at the University of North Dakota in 2014. He was diagnosed with a very aggressive form of acute myeloid leukemia (AML). The mutation that seemed to be the primary driver of his cancer was FLT3, which was treated with the targeted therapy, sorafenib (Nexavar®) plus an experimental drug identified as 5-azacitidine. Those drugs were effective enough that he could have a stem cell transplant. However, the stem cell transplant failed, and he then endured six different drug regimens, four relapses, and multiple life-threatening side effects. At nine months, his leukemia developed a new mutation, one that could be identified because tumors can be routinely genetically sequenced at major medical centers today. This is known as the "Philadelphia chromosome," usually associated with CML. Imatinib (Gleevec®), as we saw earlier, is very effective in treating that form of leukemia. Mr. Johnson was given the next-generation version of that drug, dasatinib (Sprycel®). However, he suffered a relapse. He was switched to ponatinib (Iclusig®), again targeting

FLT3, which had the desired effects. This permitted a second stem cell transplant, which has resulted in a remission of unknown duration. The cost of Mr. Johnson's 17 months of care at the Mayo Clinic was more than $4 million.

Mr. Johnson's story is different in important respects from Dr. Hillard's story. We can say that Dr. Hillard's story has a happy ending. We have no idea at this point that Mr. Johnson's story will end happily as well. The aggregate cost of Mr. Johnson's care was four times greater than Dr. Hillard's. Put another way, each year of life gained for Dr. Hillard cost $150,000, while each year of life gained so far for Mr. Johnson cost $2 million. Does every cancer patient have a presumptive just claim to $4 million worth of care, if they are able to derive *some degree* of benefit from that care? Perhaps we should say that this is not a matter of justice; this is a matter of social beneficence. That hardly erases the moral challenges raised by cases such as this. The obvious ethical question to ask is: Why was *he* picked to be the object of such generous beneficence?[15]

Is it of ethical relevance that Mr. Johnson is a young man, as opposed to an 80-year-old? If so, where would we imagine the cutoff might be? What would be the ethical justification for drawing the line at any particular age? Perhaps what is ethically significant is not the age of anyone needing this life-prolonging therapy but the fact that there is a substantial gain in life expectancy measurable in years, even though the cost of achieving that gain might be very high.

One practical conclusion to draw would be that more research needs to be done that might tell us before the fact that this particular patient will experience a gain in life expectancy measurable in weeks or no more than three months. What then? Do we then conclude that such patients would have no just claim to these very costly drugs at social expense; they would always be free to use personal resources to secure access to these drugs if they were so motivated. This is clearly not a conclusion that a strong egalitarian such as John Harris (1985) would endorse. From his perspective, patients on the lower side of the median for survival or progression-free survival have just as strong a claim to these targeted therapies at social expense as those patients

---

[15] We might be tempted to say that these are private resources which companies are ethically free to provide or withhold as they wish. However, that is not accurate. These resources do not represent personal wealth. Whether Mayo or the insurance company "absorbed" those costs, what that means in practice is that everyone else attached to Mayo or that insurance plan "accepted" higher premiums or higher charges to cover this act of beneficence. That leaves untouched our original ethical challenge: Can I expect a comparable act of generosity should I find myself in comparable circumstances (since I contributed unknowingly to that generous act)?

on the upper side of the median for survival. If we take that perspective as a conversation stopper, then it seems we will never be able to effectively, or fairly, address the problem of escalating health care costs.

1.5. Precision Medicine: Is Rough Justice "Just Enough"?

The European Medical Agency has approved panitimumab (Vectibix®) and cetuximab (Erbitux®) as first-line chemotherapies for patients with metastatic colorectal cancer "with no mutations in the codon 12 and 13 of the KRAS gene" (Ruzzo et al., 2010). Both these drugs are extraordinarily expensive: more than $100,000 for a course of treatment. Neither drug will effect a cure for the cancer. If everyone with metastatic colon cancer receives these drugs, then the average gain in life expectancy will be a few weeks. If these drugs are given only to patients lacking the specified mutations, some of those patients might gain two extra years of life (Van Cutsem et al., 2010). About 40% of these patients have a KRAS mutation predictive of non-response to these drugs. Another 35%–40% with wild-type KRAS will have an objective response to these drugs (i.e., some degree of tumor shrinkage), though it might be very marginal from a therapeutic perspective.[16]

To put all of this in context, about 55,000 patients in the United States died of colorectal cancer in 2018. If all these patients had access to these drugs at $100,000 for a course of treatment, that would add about $5.5 billion per year to the cost of caring for these patients. In theory, several billion dollars could be saved if access to these drugs were restricted to individuals with a genotype that was most likely to be responsive to these drugs (the 35%–40% with wild-type KRAS). Individuals with wild-type KRAS do not all show the same "objective response." Only some will achieve maximal gains in life expectancy (Ortega et al., 2010). Others will only gain extra months. We do not know whether additional genetic factors identified through future research will yield a picture of enhanced median survival. Would it be unjust to do the further research that will yield some basis for more restrictive access to these

[16] Treatment options for metastatic colorectal cancer with KRAS mutations remain extremely limited. Consequently, these patients have a very poor prognosis. *KRAS* is the most frequently mutated oncogene in cancer. The pharmacological drugging of *KRAS* remains a key challenge for cancer research. However, the drug sotorasib has proven effective against KRAS (G12C) mutated colorectal cancer (Hong et al., 2020). Unfortunately, this very specific mutation occurs in only 1%–2% of metastatic colorectal cancers.

expensive drugs for patients with marginally responsive genotypes?[17] What can be said to them, morally speaking, that would justify denying them that desired benefit?

Would it be unjust to deny the whole cohort of patients access to these drugs at social expense who would only gain extra months of life (less than a year), especially when current practice often provides aggressive and expensive therapies to many sorts of end-stage patients who will gain only weeks or months of additional life? However, is it reasonable to ask whether such current practices should be given ongoing moral authority simply because they are current practice? This is again Callahan's (1990) "ragged edge." We are faced with "rugged moral terrain" because this sort of issue will become ubiquitous as the field of precision medicine advances over the next decade. The complexity and uncertainty associated with both the basic science and clinical judgment will allow us to achieve no more than "rough justice." That in turn raises the question of how rough "rough justice" can be and still be "just enough." Age, for example, appears to be a prognostic marker for a poorer outcome with colorectal cancer. About 70% of deaths from colorectal cancer occur among those more than 65 years old (Van Cutsem et al., 2010). Should we distinguish among older patients who have more or less promising outcomes for purposes of determining who among them should have access to these expensive drugs at social expense as a matter of justice? And if we were to adopt such a policy for these cancer patients, what policies would we be morally obligated to adopt for patients in their 80s and 90s who today are routinely provided with dialysis and open heart surgery (Caceres et al., 2013; Thorsteinsdottir et al., 2015; Kurella et al., 2007)?

If there were a neat division between responders and non-responders identifiable through some form of genetic testing, then we might well be able to make a strong moral and economic case for providing the drug only to the responders. This will be true in some cases. However, the more common medical reality is a gradient between the two ends of the spectrum. How then can we possibly justly create a bright line determining access to these extraordinarily expensive drugs and their promised medical benefits? Recall that survival gains for each genotype are expressed in terms of *median survival.*

[17] More evidence regarding expected medical outcomes (the right measurement, the right biomarker, the most effective drug combination) will rarely yield bright lines in place of the ragged justice edges. Caplan (2011) has argued persuasively that this is a pipe dream. The interpretation of evidence "depends much upon one's circumstances and values." A desperate cancer patient sees a 1% chance of an extra month of life from a $100,000 drug as a ray of hope, while a managed care plan administrator sees it as a mirage of waste.

That means there is a range around that median, and physicians might not have a clear idea regarding the boundaries of that range. Half the patients are below that median, and half are above. How far above? What are the just claims of those "far above" patients, who we know statistically are there?

Again, we ask the question: How rough can "rough justice" be that we ought to accept? We might be tempted to say that rough justice is not "just enough" and that it must be resisted. What would the alternative be? Surely, we should not defend the status quo in the United States as being morally preferable. The status quo means that individuals who are fortunate enough to have excellent health insurance provided through an employer would have access to these extraordinarily expensive cancer drugs at relatively little direct expense to themselves. If nothing else, this has the psychological effect of solidifying the idea that they "have a right" to these drugs. This, in turn, makes it much more difficult to generate sustained political support for health reform aimed at covering the remaining 30 million uninsured in our society with a reasonably comprehensive benefit package. This is because we could not afford to provide unlimited access to these very marginally beneficial non-costworthy cancer drugs as part of a national benefit package.

Health reform, as noted earlier, will require defining a benefit package that will be guaranteed to all. How should such a benefit package be defined *in clinical practice* in the light of the "ragged edge" problem? Consider again the patients with metastatic colorectal cancer and the BRAF V600E mutation. Should such judgments be made at the bedside by individual clinicians responsive to the distinctive clinical circumstances of an individual patient? Should this be a matter of shared decision-making? If so, what assurances would patients have that they would be treated justly (not denied very expensive life-prolonging care arbitrarily)?

We said earlier that "rough justice" was all that we could reasonably expect, given the complexity of our health care system. Would this clinical judgment approach yield outcomes that were within the bounds of "rough justice"? Or would outcomes tied to individual clinical judgment be "too rough," morally speaking—too arbitrary, too idiosyncratic, or too costly? Should we rely instead for these judgments upon panels of clinicians in a range of specialty areas? Alternatively, should we rely upon managers and administrators of health plans and health facilities to trim the ragged edges and establish limits? What should be the role of current patients in making these judgments? Must we rely instead upon future possible patients who are currently ignorant of their future possible health needs, and therefore better positioned to make such judgments more impartially? What I am referring to here would be some broad and inclusive process of rational democratic deliberation (which we discuss in Section 1.6).

1.6. Precision Medicine: Key Ethics Issues

Our key question: What are the just claims of cancer patients to these expensive cancer drugs when the genetic characteristics of their cancer predict only a very modest gain in life expectancy from being given these drugs? Alternatively, what are the just claims of cancer patients to these expensive cancer drugs when the genetic features of their cancer would predict a substantial gain in life expectancy from being given these drugs? More specifically, is there a "just enough" way of establishing limits with regard to accessing these drugs when there is something approximating a seamless continuum of responses to these drugs from very strong to relatively weak responses? That is, can this specific version of the "ragged edge" problem be addressed "fairly enough"? I will ultimately argue that "rough justice" (with its ragged edges) can be achieved and legitimated through suitably managed processes of rational democratic deliberation.

Does every patient faced with a potentially deadly cancer have a just claim to whichever of these targeted therapies offers some promise of benefit to them? One justification for an affirmative answer would be that these represent "last chance" therapies; these patients are faced with a terminal prognosis, and they have no other options that are more promising than what these targeted therapies might offer. An implicit premise in this line of argument would be that it would be indecent and unjust to deny such desperate patients the only medical intervention that offered any hope of prolonged life. Other rationales can be combined with this one. One such rationale would be that these patients are clearly among the "medically least well off," and consequently, they ought to have very high priority for whatever medical interventions might benefit them.[18] A prioritarian theory of health care justice would advocate for this point of view. Of course, these interventions are extraordinarily costly. An oft-invoked response to that line of argument will be that human life is priceless. That is, if we have the medical or technological capacity to save or prolong a human life, then no amount of money

---

[18] A critical assessment of this point of view is offered by Brock (2002).

should stand in the way of our using that technology for that purpose. The practical embodiment of that perspective is what is usually referred to as the "rule of rescue," which we see acted on whenever individuals have managed to get themselves stranded at sea or on a mountain or in a cave in Thailand, and so on.[19]

I have bundled all these apparently disparate rationales together because they all have the same practical consequence. Specifically, they would result in a distortion of our health care priorities that would be unjust, imprudent, and unaffordable. As noted already, if all end-stage cancer patients had a just claim to these expensive targeted cancer therapies, the cost to our health care system in the United States would be at least $50–$60 billion each year (which is a very conservative figure). In theory, we could actually afford to do this. However, no persuasive moral argument would justify restricting such social largesse to cancer patients. Virtually all end-stage patients would have the same moral right to whatever medical interventions could offer them any gain at all in life expectancy (at least if we are inclined to embrace an egalitarian theory of health care justice). If this were really a moral obligation in some very strong sense, we would have little ability to provide any form of somewhat expensive health care that "merely" improved quality of life as opposed to improving length of life, such as somewhat expensive medications that relieved pain or various technologies that restored functional abilities otherwise lost to disease or accident. An outcome such as this would have nothing to recommend it from the perspectives of justice, prudence, or compassion. This conclusion will be true whether we have in mind egalitarian, utilitarian, prioritarian, sufficientarian, or luck egalitarian theories of health care justice.

To be clear, I am not arguing that considerations of health care justice would *never* warrant providing patients with terminal diseases "last chance" therapies. Effectiveness matters. AIDS patients in 1995 were doomed to die within two years once they were faced with opportunistic infections because of their severely compromised immune systems. However, protease inhibitors were discovered in 1996, and, more recently, fusion inhibitors. The cost of four-drug combination therapy is now about $35,000 per patient per year, but these drugs are very effective in restoring a reasonable quality of life for additional decades in most cases. At some point HIV might mutate

---

[19] Critical assessments of the appeal to the rule of rescue may be found in McKie and Richardson (2003). See also Cookson et al. (2008).

around these drugs and render them ineffective. AIDS patients would then be faced with very limited life expectancies and, very likely, the same kinds of extraordinarily expensive, marginally effective life-prolonging interventions as end-stage cancer patients. At that point, if we were denying (at social expense) these expensive cancer drugs to patients who would gain only extra weeks or extra months of life from them, then the same morally relevant considerations that justified those denials would justify comparable denials to end-stage AIDS patients.

This same line of argument would apply if the rationale we invoke for providing these expensive cancer drugs to end-stage cancer patients is that they are among the "medically least well off." There are many kinds of patients who can be correctly described (for moral purposes) as being among the "medically least well off." Some of them can be treated at very great expense very effectively for years. That, of course, removes them from the category of the "medically least well off," at least as long as a specific therapeutic intervention continues to be provided. Thus, very young individuals may be diagnosed with Gaucher's disease, which will be fatal if nothing is done for them. However, if they receive the drug imiglucerase at a cost of $300,000 per year, their lives will be saved for an indefinite period of time at a cost of $300,000 for each saved year. This is very far outside the range of what is usually thought of as a reasonable cost-effectiveness ratio. What makes the difference, morally speaking, is that these are young lives of high quality that are sustained by this drug for long periods. This is the exact opposite of the outcomes associated with the expensive cancer drugs where the life sustained is of diminished quality for a relatively brief period of time before death.

We should add that the logic of the moral argument being made here does not put at risk the lives of persons with various disabilities, such as individuals who may have become vent-dependent quadriplegics due to an accident. Those individuals will often incur medical expenses approaching $1 million for the first year after an accident. Still, substantial functional restoration is usually possible through intense rehabilitation and reliance upon a range of assistive technologies. If one reasonable basis for determining fair allocation of health care resources is reliance upon a fair equality of opportunity principle (Daniels, 1985), then persons with these sorts of disabilities will have strong just claims to the services and technologies that will protect for them access to a broad range of functional opportunities for many years. That range of opportunities (regrettably) is no longer available to individuals with end-stage cancers likely to be only very marginally responsive to any of these targeted therapies. What these individuals do have a strong just claim to is high-quality palliative care that will ease their dying and sometimes prolong their lives (Temel et al., 2010).

This brings us to a second type of moral argument that might be invoked by these end-stage cancer patients with a genetic signature in their cancer predictive of only marginal benefits. They might say, "I do not want high-quality palliative care to ease my dying; I want these drugs that might prolong my living." However, respect for patient autonomy is often justifiably constrained by considerations of health care justice. That a patient desperately wants some scarce or expensive form of life-prolonging medical care does nothing to justify that claim as far as health care justice is concerned. To be clear, in the case of non-scarce health care resources, such as these cancer drugs, justice will not absolutely deny access to these drugs for these patients. What justice denies is that access would be *at social expense*. If individuals have the personal resources to purchase these drugs (without any type of social subsidy), no weighty moral considerations will justify a policy that denied them access to those drugs. This is because no other patients would have their just claims to these drugs (or other high-priority health care) compromised by allowing the financially well off to buy these drugs. The assumption here is that a fair and reasonable societal judgment will have been made that these drugs for particular types of individuals in particular medical circumstances yield too little benefit at too high a cost relative to limited social resources.

This brings us to the third type of argument regarding individuals denied these expensive cancer drugs because their cancer has a genetic signature only marginally responsive to these drugs. This would be an egalitarian argument. We earlier called attention to Harris (1985), who argued (in effect) that the size of the gain in life expectancy from these drugs was irrelevant to determining who would have a just claim. His view would seem to be that if anyone had a just claim to access these cancer drugs at social expense, then everyone who might benefit with only a few extra days of life would have an equally just claim to access those cancer drugs at social expense. He sees himself as defending a principle of equal concern and respect. In another of his essays, Harris (1987) calls our attention to seven individuals who will all die in a matter of days without medical treatment. However, if they have treatment, then six of them will live for a year. George, however, can live for seven years if he has access to a treatment that costs five times as much as the treatment for any of the six other individuals. That means we could save more life-years at a lower cost per life-year saved by saving George and allowing the others to die. Harris then comments, "It does not follow that even if each person, if asked, would prefer seven years' remission to one for themselves, that they are all committed to the view that George should be treated rather than that they should. Nor does it follow that this is a preference that society should endorse. But it is the preference that QALYs [quality-adjusted life-years] dictate" (1987, at 118). What Harris is rejecting in this passage is the utilitarian principle that he sees underlying the use of QALYs as well as cost-effectiveness analysis. Harris adds to his earlier point, "A society which values the lives of its citizens is one which tries to ensure that as few of them die prematurely (that is when their lives could continue) as possible" (at 118). Finally, he writes, "The principle of equal access to health care is sustained by the very same reasons that sustain both the principle of equality before the law and the civil rights required to defend the freedom of the individual. They are rightly considered so important that no limit is set on the cost of sustaining them" (at 122).

In theory, the principle of equal concern and respect would be satisfied if everyone with end-stage cancers were denied access to these drugs. Harris clearly rejects that view since he sees a society such as our own as obligated to save all the lives that can be saved. And in the last quoted passage he clearly rejects the view that monetary considerations should be used to make any distinctions or set priorities with regard to which lives to save. All such distinctions in his view represent disrespect for the rights of some individuals who would then die "prematurely." Should I be more charitable in my reading of Harris, given these were his views in the late 1980s? However, in 2008 Harris (Daily Mail Reporter, 2008) expressed essentially the same views in a newspaper interview where he criticized the National Institute for Clinical Excellence (NICE) for recommending against having the British National Health Service pay for the same cancer drugs we are discussing.[20] He contended there that if such decisions absolutely had to be made, it would

---

[20] I discuss later the work of NICE and the ethics issues raised by its work. The United Kingdom has the National Health Service, which provides a reasonably comprehensive set of health benefits to all British citizens. NICE is a non-governmental body charged with determining which new health services ought to be incorporated into that national benefit package. NICE uses multiple criteria to make these judgments, but cost-effectiveness is a preeminent consideration. NICE has approved a number of these targeted cancer drugs for limited specific use, but it has also rejected others judged to yield too little medical benefit at too high a price. There have been proposals for a comparable entity in the United States. Those proposals have been soundly rejected by Congress, largely because it would make rationing decisions explicit and publicly visible.

be fairer to make them with the toss of a coin rather than the guidelines used by NICE.

In commenting on Harris' views, we should note that a reasonable or moderate egalitarianism has much to commend it, morally speaking. However, an unqualified egalitarianism is not morally defensible. Individuals with the same health needs and roughly the same likelihood of having those needs effectively addressed ought to have the same just claims to health care resources. Likewise, the quality of life of an individual (where we have in mind persons with a range of disabilities) should not justify differential access to these interventions, so long as none of those disabilities diminish the likelihood of the effectiveness of that intervention below some threshold of marginal benefit. Harris would likely not endorse my qualifiers. Nevertheless, I will argue they are reasonable and not unjust.

If resources for funding access to these drugs were absolutely restricted, then we could follow Harris' advice and flip coins or use a lottery system to achieve an outcome that was reasonably just. We would have no justified moral alternatives for doing something other than a lottery because of our prognostic ignorance. This would be a reasonable egalitarianism. It is doubtful that Harris would actually endorse this idea in the real world. Instead, what he has written would suggest that he would demand that the dollars be available to fund access to these drugs for everyone with a relevant cancer diagnosis. Ultimately, the logic of this position assumes that human life is priceless and that the need for health care rationing is escapable. However, we have already shown that there is nothing realistic or fair in practice about this position (Fleck, 2009, chap. 3).

If we consider one medical condition at a time and ask whether we (in the United States) can afford to provide medical interventions to treat that condition for all who have that condition with any degree of effectiveness for whatever it might cost, we will almost always have to answer in the affirmative. The real world, however, is one in which there are endless health needs and a correspondingly enormous range of health care interventions that *might* positively effect a therapeutic outcome for those who have those needs. Making no discriminations among all those needs and interventions in order to protect the integrity of an ideological egalitarianism is neither rational nor just nor affordable. Reasonable egalitarian commitments must be bounded by some utilitarian considerations (cost-effectiveness and QALYs), by some prioritarian considerations, by some libertarian considerations, and by some sufficientarian considerations. In short, I will argue that a pluralistic conception of health care justice will be needed to address the real-world complexities of our health care system, and then the most it will be reasonable to expect will be "rough justice with ragged edges."

When Harris advocates that everyone with an advanced cancer have access to these expensive cancer drugs, he is in effect saying that he has gotten rid of the morally troubling (potentially discriminatory) ragged edges. However, this has no relationship to the real world. In the real world, individuals will have a cancer and some other life-threatening co-morbid conditions. An individual may be at risk of dying from their cancer in two years, but what is immediately threatening to end their life in the next three months is an advanced heart condition requiring a $500,000 artificial heart transplant. If we are committed to Harris' strict egalitarianism, then it seems we would be morally obligated to treat both the cancer and the heart disease (or the kidney failure, or the chronic obstructive pulmonary disease, or the end-stage liver disease, etc.). This is another ragged edge.

Diseases overlap in persons in all sorts of complex ways. If we were very strict egalitarians, we would hardly be justified in treating only the life-threatening heart disease of those with cancer. Again, the logical implication of this position is that the entire expanding universe of health needs would have to be treated, no matter what the cost, no matter how minimal the benefit. In theory, this would eliminate ragged edges as well as the risk of morally troubling discrimination. However, this is unreal, unwise, and unfair (given that we have numerous non-health social needs as well). Trade-offs must be made; health care priorities need to be established. How can such choices be accomplished as fairly as possible?

1.7. Summary and Conclusion

In this chapter we have only begun to introduce precision medicine in the context of cancer care. As popular literature about precision medicine puts it, the goal of precision medicine is to provide the right drug in the right dose for the right reason at the right time. Precision medicine seeks to take advantage of our rapidly evolving understanding of genetics to provide very refined, somewhat personalized therapeutic interventions. In many respects the treatment of cancer is currently the paradigm of what precision medicine aspires to be. That is, by making medical therapy as precise as possible, using the dominant distinguishing genetic features of a cancer to guide choice of an anti-cancer drug, the goal is to minimize harmful side effects, maximize intended benefits, and reduce the overall costs of treating that specific medical condition. Given this description, it is hard to imagine that there could be significant ethical challenges attached to this endeavor. However, as we have seen, there are such ethical challenges.

Our challenges for the present are focused on the problem of health care justice. The 150 or so targeted cancer therapies currently on the market typically have costs of $100,000 or more for a course of treatment (with many now in the $150,000 to $200,000 range). These drugs are typically used with advanced or metastatic cancers. If these drugs could effect a cure of these cancers, or at least provide many years of reasonable quality of life for that price, then the $100,000 might represent a reasonable expenditure of social resources, and we might be able to determine a way to accomplish that equitably. However, the reality is that none of these drugs literally cures a metastatic cancer. Moreover, only a small percentage of patients can hope to be super-responders, such as Dr. Hillard. For the vast majority of patients, expected gains in life expectancy will be measured in weeks or months, sometimes a year or two. The obvious hope of medical researchers is that this will change with time and successful future medical research. That hope is imagined as a world in which advanced or metastatic cancer has become a managed chronic disorder, much like AIDS, as opposed to being a terminal disorder. However, as we shall see in the next chapter, that hope raises even more complicated and intractable problems of health care justice than those identified in this chapter.

2

Precision Medicine

Hope, Hype, and Hysteria

2.1. Precision Medicine: The Evolving Understanding of Cancer

Increasingly, we are approaching each patient as a unique problem to solve. Toxic, indiscriminate, cell-killing drugs have given way to nimbler, finer-fingered molecules that can activate or deactivate complex pathways in cells, cut off growth factors, accelerate or decelerate the immune response or choke the supply of nutrients and oxygen. More and more, we must come up with ways to use drugs as precision tools to jam cogs and turn off selective switches in particular cancer cells.

—Mukherjee (2016)

We start with the story of Kellie Carey, as reported in the *Wall Street Journal* (Winslow, 2013). In 2010, at the age of 45, she was diagnosed with lung cancer. Her physician informed her that she might have only three months to live. However, she was persistent. She was able to enter a clinical trial for the drug crizotinib (Xalkori˚) because an ALK gene mutation was the primary driver of her cancer. Crizotinib is an ALK inhibitor. Roughly 5% of lung cancer patients have that as the driver mutation of their cancer. Crizotinib did work for about 18 months, but then her cancer again progressed. The cost of that drug in 2013 was $10,800 per month. She was put on another drug in the same class as crizotinib, which still seemed to be working somewhat in July of 2013. That other drug was not named in the article. However, it was likely ceritinib (Zykadia˚) (Masters et al., 2015), which is described as a second-generation ALK inhibitor and is just as expensive as crizotinib. In mid-2013 ceritinib seemed to be becoming less effective for Ms. Carey, likely as a result of cancer drug *resistance*.

Precision Medicine and Distributive Justice. Leonard M. Fleck, Oxford University Press. © Oxford University Press 2022.
DOI: 10.1093/oso/9780197647721.003.0002

Cancer drug resistance is a complex phenomenon. It is related to what we mentioned in Chapter 1 as the heterogeneity of cancer. Tumors are described as being "heterogeneous" when they contain cells that have multiple mutations. This is in contrast to what might be regarded as normal biology wherein each cell in our body has essentially the same DNA. Mukherjee (2016) writes:

> No other human disease is known to possess this degree of genetic heterogeneity. Adult-onset diabetes, for example, is a complex genetic disease, but it appears to be dominated by variations in only about a dozen genes. Cancer, by contrast, has potentially unlimited variations. Like faces, like fingerprints — like selves — every cancer is characterized by its distinctive marks: a set of individual scars stamped on an individual genome.[1]

Intertumor and intratumor heterogeneity are both common phenomena in cancer (though this is something that was not medically well understood until somewhat recently) (Gerlinger et al., 2012; Raspe et al., 2012; Longo, 2012). Both contribute to the problem of cancer drug resistance. "Intratumor heterogeneity" means that within any given tumor the cancer cells will have multiple genetic identities. That is, the cancer cells will not be genetically identical with one another, though they are all part of the same tumor. "Intertumor heterogeneity" means that multiple tumors (as in metastatic cancer) will be genetically distinct from one another. The heterogeneity matters for therapeutic purposes because these targeted therapies are always targeting some specific genetic mutation in these tumors, such as an ALK rearrangement or an EGFR mutation of a specific sort. However, as Gerlinger et al. (2012) have pointed out, the practical implication of this heterogeneity is that no single biopsy of a tumor will necessarily yield an accurate picture of the genetic mutations that characterize that tumor. A single biopsy will likely yield an overly simplistic picture of that tumor and tell a physician virtually nothing about the distinctive genetic characteristics of all the other tumors that are part of that cancer diagnosis. Consequently, multiple biopsies and genetic sequencing will be needed to obtain a roughly accurate overall picture of that cancer, still with no guarantee that this represents a complete

---

[1] Readers might recognize the name of Siddhartha Mukherjee as the author of *The Emperor of All Maladies: A Biography of Cancer* (2010).

picture. Further, the genetic characteristics of a cancer evolve over time with the progression of the cancer (Jamal-Hanjani et al., 2017).

The current medical belief is that tumors grow because of "driver" mutations. Targeted therapies are aimed at disabling those driver mutations (assuming that clinician researchers can correctly identify the driver mutation in the midst of this genetic complexity). These targeted therapies are often successful in disabling a correctly identified driver mutation. This is where cancer drug resistance comes in. Researchers believe that something like Darwinian evolution occurs when a driver mutation is disabled. That is, one of the other mutations becomes the new driver mutation and allows the cancer to progress. This is why disease progression occurs typically after a few months of treatment with one of these targeted therapies. Again, those few months represent a median. Ms. Carey did better than that. She seems to have gotten a bit more than a year of progression-free survival (PFS) with each of those drugs. However, the point is that these drugs are not curative; their therapeutic efficacy is limited. Moreover, use of these drugs in succession has resulted in escalating costs for cancer care without consistent corresponding gains in clinical outcomes that would justify those costs. In a world with limited resources and unlimited non-cancer health care needs, this is a moral problem as well as an economic problem.

More recently, research efforts have turned to combinatorial approaches with targeted therapies to address the resistance problem and genetic heterogeneity (Castro et al., 2013; Al-Lazikani et al., 2012; Yap et al., 2013; Garraway, 2013). That is, researchers are adopting the AIDS paradigm wherein three- or four-drug combinations are used to contain (not defeat) HIV. There is no question that this has yielded dramatic success in the case of HIV. Hundreds of thousands of HIV-positive individuals have lived 20 or more years because of this therapy, which would never have been possible in the early 1990s. For four-drug combinations, the cost per life-year saved has been about $35,000. However, there are moral and medical dis-analogies here that ought to temper the enthusiasm of cancer researchers for this approach.

First, cancer has proven to be enormously more complex and devious in its capacity for transmutation than the AIDS virus. It is impossible to overstate that complexity and the consequent ability of a cancer to survive the onslaught of chemotherapeutic agents aimed at destroying that cancer. Shi-Ming Tu (2010) is one researcher who attributes the wiliness of cancer to its "stemness," the fact that many cancers possess (or come to possess) the versatility of stem cells. He writes, "Can it be just incredible coincidence that many of the same essential and relevant characteristics of a cancer cell that command and deserve such attention also happen to comprise the very basic features of a stem cell?" (at 56).[2]

Second, Al-Lazikani et al. (2012) have noted that the theoretical drug combinations for attacking cancer are vast. They call attention to about 250 approved cancer drugs. That yields 31,000 two-way combinations and 2.5 million three-way combinations. Moreover, 1,200 cancer drugs are in various stages of development, which would yield 287 million possible three-way combinations. Many of these mathematically possible combinations would not make clinical sense. Still, it will require enormous investments in research to sort out all these possibilities, never mind clinical trials and the risks of unanticipated toxicities from these combinations.[3] This sort of

---

[2] It should be noted that the cancer "stem cell hypothesis" advocated by Tu (and many others) also has its critics, such as Rahman et al. (2011). One of the virtues of the stem cell hypothesis is that it does help to explain the very limited effectiveness of targeted therapies that attack only one mutation or pathway at a time, thereby failing to disable the complex regenerative capacity of many cancers, what Tu (2010, chap. 12) refers to as the "intrinsic pluripotency" of these cells (see also Makena et al., 2020). The take-home message is that it will be extremely difficult to defeat any metastatic cancer with any single drug or combination of drugs because of the biological complexity and elusiveness of these cancer stem cells (Lathia et al., 2020). At present, there are no targeted therapies that can effectively attack these cancer stem cells (Clarke, 2019).

Why does it matter whether or not there are cancer stem cells? The short answer may be that cancer may never be defeated in an individual if researchers cannot develop drugs that directly attack and disable these cancer stem cells. The hope of some researchers is that if these stem cells can be destroyed, the result will be a cure for cancer. However, some research suggests that "normal cancer cells" can revert to a stem cell state, thereby replenishing the supply of stem cells that had been killed off (Kaiser, 2015). More recently, the concern is that cancer stem cells are "too similar" to other stem cells in the body, which would also be damaged or destroyed by any drug that killed cancer stem cells (LeMieux, 2018).

[3] Philosophers might wonder why all this detail regarding the biology of cancer is necessary when the ethics issues are what is primarily important. They might frame their frustrations this way: "Isn't the really fundamental ethics question whether a cancer patient has a just claim (a moral right) to use hundreds of thousands of dollars worth of these cancer drugs to achieve a few extra months of life? Just address that question and skip all the distracting details." Maybe that makes ethical analysis easier. There are thousands of ways of committing murder, but all those murderous details may be ignored for purposes of concluding that murder is ethically wrong. Perhaps that way of thinking has ethical utility for the policymaker or health care administrator with responsibility for controlling health care costs. However, physicians are in a very different moral position. They are caring for individual patients with very distinctive variations of cancer. They need to deal with conflicting evidence in the medical literature regarding the efficacy of various possible targeted therapies. Physicians have to deal with multiple complex forms of uncertainty. There is diagnostic uncertainty: Has the genetic makeup of this cancer been correctly characterized? There is therapeutic uncertainty: Is this the right drug in the right dose for this genetically distinctive cancer? There is prognostic uncertainty: Is this therapeutic choice, rather than some other possible choice, going to yield the most benefit and do the least harm to this patient? These clinical details make a difference to the very fine-grained ethical judgments physicians must make in clinical practice. Ultimately, policymakers and health care administrators must be sensitive to this level of detail as well, lest their judgments threaten the ethical integrity of physicians. The same will be true for moral philosophers such as myself.

clinical complexity is not true of efforts to identify effective therapeutic combinations for treating HIV.

At this point, I ask the reader to pass over these practical challenges to consider the moral and economic challenges that success would yield. Recall that the goal of this combinatorial strategy is to permit patients with metastatic cancer to achieve extra years of reasonable-quality life. Assume that researchers are aiming for five extra years not now available to these patients. If each of those years cost "only" $100,000 for two or more of these targeted drugs, and if these drugs would need to be taken in reduced doses for the rest of an individual's life (as with the AIDS drugs), and if there are about 600,000 individuals who die of cancer each year in the United States, that yields an annual cost of $60 billion.[4] If there were a five-year gain in life expectancy for each cohort on average, then in Year 5 we would be sustaining 3 million lives with metastatic cancer at a cost of $300 billion.[5] This is *only* for treatment of metastatic cancer in these cohorts, not for cancer in anyone else, not for any other medical problems of these individuals, such as side effects related to this therapeutic approach. To put this in context, I will mention that 1.8 million individuals were diagnosed with cancer in the United States in 2020. All the costs associated with diagnosing and treating those individuals would need to be added to that $60 billion Year 1 figure. Further, because of the aging out of the post–World War II generation, projections are that 2.2 million individuals will be diagnosed with cancer in 2030 (Rahib et al., 2014). As these statistics suggest, future cancer costs will be increasing dramatically.

Some researchers, furthermore, imagine a future in which this combinatorial therapy would be highly individualized. Targeted cancer drugs would be combined and recombined in numerous ways in response to repeated deep genomic sequencing of specific cancers at various stages of the disease

[4] In 2018, the actual cost of some of these combinations was $250,000 for a year, as we discuss below. However, the comforting economic news, as things are now with health insurance in the United States, is that less than half of those 600,000 individuals would have the financial ability to pay for those therapies because they are uninsured, are underinsured, or have various insurance limitations (co-payments, deductibles) that leave them with unaffordable personal expenses for these drugs. This is hardly ethically comforting. I recently encountered a patient I will call "Stan." He was diagnosed with myelofibrosis six years ago. He is taking a drug called ruxolitinib (Jakafi'). He told me he has great insurance because it pays $8,000 per month for that drug. The problem is that he pays an additional $3,500 per month. He has almost spent down his retirement savings. How should we assess that from a moral point of view? This is now described as the "financial toxicity" associated with cancer care (Zafar, 2016).
[5] By way of comparison, there were in 2020 about 1.1 million Americans who were HIV-positive. That cohort is growing very slowly, in spite of the effectiveness of protease inhibitors, fusion inhibitors, and other drugs in the AIDS armamentarium. Preventive efforts have been reasonably effective in reducing new HIV infections.

process (Castro et al., 2013). Such repeated sequencing would be necessary and costly because of recurrent cancer drug resistance related to intratumor and intertumor heterogeneity as well as genetic evolution of the tumors. This raises yet another question of health care justice. How many of these combinatorial modifications is each and every advanced cancer patient entitled to? Are they entitled to as many as they can tolerate before death, no matter how marginally effective or costly each iteration might be? What should be the moral and economic limits? Does comparison with our treatment of HIV-positive individuals yield any helpful moral insight?

Yet another morally relevant factor must be noted. Cancer is predominantly a disease of older patients, patients covered by Medicare in the United States. Because of advancing medical technology and the aging out of the post–World War II "baby boom" generation, the Medicare population will double to 80 million by 2030, and the cost of the program in 2022 is expected to reach $1 trillion (Keehan et al., 2020). Moreover, the 10-year cost of Medicare (2019–2028) is projected to be about $8.3 trillion.[6] Medicare is forbidden by law from using cost-effectiveness to make coverage decisions. That means that any of these targeted cancer drugs found to be safe and minimally effective would be covered by Medicare.[7] Private employers offering health insurance as a benefit would be under no comparable obligation, and the uninsured and underinsured would have no reliable access to these drugs either. What this would mean is that non-elderly metastatic cancer patients would generally not have assured access to the future possible benefits of these combinatorial cancer therapies, though they would be paying increased taxes to support such access for elderly Medicare recipients. Should a just and caring society accept such a state of affairs as "just enough"? Can it be argued that this is the same moral, political, and economic logic that applies to Social Security? In other words, as workers we all pay into Social Security, hoping to live long enough to enjoy that investment in retirement. No one has a just

---

[6] These 10-year projections do not include the potential costs associated with successful implementation of a targeted combinatorial cancer strategy. The assumption is that the majority of future cancer patients, faced with the cost of these $100,000 drugs (even with health insurance) will not be able to afford to access them.

[7] Big Pharma was successful in 2006 in having incorporated into the legislation that authorized Part "D" of Medicare a prohibition on Medicare negotiating drug prices using its 55 million covered lives to extract large discounts from pharmaceutical companies. That was nakedly self-serving. Both Democrats and Republicans have opposed Medicare's use of cost-effectiveness in making coverage decisions "for reasons of compassion," that is, not wanting to deny desperate patients facing death access to drugs that "might" save or prolong their lives. Put another way, Congress and Medicare could not be accused of making rationing decisions.

grievance if they fail to live to retirement age due to bad luck and bad health, as opposed to a socially correctable adverse social determinant of health. Is our fragmented system for financing access to health care for the non-elderly a socially correctable adverse social determinant of health that ought to be corrected? How can cost control judgments be justly determined in the fragmented and inequitable system we have in the United States for financing health care? Is that just a quixotic hope?

2.2. Immunotherapy: More Resistance and More Ragged Edges

We return to the story of Ms. Carey. In late 2013, she was considering entering a trial with a new class of drugs known as checkpoint inhibitors. The immune system is designed to attack foreign biological "stuff" within our bodies (i.e., bacteria, viruses, fungi, and cancer cells). However, if this immune response is not effectively controlled, we have autoimmune disorders. The body uses molecules known as immune checkpoints to control the strength and dura- tion of the immune response. Some tumors are able to produce these check- point molecules, thereby preventing the immune system from attacking these tumors. The drugs known as immune checkpoint inhibitors are designed to release the tumor-induced brakes on the immune system. At this writing (2021) six major checkpoint inhibitors have received US Food and Drug Administration (FDA) approval: ipilimumab (Yervoy˚), a CTLA-4 inhibitor that downregulates the immune system; pembrolizumab (Keytruda˚), a PD-1 (programmed death) inhibitor; nivolumab (Opdivo˚), also a PD-1 inhib- itor; atezolizumab (Tecentriq˚), a PD-L1 inhibitor; durvalumab (Imfinzi˚); and avelumab (Bavencio˚). These six drugs are used with a variety of cancers. Some of them have had some initial success with non-small cell lung cancer (NSCLC) as well as melanoma.

Ms. Carey was likely put on one of these drugs for her ALK-mutated lung cancer. Let us assume that she was placed on nivolumab. One impor- tant clinical trial for squamous-cell NSCLC reported that, compared with second-line chemotherapy, median survival with nivolumab improved from 9.4 months to 12.2 months (Brahmer et al., 2015). We will note in passing that the cost of nivolumab is $156,000 per year or, in cost-effectiveness terms, $600,000 per quality-adjusted life-year. This is because the incre- mental gain from nivolumab is a bit under three months. Pembrolizumab is another checkpoint inhibitor used for NSCLC. It yields comparable results with a median survival of about 12 months. The cost of this drug is about $150,000 per year, $8,800 for an infusion every three weeks. Two things are noteworthy about this drug: (1) tumors shrank in about 20% of patients and (2) half the patients with high PD-L1 levels experienced tumor shrinkage and lived longer before the cancer worsened (Gettinger et al., 2015).

Point 1 is significant because, despite the hype that immunotherapy has received recently, it is a relatively small percentage of patients who are actually responsive.[8] This certainly seems relevant as a problem of health care justice, given the very high cost of these drugs. Point 2 might be a little surprising because what is being said is that individuals who have a higher mutational burden actually have a greater likelihood of a more sustained therapeutic response. The working hypothesis is that this higher mutational burden actually triggers a more vigorous response from the immune system because it has been primed by one of these checkpoint inhibitors.[9] The other significant point is that if effectiveness were relevant to making health care justice judgments, then patients with that higher mutational burden would have a prima facie stronger just claim to these checkpoint inhibitors.[10] Still, the larger overall point is that these drugs are not curative in the case of

[8] For the reader interested in achieving a basic understanding of the immune system and current use of the immune system to attack cancers, I recommend *The Beautiful Cure: The Revolution in Immunology and What It Means for Your Health* (2018) by Daniel Davis, an immunologist in the United Kingdom. He writes that, "we don't yet know which molecules on a person's cancer are the best to target, we don't yet know whether or not every cancer cell would have to possess the same genetic signature, we don't yet know how to limit the possibility of healthy bystander cells being attacked, causing unwanted side effects, and so on" (at 194). See also Graeber (2018).

[9] That "more vigorous" response is actually a mixed blessing. An amplified immune system can trigger a range of autoimmune disorders. Schrag and Basch (2018) write: "For non-oncology subspecialists, the increasing use of immune therapies generates more cardiology consultations for immune-mediated myocarditis, more gastroenterology consultations for colitis, more endocrinology consultations for pituitary disorders, and more pulmonary acute care visits for cytokine release syndrome and myriad other consequences of manipulating the immune system to treat cancer" (at 2203). This outcome exemplifies what we discuss in Chapter 3 as a "wicked problem," medically, morally, and economically.

[10] Patients with low levels of PD-L1 experienced no gain in survival from atezolizumab, which is just as expensive as the other checkpoint inhibitors ($12,500 per month). This certainly seems like one reasonable biomarker for limiting access to this drug. There were also patients with middling levels of PD-L1, which raises once again the "ragged edge" problem and what would count as a "just enough" response to that problem. To illustrate, when atezolizumab was used to treat bladder cancer, 26% of patients with high levels of PD-L1 experienced significant tumor shrinkage and 12% had complete remissions. However, among patients who had low or undetectable levels of PD-L1, 9.5% had tumor shrinkage and 2.4% had complete remissions (Pollack, 2016). However, just knowing who would benefit "the most" does nothing to address the ragged edge issue of what is a "just enough" response to those who would benefit "somewhat," such as the bladder cancer patients.

metastatic lung cancer. Further, for the vast majority of these patients gains in life expectancy are marginal at best.

Melanoma is another form of cancer that has sometimes been dramatically responsive to these checkpoint inhibitors. Winslow (2014) reports the stories of several individuals who each gained more than five extra years of life from these checkpoint inhibitors. These were all amazing stories about individual super-responders. These results may raise some hope. However, they also raise more difficult ethical issues, given the overall cost of significantly prolonging the life of one individual. When is it the case that "too many" individuals need to be treated at extraordinary expense in order to prolong the life of that super-responder? Are 10 treatment failures "too many" to save that one super-responder? Is that too low a number? Should that number be 20, 50, or 100?

Let us return briefly to the results of recent clinical trials associated with melanoma and treatment with these checkpoint inhibitors. Ipilimumab was the first checkpoint inhibitor used to treat advanced melanoma. However, pembrolizumab and nivolumab or ipilimumab may yield better results (Asher et al., 2020; Olson et al., 2021; Robert et al., 2019; Wolchok et al., 2017) than any one alone. The objective response rate of 64% was for the combination therapy compared to 11% for ipilimumab alone. This is an example of the AIDS combined therapy strategy mentioned earlier. Further, median PFS was only 4.4 months for ipilimumab alone. However, the cost for this combination therapy would have been much greater than that of either drug alone. One article put that combination cost for a course of treatment at $252,000 (Workman et al., 2017). More problematic is that drug-related adverse events of grade 3–4 were much greater in the combination therapy than treatment with either drug alone (54% to 24%), and many of those adverse events would themselves generate substantial costs, especially if those adverse events required hospitalization. These latter costs are typically not included when reporting the "costs" of treatment for a specific cancer, which results in underestimating the true cost-effectiveness of the intervention as well as the all-inclusive cost to Medicare, Medicaid, or some other insurance plan.[11]

---

[11] An example of these "extra costs" associated with treating a cancer is that of Hedda Martin, age 60, from Grand Rapids Michigan. She was treated for breast cancer in 2005 with powerful chemotherapeutic agents that initiated heart failure as a side effect. By 2018 her heart failure progressed to the point that she would need a heart transplant. She could not be certain that a heart for transplantation would be available quickly enough, which meant she would need a left ventricular assist device (LVAD) as a "bridge to transplant." The cost of the LVAD procedure would be $250,000. The cost of

The trial reported above is the Checkmate 067 trial. The results of that trial were updated two years later by Wolchok et al. (2017), the same group of researchers as above. What we now have are three-year survival rates for previously untreated metastatic melanoma patients. I remind the reader that the most ethically relevant statistics will be overall survival (OS) and PFS. In the nivolumab-plus-ipilimumab group, OS was 58% at three years, compared to 52% in nivolumab monotherapy and 34% in ipilimumab monotherapy. Those are significant differences compared to ipilimumab monotherapy. However, treatment-related adverse events were at 59% (grade 3–4) for the combination therapy compared to 21% in the nivolumab group and 28% in the ipilimumab group. The rates of PFS at three years were 39% in the combination group, 32% in the nivolumab group, and just 10% in the ipilimumab group.

The combination therapy made a significant difference in PFS. However, the same ethics issues are again raised, as above. Does the higher cost of the combination therapy yield enough in the way of medical benefit to justify that allocation of health care resources? Further, the adverse event rate was very significant and costly. The other point to note is that PD-L1 positivity or negativity made a substantial difference in clinical effectiveness when comparing combination therapy to nivolumab alone. The obvious clinical conclusion is that patients who are PD-L1-positive should get the costlier combination therapy. The problem, however, is that positivity is on a continuum. If 50% or more of tumor cells are PD-L1-positive, then that represents "high" positivity. Technically speaking, if only 1% of tumor cells are PD-L1-positive, they are rated as "positive." However, is it correct to believe that tumors that are 1% or 5% or 10% PD-L1-positive will yield the same degree of clinical effectiveness as tumors that are 50% PD-L1-positive? If that is unlikely to be true, then would it be "not unjust" to deny the combination therapy to advanced melanoma patients whose tumors were only marginally PD-L1-positive? This is again the ragged edge problem.

According to one trial, patients lived at least twice as long after treatment with pembrolizumab when compared to historically treated patients. There were 655 patients in the trial. Those patients had a median survival of 24.4 months and an estimated three-year survival of 40% (Bankhead, 2016). Only about 33% of that patient cohort had an objective response,

---

the heart transplant would be $500,000. Another $30,000 would be needed for immunosuppressant drugs for six months, then $2,500 per month for these drugs for the rest of her life (Reindl, 2018).

judged "durable," as opposed to a very minimal short-term response. Why did that other 67% not have a durable response? Moreover, if further research were done that resulted in likely reasons for that marginal and ephemeral response, would those reasons be sufficient to justify (ethically speaking) not offering pembrolizumab as a treatment option? Alternatively, does the fact that pembrolizumab might well represent a "last chance" therapy give it some sort of special moral status that would exempt it from normal justice-relevant allocation criteria?

At a 2016 meeting of the American Association for Cancer Research investigators reported a 5-year survival rate of 34% for patients with advanced melanoma who had been treated with nivolumab (Bankhead, 2016). What was not formally reported, but could be ethically relevant, would be the shape of the survival curve for that cohort. The survival curve might have been a smooth, gradually descending curve. Alternatively, the "curve" might have actually displayed a steep drop around the one-year mark, followed by a fairly flat survival line for the 34% of patients referred to above. If this latter scenario were true, it would be reasonable to ask whether the shorter-term survivors had as strong a just claim to the nivolumab as the long-term survivors. As things are now, investigators do not know which individuals might be in either of these groups. However, if future research were able to reveal those differences before the fact, would that justify denying access to nivolumab for those judged to be short-term survivors?

To add to the ethical complexity behind that question, current medical practice would continue to provide the drug to these patients as long as the toxicities were tolerable or until evidence emerged of cancer progression (Robert et al., 2016).[12] What that means from the perspective of health care justice is that spending per patient would be proportional to survival. It would cost about $150,000 for one-year survival patients and $750,000 for five-year survival patients. Does this imply, ethically speaking, that patients able to survive five years have as strong a just claim to the resources needed to achieve that goal as patients who will survive only one year, despite the fact that those aggregated costs for longer-term survivors might

[12] Robert et al. (2016) reported that some patients were on pembrolizumab for 3.5 years and that 21% were still receiving the drug at last follow-up. Some researchers wonder whether immune therapies might be discontinued after some limited period of time. The thought is that the immune system might have been sensitized sufficiently from a limited course of treatment with one of these checkpoint inhibitors so that it would continue to destroy cancer cells without constant reinforcement from this drug. I will just comment that trying to test this hypothesis strikes me as being medically and ethically risky, given the phenomenon of cancer drug resistance.

have disruptive allocational consequences for larger institutional budgets (Medicare, Medicaid, accountable care organizations). Another way to ask a potentially ethically relevant question would be: Do short-term survivors have less of a just claim to these resources because they have "less to lose" compared to potential long-term survivors who would have "more to lose"? I am certain that raising that question would leave many of my readers ethically uncomfortable, especially if their fundamental ethical commitment is to some version of egalitarianism. For them, it would be ethically obligatory to save all of those $150,000 life-years by providing access to nivolumab for these patients with advanced melanoma. However, if we take seriously the central implication of the "just caring" problem (limited resources to meet unlimited health care needs), then funneling resources to nivolumab and these melanoma patients will mean taking those resources away from some other patient group.[13] If this were what must happen in the real world, then would it be incumbent upon egalitarians to know from where those resources were taken and to provide sufficient ethical justification for that trade-off?

This last question is not a speculative ethical question. It has been a matter of urgent practicality in the Netherlands (just to put this in a comparative perspective). Sleijfer and Verweij (2016) call attention to the fact that the Dutch have included these novel anticancer agents in their standard package of health benefits. However, nivolumab has caused the Dutch to rethink that acceptance. Sleijfer and Verweij point out that the cost of nivolumab is projected to be €200 million per year "which would account for almost an eighth of the Netherlands' total expenditures on drugs for inpatients." The authors conclude, "This situation creates a new precedent, and the era of automatic inclusion of new anticancer drugs to the Netherlands' standard health-insurance package is now over."

It is not just an economic problem that a single drug could commandeer that large a portion of the inpatient drug budget. It is an ethical problem, a problem of health care justice. For a moment let us put this into the context of health care in the United States. Some drugs are twice as expensive as nivolumab. In Chapter 1 we discussed the cystic fibrosis drug ivacaftor, which costs $300,000 per person per year. While that is an extraordinarily

---

[13] More recently, nivolumab has been combined with ipilimumab to treat advanced melanoma. The result has been median long-term survival greater than 60 months (Larkin et al., 2019). I call attention to this research because it does involve a combination of these immunotherapies, which means it is a much more expensive option on both an annual basis and an aggregated survival basis. These are significant (and costly) gains in life expectancy, albeit at present for only a small segment of the late-stage cancer population.

high cost per person, the number of persons needing that drug is approximately 2,000. In contrast, 234,000 individuals will be diagnosed with lung cancer in the United States annually, and 160,000 will die of their lung cancer. That latter group is the patient population for nivolumab. Unlike the Netherlands, there is no national health care benefit package in the United States, except for Medicare. Consequently, the number of individuals with advanced lung cancer who would be candidates for the drug will be greatly diminished because a large portion of our population remains uninsured. Moreover, an equally large portion is underinsured. In addition, many insurance plans require co-pays for a drug such as this in the 30%–50% range (effectively excluding individuals from accessing this drug who are not very well off financially).[14] State Medicaid programs may or may not include coverage for this drug. These state programs are free to make such choices, mostly in accord with state budgetary limitations constrained by the relative wealth of the state and the willingness of taxpayers to raise taxes.

These limitations reduce considerably the "societal economic burden" associated with these targeted cancer therapies. From an egalitarian ethical perspective, however, this would hardly be cause for elation. If the financially well off see their having access to this drug as welfare-enhancing, then we would have reason to believe that those financially less well off with advanced lung cancer would also see such access as being welfare-enhancing.

Libertarians, of course, would see things very differently. Life is about trade-offs. No one has unlimited resources. Individuals should be free to make trade-offs within their resource bundle which they see as being congruent with their own welfare goals. Libertarians would generally not be very supportive of the Medicaid program. They object to extracting dollars from taxpayers to pay the extraordinary costs associated with these targeted cancer therapies, especially if many of those taxpayers could not afford the drugs themselves if they were faced with metastatic cancer. Further, some libertarians will argue, the poor themselves might regard spending Medicaid dollars on these targeted therapies as an imprudent use of resources, given

---

[14] Szabo (2018) reports the case of Mary Anne DiCanto, whose breast cancer became metastatic four years earlier at age 55. Her husband, Scott Primiano, put his faith in precision medicine. Still, she died in 2017 at age 59. She tried one targeted therapy that matched a genetic feature of her cancer, but that failed after a while. She tried a second drug that targeted a different genetic feature of her cancer, but that almost killed her. Over 13 years Mr. Primiano reports he spent $500,000 out of pocket for her care, not an option for most Americans. Maybe we (ethically concerned citizens) should just accept this. However, Szabo points out that "hospitals promote their precision-medicine programs by showcasing the stories of long-term survivors." Szabo comments, "Against this backdrop of hope and desperation, how are patients (or democratic deliberators) supposed to make informed choices?"

their limited benefits. They might argue that if taxpayers were willing to spend more money on Medicaid, other health care needs should be funded instead that yielded more health good at a lower cost. Apart from Medicaid, libertarians would oppose including coverage of these drugs in any mandated health plans for the uninsured. They would object that such enriched health benefit packages would be commandeering resources from the currently uninsured (often living at economic margins) for purposes that they did not see as advancing their welfare significantly.

In fairness to these libertarian concerns, we should say that these concerns are not irrational or so obviously unethical that they are not worthy of ethical analysis and argument. However, egalitarian and utilitarian concerns need to be fairly addressed as well. Let us assume that it is at least ethically desirable that everyone in our society ought to have access to medically necessary, effective health care. We make this assumption for reasons of compassion that all would endorse. Given that, what sort of universal health care benefit package should be created that can effectively balance egalitarian, utilitarian, and libertarian core values, especially with respect to the inclusion or exclusion of these very expensive targeted cancer therapies? We should also inquire how prioritarians and sufficientarians might assess access to these targeted cancer therapies. This is a wicked problem, as we discuss in Chapters 3 and 4.

2.3. Biomarkers: Seeking Therapeutic Precision

We have called attention to the complexity of cancers: the complexity of their biological environment, the complexity of their evolution, and the complexity of their molecular composition (i.e., their genetic signature). Given that complexity, how are physicians supposed to achieve a precise therapeutic response? How are they supposed to know which of 150 targeted therapies is the right therapy for the molecular features of a particular cancer? This is where biomarkers are supposed to have a role.

What exactly is a biomarker? The National Institutes of Health (Biomarkers Definitions Working Group, 2001) defines a biomarker as a "characteristic that is objectively measured and evaluated as an indicator of normal biologic processes, pathogenic processes, or pharmacologic responses to a therapeutic intervention." Broadly speaking, biomarkers can be used for prognostic, predictive, or pharmacodynamic purposes (Blanchard and

Wik, 2018). Prognostic biomarkers are supposed to identify specific groups of cancer patients who are likely to have a shorter survival due to specific features of their cancer. Prognostic biomarkers might also identify patients who are likely to have a robust response to an appropriate targeted therapy, again because of specific features of their cancer. Predictive biomarkers predict a patient's likely response to a specific therapy. Women who have breast cancer that is HER2$^+$ will have a positive response to the drug trastuzumab (Blanchard and Wik, 2018). Pharmacodynamic biomarkers are intended to help identify the optimal dose of a drug to achieve a strong therapeutic outcome with minimal side effects.

What is most important about biomarkers is their clinical utility. As we noted in Chapter 1, genetic features of an individual's DNA will tell a clinician whether a patient will be a normal metabolizer of a drug, as opposed to a fast or slow metabolizer. Knowing this will prevent either a harmful or an ineffective response to a particular drug. Serious side effects can also be prevented if the genetic features of some individuals render them particularly vulnerable in the case of a specific drug. Some biomarkers can also inform a clinician whether or not a particular drug will be effective in a particular patient, thereby both sparing that patient the unnecessary risk of nasty side effects and sparing society costs without any benefit (or unnecessary costs associated with treating unnecessary side effects). Biomarkers that permitted such clear clinical judgments are ideal. However, that is really the exception rather than the rule when it comes to cancer. Blanchard and Wik write, "However, the complexity, plurality, and uncertainties around the mechanisms of cancer should make us cautious when biomarkers are depicted as able to allow both comprehensive and robust insights into cancer, and better, safer, economically sustainable medical decision making and therapies" (2018, at 10). This comment is especially true in the case of metastatic cancer. A theoretically simple case would be HER2 in breast cancer. However, it turns out there are degrees of HER2 positivity. At the far end of the spectrum clinicians can be confident that trastuzumab will have a beneficial effect for the patient. In the middle of the spectrum, with marginal HER2 positivity, it will be unclear whether trastuzumab will yield any benefit at all; and, for some patients, trastuzumab will have cardiotoxic effects.

Much cancer research has results reported in the form of median gains in PFS, as opposed to OS. I assume that what ultimately matters for metastatic cancer patients is OS. Obtaining timely approval for new drugs is facilitated by using PFS as a surrogate endpoint. Sometimes there will be a good correlation between PFS and OS; at other times that will not be true. Maj et al. (2016) report that with anti-angiogenic cancer treatment withdrawal of the anti-angiogenic agent (due to progression) results in rapid tumor regrowth and no gain in OS. From the perspective of the just allocation of health care resources, what should be concluded? Assume, for hypothetical purposes, that this is true across the board. That would make it easy to deny future patients these drugs for this cancer because there was no net gain in life expectancy, and hence no just claim to one of these $100,000 drugs. But what if, hypothetically, median PFS was nine months and gain in OS for 30% of the cohort was three months, with zero gain in OS for the remainder? Would our sense of health care justice require that all in the cohort have access to that angiogenic inhibitor at social expense? Or would it be "not unjust" if all in that cohort were denied that drug at social expense? Or should such decisions be left to individual clinicians caring for individual patients, as opposed to having an entity such as the National Institute for Clinical Excellence in the United Kingdom make such decisions for whole categories of patients potentially offered a particular cancer drug, using as a basis for a decision medical and economic data and ethical judgment?

Another provocative piece of research is provided by Salas-Vega et al. (2017). They reviewed all new cancer drugs licensed between 2003 and 2013 by the FDA in the United States or by the European Medical Agency. Median OS gains came to 3.43 months. They note that there have been larger survival gains on the other side of that median but that these "are unevenly distributed across all newly licensed medicines, often . . . at the cost of safety, and may not always translate to real-world practice."[15] I would call attention, in particular, to the issue of real-world practice wherein patients with all manner of co-morbidities atop their metastatic disease often have outcomes from these drugs that are far less positive than suggested by clinical trial results. This too is part of the challenges associated with ragged edges in clinical practice that generate comparable ragged edges for ethical judgment regarding resource allocation.

What should be the appropriate ethical response to the OS results reported above? One response might be that what is most ethically important are those patients whose OS is on the "far side" of the median. Granted that half the patients for many (not all) of these cancer drugs gained less than four

---

[15] Salas-Vega et al. (2017) also note that 30% of these new cancer drugs are associated with no gain in OS. Their work is corroborated by Prasad et al. (2018).

months in OS, the other half gained more than that, perhaps years in a small number of cases. The claim would be that it would be unjust and uncaring to deny those patients those extra gains in survival, even if we collectively have to bear the costs of the marginal survivors. So far as health care justice is concerned, we might think of this as an egalitarian argument. That is, if anyone has justified access to some very expensive cancer drug at social expense because some biomarker predicts some degree of likely benefit, then everyone in those same clinical circumstances should have access to that drug at social expense. After all, as things are now, we have no way of knowing which individuals will be weak responders rather than stronger responders. Granted, cancer biomarkers were used to identify some subset of patients with a particular cancer who were likely to respond to some degree to one of these targeted therapies. But we have no reason to believe that successful biomarker research in the future will yield some complex set of biomarkers at the level of an individual patient that will reliably predict substantial gains in survival from this drug rather than that drug. That is a utopian mirage according to the egalitarian.

We need to grant that this egalitarian perspective has considerable ethical attractiveness. We might even think of this view as being very congruent with the European norm of solidarity. However, some critical ethical distance is needed. Our critical question is this: What precisely is the scope of our egalitarian commitment? Ethically speaking (health care justice), can that commitment be limited to these patients with NSCLC who are being treated with nivolumab? Or must our egalitarian commitments extend to NSCLC patients treated with pembrolizumab as well, though the therapeutic response might be less dramatic overall? Drawing a distinction would seem ethically arbitrary. All the drugs listed above are checkpoint inhibitors. So what should be the ethically appropriate response when Hirsch et al. (2016) report that "the benefit from the checkpoint inhibitor was higher in patients with PD-L1-positive tumours than in patients with PD-L1-negative tumours, although some patients with PD-L1-negative expression responded to nivolumab and atezolimumab" (at 1019). At this time, we have no way of knowing before the fact who those "some patients" will be. What then should our egalitarian ethical commitments require of us by way of response, at least with regard to the use of social resources?

Perhaps we need to include metastatic melanoma patients and breast cancer patients and patients with gastric cancers to satisfy our egalitarian commitments. But once we start this list there is no obvious ethical reason why we should not include patients with any form of cancer at all, as long as they are somewhat likely to achieve some degree of clinical benefit from any of these targeted cancer therapies. This, someone might argue, is what solidarity is all about. But then why should our egalitarian commitments be restricted to cancer patients, our egalitarian philosopher and pharmaceutical representative ask? Patients with heart disease or rheumatoid arthritis or non-cancerous forms of liver disease or renal disease or lung disease all deserve equal care and concern (i.e., access to expensive drugs at social expense), even if only marginal gains in health or survival are possible. This conclusion permits us to bypass the ragged edge problem and the ethical challenges associated with having to make fair rationing decisions or having to do fair priority-setting among health care needs. But this is entirely unrealistic. No society endorses this conclusion in practice.

No society can endorse allocating unlimited social resources to meeting unlimited health care needs. So where exactly is the ethical problem? The most fundamental ethical problem is that there is no public rational conversation about health care rationing as a problem of health care justice. Instead, economic, political, and social forces (often using pseudo-ethical language) capture and direct social resources toward a favored health care need. In this case that favored need is cancer research and the needs of cancer patients. To be clear, the needs of cancer patients make just claims on social resources; but, I argue, not all cancer needs make *equally compelling* just claims on social resources. One would never know that was the case from the way in which discoveries regarding cancer biomarkers are presented to both the medical and non-medical public. Those biomarkers are presented as "credible evidence" to the public of "a chance to live longer"[16] for desperate patients with metastatic cancer who have no other options. Those biomarkers are used to identify *that drug for that cancer* "precisely." This is cutting-edge medicine dedicated to saving and prolonging lives. "How," it is rhetorically asked, "could any just and caring society not provide assured access to such drugs?" However, by focusing social ethical attention on this question, attention is

---

[16] This phrase is actually used in television and print commercials in the United States for nivolumab (Opdivo) for NSCLC. Those words are portrayed in the form of 30-foot-high letters on the side of skyscrapers with awestruck crowds gazing up in complete astonishment. In the print version of these ads, attention is called to "patient assistance" programs that will underwrite the cost of co-pays that many insurance plans might require. A course of treatment with that drug costs about $156,000. Those programs would be better characterized as "paytient" assistance programs since their intent is only to help insured patients. That dulls any moral luster such programs are designed to project (see iSpot.tv, 2015).

diverted from seeing numerous other health care needs at risk of being neglected or short-changed, especially if those individuals with those needs are socially or financially less well off. In essence, those other needs are ethically invisible. The practical implication is that rationing is thereby accomplished invisibly. Such invisible rationing efforts, I have argued elsewhere (Fleck, 2009, chaps. 1, 3), are intrinsically unjust because they violate the publicity condition that is a core element of our sense of social justice (Rawls, 1971).

Very problematic are "successes" that are announced in prominent medical journals, along with national news coverage, that might turn out to be premature and greatly misleading. In the week December 3–10, 2016, an article was published by Eric Tran et al. (2016) in the *New England Journal of Medicine* discussing a breakthrough in targeting mutant KRAS in cancer, followed by a somewhat glowing editorial by Carl June, "Drugging the Undruggable Ras—Immunotherapy to the Rescue?" (2016). To quote the abstract from the original article, "We identified a polyclonal CD8$^+$ T-cell response against mutant KRAS G12D in tumor-infiltrating lymphocytes obtained from a patient with metastatic colorectal cancer." This patient was identified as Patient 4095. Patient 4095 is actually Celine Ryan, age 50, an engineer and database programmer. She was the focus of a *New York Times* story the same week by Denise Grady (2016), who writes, "Her treatment was the first to successfully target a common cancer mutation that scientists have tried to attack for decades. Until now, that mutation has been bulletproof." The question that June himself raises is whether this case is utterly unique (or nearly unique) or something that can be replicated in subsequent research for a significant number of patients. In the meantime, colorectal cancer patients with KRAS mutations will have their hopes raised and demand access to this therapy on a compassionate use basis. Is this a sufficient basis for a large and costly clinical trial? This is one place where there is the potential for a misallocation of health care resources. What if 10% of the patients in such a clinical trial achieve an outcome comparable to that of Celine Ryan, but no one knows precisely why that 10% achieved that remarkable outcome while others gained only marginal benefit? As a just and caring society, are we then ethically obligated to provide this same therapy (no doubt for more than $100,000 each) to all colorectal cancer patients identified by the same biomarker, even though only 10% of them are likely to achieve substantial life-prolonging benefit? This is the egalitarian problem noted earlier.

This is also the super-responder problem we introduced in Chapter 1. There are often very small numbers of patients who are described as super-responders to various forms of precision medicine. These are patients who survive for years, whereas almost everyone else in their treatment cohort has died in a matter of months to a little over a year. Celine Ryan might be one of them, along with Dr. Hillard. Again, what should we conclude from an ethical perspective? If we can identify such patients before the fact, do they alone have a just claim to these $100,000 drugs because for them these drugs are cost-effective? By way of contrast, if an NSCLC patient is treated with nivolumab and gains only three months in OS at a cost of $140,000, then the cost-effectiveness of that drug would be $560,000 for one quality-adjusted life-year.

As things are now, we have no reliable mechanism for identifying those patients who would be marginal responders. But if future research identified other biomarkers that indicated no more than a likely marginal response (survival gain of less than three months, 90% confidence), would that justify withholding these drugs from these patients, at least at social expense? A more concise way of asking the same question would be: Should cost-effectiveness matter when it comes to health care justice and resource allocation? This is the utilitarian challenge raised to egalitarians. It can be summarized in this way: If we have only limited resources to meet virtually unlimited health care needs, then is it not rational and reasonable and just that those resources should be used to purchase the most health good possible (i.e., additional high-quality life-years)? This is another example where we are faced with ethical ambiguity. Both egalitarian and utilitarian considerations appeal to us for purposes of making just resource allocations among unlimited health care needs.

Here is a slightly different example. Sparano et al. (2015) reported on a 21-gene expression assay in breast cancer. The trial included more than 10,000 women (HER2-negative, axillary node–negative). The assay was used to assess likelihood of recurrence: 1,626 women had scores of less than 10, which meant that they could avoid chemotherapy because they were at very low risk. At five years 93.8% of these women had invasive disease-free survival. OS was 98.0%. The justice-relevant ethics issue would be this: Could we (Medicare, Medicaid, private insurance companies) have a policy of not paying for chemotherapy for these women because risk of recurrence was so low? Or should they be offered the choice, and have it paid for from social resources, no matter what they chose? Is this a situation where the ethically appropriate choice is to respect whatever choice a suitably informed patient autonomously makes in the context of the doctor–patient relationship?

Cancer biomarkers have proven very useful in redirecting therapy with metastatic disease progression. In many respects this is a commendable outcome. But this also adds to the problems of health care justice for the health care system as a whole. We noted earlier the problems of cancer drug resistance and heterogeneity. Recognition of this problem by researchers has resulted in more complex (and still more expensive) strategies for attacking specific cancers. The realistic goal is to manage the disease process and postpone death for as long as possible. In other words, the goal is to achieve imatinib-like results. In the case of advanced melanoma, for example, clinical trials are combining nivolumab and ipilimumab compared to either of these drugs alone.

Hassel (2016) comments, "Reliable biomarkers are still needed to enable prediction of response, which might be used to select patients in clinical practice." That takes us back to the problem of ragged edges. How much of a positive predicted response is necessary in order to justify providing these extraordinarily expensive drugs? In addition, there are the ethical and economic issues associated with the aggregation of these costs. It is one thing to provide imatinib at $120,000 per person per year to 10,000 patients. It is quite another to provide a drug like that to the 610,000 cancer patients who die of their cancer each year in the United States or to provide a drug like that for multiple years of survival with various cancers or to provide drug combinations at a cost of $250,000 per person per year for multiple years for a population of patients that increases from year to year as a result of survival.

As we discuss in the next chapter, the questions posed here are not simply difficult and complex. They are more correctly characterized as being "wicked." The precise implications of being so characterized will be analyzed in detail.

3
Precision Medicine, Diffuse Wickedness

3.1. Precision Medicine: Wicked Ethical Issues as Resistant to Ethical Analysis as Any Cancer to Targeted Therapies

3.1.1. Wickedness: A Conceptual Description

Some of my readers may not be familiar with the term "wicked problems." The term actually emerged from the urban planning literature (Rittel and Webber, 1973). It refers to the sort of problem for which every proposed solution generates more problems that are at least as difficult, sometimes more difficult, than the original problem. In addition, (1) formulating the problem itself may be controversial because of inherent complexity; (2) knowledge needed to address the problem may be uncertain and incomplete; (3) conflicting social values of disputed weight and relevance may be integral to the problem; (4) the social, political, economic, and technological landscape may be changing too quickly for the implementation of any proposed resolution; (5) considerable disagreement may exist regarding criteria for recognizing what would count as an acceptable resolution of the problem; and (6) organizational boundaries and responsibilities for addressing the problem may be unclear, perhaps related to the multi-causal nature of the problem.

Wicked problems (7) will also typically require changing behavior, whether at the individual level, the institutional level, the professional level, or the governmental level. That behavior might be health-related or ethically related or politically related or economically related—the take-home point being that behavioral change is never easy, especially if self-interests are at stake. Still, something must be done; passive acceptance of the status quo is not an acceptable option. I believe the problems of health care justice in relation to precision medicine as it is evolving are of the wicked variety, as I shall demonstrate in the remainder of this chapter. This is because of both the nature of precision medicine and the economic structure of the US health care system.

Precision Medicine and Distributive Justice. Leonard M. Fleck, Oxford University Press. © Oxford University Press 2022.
DOI: 10.1093/oso/9780197647721.003.0003

3.1.2. The Beginning of Wickedness: Cost Matters

We start with the reasonable, almost universally endorsed premise, that we have *only limited resources* to meet virtually unlimited health care needs. This implies we have to make choices. Given the consequences for individuals (premature death, substantial disability, greatly diminished quality of life due to not having serious health needs met adequately), we also recognize that considerations of justice and compassion should govern how these choices are made at a societal level. Let us start with the notion of limited resources.

Cost matters. How much is "too much" for any particular therapeutic intervention? If cost matters, then saving human lives or life-years cannot be priceless. That is, we cannot be willing to spend unlimited sums to save a life or a life-year or some portion of a life-year. If I were to ask whether some insurance company or Medicare or Medicaid were ethically obligated to spend $1 million in order to extend an individual's life for one day (knowing for certain it was just one day), I am confident that no ethically thoughtful individual (responsible for paying taxes or insurance premiums) would endorse spending that much money to prolong a life for one day as an ethical obligation. We could expand that scenario to a week, and I would still be confident that virtually no one would change their mind about spending that money.

If we were to expand that scenario to a month, some individuals might be tempted to alter their judgment. Perhaps those individuals are imagining the scenario this way: This patient will be dead in the next 24 hours if we fail to provide this million-dollar therapy. Otherwise, this patient would know they would have just one more month to live. That would be a very precious month. For many people it might feel cruel to deny that individual that month of life "just to save some money." Of course, this version of our scenario has all the marks of a "philosopher's" scenario, the suggestion being that it is too unrealistic. A more realistic scenario would be one in which an individual is told with confidence that they have only six months to live. However, we have a therapy that costs $1 million and will give them one more month of life on top of the six months. In this alternate description, it is much harder to elicit the emotional-ethical judgment that it would be cruel to deny this individual that extra month of life. After all, they still have six months to fulfill whatever hopes and dreams they judge are most important.

We can try one more version of our scenario. Imagine that for $1 million we can provide an individual with one extra year of life. This is getting closer to what we actually find today in the world of precision medicine.

As noted in Chapter 1, chimeric antigen receptor (CAR) T-cell therapy for some cancers can cost as much as $1 million, once we take account of the costs associated with the side effects of that intervention (Rosenbaum, 2017). However, some of those individuals will gain several extra years of life of reasonable quality. Hence, the actual cost per life-year saved might be closer to $250,000. Consequently, we will put that example aside and stick with our one-year scenario. Notice that I have presented this example as being about "an individual." This is just an abstract individual, no name, no face. Still, it is just an individual. Hence, I can readily imagine many individuals judging that it would be unjustifiably stingy to deny that individual that extra year of life. I suppose I myself would endorse that conclusion if we were only talking about that one individual. However, that again has all the features of a "philosopher's" example. In the real world, we would have to ask: What would make that individual so utterly unique that no one else would ever be in an ethically comparable situation where they could justifiably demand $1 million for an extra year of life? I cannot imagine any plausible answer to that question.

Recall that the context for this discussion is metastatic cancer and precision medicine. Recall that roughly 610,000 individuals in the United States die annually of some form of cancer. Recall that the annual cost of any one of these targeted therapies or immunotherapies is in excess of $100,000, with costs for a course of therapy in some cases approaching half a million dollars. Granted, as things are now in the United States, access to these cancer therapies is very dependent upon insurance status and individual ability to pay. We will put aside for now arguments about whether such a state of affairs is ethically acceptable. Instead, we can just think about this issue in the context of Medicare, which is essentially universal health insurance for the elderly.[1] We can see this as the political expression of equal concern and respect for each and every elderly person as far as access to needed health care is concerned.

---

[1] The "universal" quality of the Medicare program has been subverted to some extent as a result of the availability of the somewhat privatized "Medicare Advantage" options. Individuals who want lower monthly payments (sometimes no monthly payment) and a somewhat enhanced benefit package and who are willing to accept a $5,000 deductible (because they believe they will be completely healthy for the year) may choose a Medicare Advantage plan. There are pros and cons that can vary with the plans. From a system perspective Medicare Advantage plans are attractive (less costly) to the healthy elderly, which means traditional Medicare must cover sicker, costlier patients, such as our cancer patients.

In 2018, there were 440,000 cancer deaths among the Medicare population. In that same year, roughly 1.5 million Medicare recipients would be
living with metastatic cancer and in theory would be candidates for treatment with some targeted therapy.[2] We will put aside our million-dollar question with regard to these Medicare recipients with metastatic cancer. Instead,
we will ask whether each of these patients had a just claim to $100,000 for a
targeted therapy that would yield one extra year of life for them. In the aggregate, that would potentially add $150 billion to the cost of the Medicare
program for a year, which had a total cost of $740 billion in 2018 (Cuckler
et al., 2018) ($860 billion in 2020; projected to $1.6 trillion in 2028 (Keehan
et al., 2022)).

We are talking about dozens of different types of cancer. Put aside any
questions about therapeutic uncertainty or degree of effectiveness. It seems
reasonable to assert that no one of these cancers is intrinsically "worthier"
of treatment than any other cancer. In other words, if we have a $100,000
therapy for some specific cancer that can yield an extra year of life, that fact
will be sufficient to conclude that a patient with that cancer has a presumptive just claim to that resource. If that same targeted therapy, or its therapeutic successor, can yield a second year of reasonable quality of life for some
specific cancer at a cost of $100,000, then any individual with that cancer
would have a presumptive just claim to that therapy as well. The same will
be true for a third, a fourth, a fifth year, and so on. In the abstract, this is the
moral logic of this position. In the real world, five years of these cohorts of
1.5 million individuals added to one another would equal almost the entire
Medicare budget for 2016. This is obviously unrealistic and unaffordable. We
are not going to offer any detailed ethical argument or analysis at this point.
Our only goal is to outline the contours of this wicked problem.[3]

---

[2] To avoid confusion, less than 30% of cancer patients in 2018 with metastatic disease would have a
targeted therapy or some form of immunotherapy that could be appropriate for treating their cancer.
This would be because no current drug was available that could specifically target the genetic driver
of their cancer.

[3] Sharon Kaufman is an anthropologist who has called our attention to the political-technological
logic that contributes directly to the generation of our wicked problem. The title of her book, *Ordinary
Medicine: Extraordinary Treatments, Longer Lives, and Where to Draw the Line* (2015), captures perfectly her main thesis, namely, that these extraordinarily expensive cancer treatments become part
of "ordinary medicine" through a four-step process, the end result of which is that these cancer
treatments become ethically obligatory because they have become "ordinary." Step 1: The biomedical
research industry churns out "effective enough" therapies at an unprecedented rate. Step 2: Medicare
and other insurance company committees judge that the therapy is effective enough that it ought to
be reimbursed; physicians then feel obligated to offer it, and desperate patients will demand it. Step
3: Once a therapy is reimbursable, it becomes part of the standard of care. Step 4: Once a therapy is
regarded as the standard of care, it becomes ethically necessary to provide it. Note: Kaufman does not

3.1.3. Ibrutinib and Chronic Lymphocytic Leukemia: A Paradigm of Wickedness

Lest the reader believe that I am only offering hypotheticals for consideration, I would call attention to the drug ibrutinib (Imbruvica®), which the US Food and Drug Administration (FDA) has approved as a first-line treatment for chronic lymphocytic leukemia (CLL). The median age for diagnosis of this disorder is 71, which means most of these patients are covered by Medicare. Around 130,000 patients live with CLL in the United States (Nogrady, 2016). Around 20,000 are diagnosed with the disorder each year, and about 5,200 die of the disorder each year. The five-year survival rate is 83%. The cost of ibrutinib is $156,000 per year. Patients take the drug until progression or unacceptable toxicity. Treatment-naïve patients have five-year progression-free survival of 92% (Lawrence, 2018). That means these patients are on this drug for more than five years. If 130,000 patients are on the drug in a given year at a cost of $156,000 each, that annual aggregate cost is $20.8 billion. The projections to 2025 are that 199,000 individuals will be living with the disease, in part because of increased survival, in part because of the increase in the elderly population.

To be clear, the full cost of the drug would not be borne by the Medicare program as such. Instead, patients would mostly be in Medicare Advantage plans, and ibrutinib would be a class IV drug with a 30% co-pay, roughly $57,000 per patient per year (Nogrady, 2016). That cost would reduce dramatically the number of CLL patients who could afford that drug.[4] Again, I briefly put aside the health care justice issues needing analysis. Pre-2016, therapies for CLL would still be available, though with reduced clinical benefits relative to ibrutinib. The out-of-pocket costs to Medicare recipients for that earlier therapy would be $9,200 per year. Would it be "just enough" if the vast majority of Medicare recipients with CLL only had affordable access to some pre-ibrutinib drug? After all, the following argument might be offered: Most of these patients would still experience a significant gain in life

claim to be providing a normative argument of any sort; she is simply describing (as an anthropologist) social facts.

[4] The conclusion of one research article (Shanafelt et al., 2015) addressing the cost and access issues related to ibrutinib for CLL reads: "Although ibrutinib and idelalisib are profound treatment advances, they will dramatically increase individual out-of-pocket and societal costs of caring for patients with CLL. These cost considerations may undermine the potential promise of these agents by limiting access and reducing adherence" (at 252).

expectancy from the less expensive drug. They are not being condemned to a *very premature* death, especially if the median age at onset for CLL is 71 years.

Of course, the situation is more ethically complicated than what has been presented so far. For the 40% of Medicare patients in the lower portions of the income spectrum, even that $9,200 per year co-pay for access to the less expensive drug (rituximab) would be more than they could afford. Hence, they would have no effective access to that life-prolonging drug. However, something could still be done for their CLL. They would have access to chlorambucil monotherapy, described as "relatively ineffective," with a complete remission rate of 5% and progression-free survival of one year (Shanafelt et al., 2015). Should this be sufficient to ease our collective conscience, since it is not as if we are tolerating putting these patients out in the hospital parking lot to die? This last rhetorical question puts us quite a distance, ethically speaking, from our original question about being ethically committed to spending $1 million to give a patient an extra year of life. Maybe we should just conclude this is ethically awkward or ethically embarrassing. However, there are some wicked features to this situation as well.

Everyone pays into the Medicare program during their working life, the same flat rate as a percentage of working income as opposed to investment income. If someone earns $200,000 per year, they will pay into Medicare seven times what someone who earns $30,000 per year will pay. Still, Medicare promises the same range of benefits to all. Some (wealthy libertarian individuals) may object that this arrangement is unjust. They will ask, "Why should I have to pay seven times as much for the same product as someone who earns less (and deserves less)?" However, our low-wage worker has just cause for complaint as well. All of these hyper-expensive, life-prolonging cancer drugs are "available" as Medicare-covered benefits, but a very high paywall effectively prevents our low-wage worker with metastatic cancer from accessing any of these drugs. They cannot access a Mercedes Benz either, though a significant economic distinction separates the Mercedes Benz from ibrutinib. No subsidy is available for purchasing a Mercedes Benz. Though our wealthy individual will have to pay $57,000 each year for access to ibrutinib, Medicare is paying the other 70% of the total cost of that drug, *and a portion of that 70% is being contributed by low-wage workers who will never have access to that drug*. That seems unjust. There is also something wicked here. What is the "correct" way of conceptualizing the relevant ethics issues?

Is it justice-relevant that high-salary workers would have contributed several times more to the Medicare program than would low-wage workers?

Does that give them more of a just claim at social expense to these very costly cancer drugs? Alternatively, is the justice-relevant comparable situation one in which an individual has paid for health insurance for several decades and never had a health problem that required their having to use their insurance plan? Now, however, they have metastatic cancer and want access to one of these targeted therapies at plan expense, even though their chances of actual benefit are small and remote. They want to claim they are "owed" that access because they have paid so much into the plan already, even though the plan would have an explicit rule denying everyone else in the plan access to that drug in the same situation. A fair and reasonable response would seem to be that a health plan is not a savings account; the premiums have not been accumulating with interest. Hence, this person has no just claim. Which way of thinking about our Medicare ibrutinib problem is more ethically correct? We can hardly expect to find an ethically reasonable resolution to a problem if we cannot agree on what the problem "really" is.

3.1.4. Ibrutinib: Complex Wickedness

Wickedness has many dimensions. In the most recent research that I cited regarding ibrutinib, where it was used as first-line therapy, the life-prolonging results were spectacular for the majority of patients five years out from the initiation of therapy. Some patients, however, will fail ibrutinib. This is another example of cancer drug resistance. Some patients might fail ibrutinib after one or two years. Others might fail in Year 6 or 7. Some of these CLL patients might be in their early 60s; others might be in their mid-70s. What then?

Porter et al. (2015) report a small research study with 14 CLL patients who had undergone a median of five prior therapies for their CLL. All of these patients were treated with CD19 CAR T-cell therapy. Of those 14 patients, four achieved a complete response, two achieved a partial response, and eight survived less than nine months. Two of the patients with a complete response have had a durable response of more than seven years. Recall that the base cost of this therapy is $475,000. This is a cost that is borne up front, not over some number of years. Did all of these patients have a just claim to this CAR T-cell therapy? Some of these patients survived less than three months. However, at present we have no way of identifying these short survival patients before the fact. Imagine that future research might give us the capacity to identify such patients before the fact, perhaps with 90%

confidence. Would that be sufficient to justify denying them access to CAR T-cell therapy? Alternatively, does our sense of justice or our sense of just compassion require providing this therapy to all these patients if we know that this will yield a rate of 15% long-term survival? Could we justly conclude that this was too high a price to pay for such a low yield of survival? Again, what is being reported here is a clinical trial. The numbers are small; the overall cost is manageable. What we have to ask is whether this trial would be judged a success such that this therapy would (should?) become available for treating patients with CLL more generally. Does it matter that this is a "last chance" therapy?

Treatment-naïve patients seem to do best with ibrutinib with a 92% five-year survival rate. Will that survival rate extend to seven years or 10 years, as has been the case with imatinib for chronic myeloid leukemia? No one can say right now. Each of those years will cost someone (Medicare, Medicaid, private insurance, individuals) $156,000. If someone does survive 10 years, the cost of their survival would be $1.56 million. Economically and ethically speaking, that is still quite distant from the earlier question we raised, namely, whether a just and caring society was ethically obligated to spend $1 million to provide someone with an extra year of life. However, we could be faced with the following ethically challenging scenario.

Imagine that at Year 6 or Year 7 more of these CLL patients start to fail ibrutinib. They have had a good run on ibrutinib. Would it be unjust to allow them to die at that point? Keep in mind that there would be a wide range of ages. What makes this ethically challenging is that we have the Turtle et al. (2017) research. We can offer these patients CAR T-cell therapy at a cost of $475,000, which might result in 30% of those patients gaining several additional years of life. I should also mention in that regard that 83% of the patients in the Turtle et al. research experienced cytokine release syndrome (CRS), which could add $500,000 to the cost of care for some of these patients who experience the most serious version of CRS. Is a just and caring society ethically obligated to provide CAR T-cell therapy for these "later failure" CLL patients?

In the Turtle et al. research, some of the CLL patients were relatively young, and they had failed ibrutinib relatively soon after starting the therapy. Perhaps they deserve a second chance. It would not seem fair or right to let them die with the option of CAR T-cell therapy available.[5] However, some of

---

[5] Again, this is the point of Sharon Kaufman's ethical/anthropological research (2015).

the patients in that trial were doing well enough with ibrutinib for more than three years before it failed. They were still given the option of CAR T-cell therapy. If they were given that option, how could it be ethically acceptable to deny that option to someone who failed ibrutinib after four years or five years or seven years or 10 years? What seems to be most ethically relevant is that we have this life-prolonging technology available, and it has a reasonable chance of providing a significant life prolongation benefit for at least 30% of patients like this. The aggregate cost of accomplishing this outcome for each patient who survived with CLL for 10–15 years would be $1–$2 million. Would each of these patients have a just claim to the social resources needed to achieve these gains in life expectancy?

Go back to our question about spending $1 million to gain an extra year of life for someone. If you endorsed that expenditure, then you would have to give an affirmative answer to our last question. We are only asking for 20% of that million dollars as the cost for each life-year saved. As long as we intellectually isolate each individual and each year of life in this way, it would seem stingy and uncaring to deny individuals this extra year of life. The problem, however, is that in the real world these individuals and these costs have to be aggregated. As noted earlier, about 130,000 individuals in the United States are living with CLL. It is safe to assume that virtually all of them want to live longer; that is, they do not want the natural disease process of CLL to go forward unchecked, certainly not when the technology is there to halt that progression. Ibrutinib and CAR T-cell therapy are the two best interventions for giving them extra years of life of reasonable quality. However, the aggregated cost for each of those years for this aggregate of CLL patients would be more than $20 billion.

That $20 billion is not a real number in the context of the health care system in the United States. This is because the vast majority of these patients will not have the financial wherewithal to access either of these therapies. They may be uninsured or underinsured. They may be insured but with unaffordable co-pays and deductibles related to cancer care. Their insurance may cover only a very narrow network of providers, which would almost certainly exclude the very rarefied specialists needed to provide access to these therapies. These details reflect the fragmented state of health care financing in the United States. However, our key normative question remains: Is it unjust that CLL patients, who are clearly capable of substantially benefiting from having access to either ibrutinib or CAR T-cell therapy, are denied effective access simply for financial reasons?

We could take a very pure and very stark libertarian view of health care justice and argue that no one has a just claim to needed health care if they do not have the ability to pay. If most Americans endorsed that view, that would quickly dissolve our emerging wicked problem. Medicare and Medicaid would go away. Millions of individuals would suffer needlessly and die prematurely. Given the randomness of illness and being uninsured in the United States, both self-interest and compassion would yield compelling reasons for opposing such a stark libertarian view. Still, few Americans would endorse going to the opposite end of the economic spectrum and demand that the costs of all health care be socialized, no matter how uncertain or marginal the benefit, no matter how costly the effort to achieve that benefit. A commitment such as that would be imprudent, both ethically and economically.

We are left with our basic health care rationing problems: If we are not obligated as a matter of justice to meet every health care need for everyone in our society, then when have we collectively "done enough" by way of meeting health care needs? What are the limits of our societal obligations of justice for meeting health care needs? What criteria should be used for making such judgments? When is it "just enough" to permit individual ability to pay to determine who has access to needed health care that might be very expensive and only marginally beneficial? Is the situation regarding either ibrutinib or CAR T-cell therapy for CLL patients "just enough," not open to justified moral criticism? If we took this question by itself, it would be a difficult problem of health care justice. However, this question cannot be isolated, ethically speaking, from the whole domain of health care needs and health care justice. Consequently, we must address a *wicked* problem.

3.2. More Wicked Scenarios

So far as health care justice is concerned, nothing distinguishes the ethical challenges associated with ibrutinib or CAR T-cell therapy for CLL patients from the ethical challenges associated with trastuzumab for metastatic HER2$^+$ breast cancer or pembrolizumab for metastatic melanoma or nivolumab for metastatic non-small cell lung cancer, and so on. In all these cases we have patients with a late-stage terminal cancer. These drugs are extraordinarily expensive for a course of treatment, with marginal benefits for the majority of patients, overall survival gains measurable in months, not years. Still, a small percentage of patients will gain two or three extra years of life. Further, for a tiny percentage of patients (in most cases), super-responders will gain many extra years of life but not a cure. Researchers at present have no way of knowing before the fact which patients might enjoy substantial benefit from one of these targeted therapies, though considerable research is being directed at identifying biomarkers that would yield precisely this information.[6] Assuming such information is obtained, how is that information supposed to be used? If a drug yields no benefit for a patient or a likely net harm, no problem of justice arises when denying that drug to that patient. However, if the biomarker indicates a likely gain of less than three months, is that sufficient to justify denying that patient access to that drug at social expense?

3.2.1. Wickedness: Ragged Edges and Bright Lines

This last question marks the beginning of one wicked problem, the ubiquitous problem of "ragged edges." Again, if we have relatively small numbers of patients, the high cost of providing these drugs to patients likely to benefit only marginally would be economically (and ethically) manageable. However, in 2021 160,000 patients in the United States died of lung cancer, 14,000 of skin cancer, 42,000 of breast cancer, 63,000 of genital system cancers, 160,000 of digestive system cancers, 33,000 of urinary cancers, 17,000 of brain cancers, 21,000 of lymphoma, 25,000 of leukemia, and 13,000 of myeloma (Siegal et al., 2021). In theory, if we cannot offer an ethically compelling basis for drawing a line (minimal benefit) for access to one of these targeted therapies, all these individuals would have a presumptively just claim to these drugs at social expense.

The problem of very costly marginal benefits is one wicked problem. Equally wicked, however, would be the problem of very successful targeted therapies for most of these cancers. The goal of cancer research today is to transform metastatic disease into a manageable chronic disease for many additional years of life. The medical analogy invoked is the AIDS analogy. In other words, patients would be on various combinations or sequences of

---

[6] An enormous amount of research is ongoing to identify biomarkers related to precision medicine that are expected to be both prognostic and predictive. This research is ethically and scientifically complex. See Blanchard and Wik (2018), Tranvag and Norheim (2018), and Fleck (2018).

these targeted therapies for years. This would yield extremely high aggregated costs at both the individual level and the social level. Line drawing in connection with marginal benefits is ethically very difficult. However, line drawing in connection with drugs that effectively yielded many extra years of life for patients who otherwise faced a terminal outcome after a couple of years would be ethically impossible. Imagine a representative of an insurance company saying something like this to an HIV⁺ individual in 2008: "We are really pleased that we have been able to provide you with ten extra years of life that you would never have otherwise received before protease inhibitors became part of HIV treatment. To our policyholders, who are concerned about the costs of health insurance, we have to be responsible. We feel you have benefited enough from those ten extra years of life we have paid for. We have to stop paying for those drugs now. We wish you well as you pursue other (health care) opportunities." It is impossible to imagine an ethical justification for such a statement. This is another aspect of our wicked problem.

On average, HIV⁺ patients will be much younger than most cancer patients. What does that ethically imply? Many of these patients will survive 30 years or longer because of having access to these combination therapies. If they are on a four-drug regimen, the cost will be about $35,000 per year, with potential lifetime costs close to $1 million. Do these individuals have a just claim to this much health care? If they have a moral right to $1 million worth of health care, does every American have a just claim to that same level of social resources? That would equal $330 trillion for the lifetimes of our current population. This struck me at first as an absurd amount, utterly unrealistic. However, I did some math. In 2017 total health spending in the United States was $3.5 trillion, which equals roughly $10,300 per person. If the average person in the United States lives 80 years, lifetime costs for each person would be about $830,000 (assuming health care cost escalation could be halted at today's expenditure levels). Reasonable projections of aggregate health spending to 2026 are placed at $5.4 trillion, roughly $15,000 per person, or $1.2 million per person over a lifetime. In any given year, however, 5% of the population will account for 50.5% of that aggregated health spending. By way of contrast, half the population will accumulate less than $500 in health care expenditures in a year (National Institute for Health Care Management, 2012).

The composition of that 5% will vary from year to year. Some portion of that 5% will be comprised of patients in the last year of life. Another portion will be comprised of individuals with a serious and costly life-threatening condition from which they recover.[7] Frequently, it will be virtually impossible for skillful physicians to distinguish who belongs in each of these groups before the fact. Another portion of that 5% will be comprised of individuals showing up from year to year with costly chronic conditions, such as hemophilia, cystic fibrosis, various forms of heart disease, and so on.

3.2.2. Hemophilia: Wickedly Rough Justice

There are about 20,000 patients with hemophilia in the United States, and roughly 60% of them will be diagnosed with the severe form of hemophilia (Chen, 2016). These individuals will have a life expectancy of 50–55 years today, compared to a predicted life expectancy of 20 years in 1970. That gain is entirely attributable to the clotting drugs available since the early 1980s. The overall average annual cost per patient with hemophilia is $155,136 (Chen, 2016). If we assume a 50-year life expectancy, that adds up to lifetime costs for treating that hemophilia to $7.75 million per patient. However, 25%–30% of patients with severe hemophilia develop an inhibitor problem, medically analogous to the resistance problem associated with targeted cancer therapies. The average annual cost of treating those patients jumps to $697,000 (Chen, 2016). Depending upon when that inhibitor problem arose, lifetime costs for treating those patients could be in the range of $20–$30 million per patient.

One other distinction should be mentioned: on-demand treatment and prophylactic treatment for patients with the severe form of hemophilia. "On-demand" treatment means that a bleeding episode occurs, and factor VIII is administered to stop the bleeding. "Prophylactic" treatment means that a patient is on a clotting drug before bleeding episodes occur in order to minimize the bleeding and the subsequent joint disorder problems that result from repeated episodes of bleeding. The average annual cost for on-demand treatment of patients with severe hemophilia is $184,518 compared to $292,525 for prophylactic treatment (Chen, 2016). If we again calculate 50-year lifetime costs, those numbers, respectively, would be $9.25 million

---

[7] Here is a headline from the *Lansing State Journal* that perfectly illustrates my point: "Lansing Man Celebrates Coronavirus Recovery after 90 Days in the Hospital" (Ford, 2020). This was Mr. Ernie Cabule, age 67, who suffered multiple medical complications as a result of his COVID-19 infection. Most of those hospital days were in the intensive care unit. The article did not report the cost of his care, but it was likely in the vicinity of $2 million.

and \$12–\$15 million. The benefit for patients on prophylactic treatment is reduced hospital costs and improved quality of life, though the cost reductions are less than the increased costs associated with this more expensive drug regimen.

Our questions: (1) Do all of these patients have a just claim to all of these social resources to treat their hemophilia, and (2) what does this imply with respect to limits on just claims to social resources for all other patients with very costly but treatable chronic degenerative health problems? If we assume for the sake of argument that these patients with the most severe forms of hemophilia have a just claim to more than \$20 million in lifetime health care costs, that seems to remove all limits regarding what a just and caring society must provide to patients with other very costly health care needs. If a patient with metastatic cancer needs \$1 million worth of these targeted cancer drugs for three or four extra years of life, it seems we would be ethically obligated to provide those drugs at social expense, given what we were willing to do for these hemophilia patients. This conclusion would seem to be both ethically and economically problematic. Some distinctions need to be made, though the more we try to make these distinctions, the more wicked and complicated the ethical issues become.

Hemophilia patients start life with this problem. Their overall quality of life will be diminished relative to what most people experience. None will achieve a normal life expectancy. These are all ethically compelling reasons for concluding that these patients have a just claim to extraordinarily costly health care resources. Further, the drugs that yield much improved life expectancies are clearly very effective. We are not talking about very costly or uncertain marginal benefits (compare to the targeted cancer therapies). However, prophylactic treatment costs more than \$100,000 per year "extra" compared to on-demand treatment for episodes of bleeding. Over four decades that would amount to an additional cost of \$4 million per patient. Some marginal gain in life expectancy might be associated with that prophylactic treatment. Significant improvement in quality of life is the primary benefit of these drugs since they reduce both the frequency and intensity of the bleeding episodes, thereby postponing joint damage and associated functional loss. It would be heartless to describe these quality-of-life improvements as "cosmetic," with the implication that patients had no just claims to these drugs. There is legitimate medical need here, though one is tempted to wonder if we should think about degrees of medical necessity. Another wicked problem might be detected here.

3.2.3. Rare Genetic Disorders: More Rough Justice and Wickedness

Many other patient groups require very costly drugs for years, which adds to our wicked problems. Consider patients diagnosed with paroxysmal nocturnal hemoglobinuria (PNH), who number roughly 8,000 in the United States. It is a genetic disorder (X-linked PIG-A gene) associated with 1 in 63,000 births (Coyle et al., 2014). In brief, the immune system attacks red blood cells at night. Regular blood transfusions are necessary to correct the disorder. Thrombotic events are a major problem, which can be treated with warfarin, which has its own risks. Renal failure and thrombotic events are the most likely causes of death in these patients. Median survival with PNH is 14.6 years from time of diagnosis, though 25% of patients will survive for 25 years or more.

The drug used to treat PNH is eculizumab (Soliris˚), which costs $410,000 per year (Coyle et al., 2014). The drug is not curative. It has very modest life-prolonging effects, 1.13 life-years (Coyle et al., 2014). The incremental cost-effectiveness ratio (ICER) for the drug is $4.62 million. The primary benefit of the drug is the reduction of the need for blood transfusions, which represents a quality-of-life gain for these patients. If patients were on the drug for 15 years, then the cost would be $6.15 million. Do these PNH patients have a just claim to this drug at social expense? Would a society such as our own be opened to justified moral criticism if we refused to cover it through at least our publicly funded programs, such as Medicaid and Medicare (keeping in mind that Medicare pays for renal dialysis for all non-elderly end-stage renal patients)? How are the justice-relevant circumstances associated with this drug like or unlike the circumstances associated with our hemophilia drugs?

Eculizumab is effective in that it diminishes the need for blood transfusions, which is a modest effect. The vast majority of these patients would have the same life expectancy with their PNH whether or not they received this drug. This is in contrast to the circumstances of patients with hemophilia for whom the various clotting factors (factor VIII, etc.) resulted in major gains in life expectancy. Still, it is painful (ethically and psychologically) to imagine informing these patients of the existence of this drug, then adding that our society is not willing to pay for it, given the marginal benefits.

Critics would argue that the actual costs of these drugs in the context of national budgets are miniscule. It would hardly seem ethically legitimate to describe such an expenditure as "wasteful." The lives of patients with very rare disorders do matter; they are not expendable because they are small in number (Magalhaes, 2022; Duckett, 2022). This criticism might be dismissed as being excessively rhetorical. However, how would we assess from a moral point of view a proposed social policy that strongly discouraged efforts by medical researchers to discover therapies (likely very expensive) for numerous medical disorders that afflicted relatively small numbers of patients? That should probably trigger a few twinges of conscience. On the other hand, the actual policy in the United States since 1983 has been to provide some very powerful economic incentives for precisely discovering these therapies. Consequently, that miniscule portion of the prescription drug budget associated with funding eculizumab becomes much more significant if we multiply that number by costs associated with 552 or more orphan drugs.[8]

Gaucher's is another orphan disease, a lysosomal storage disease, which can give rise to an enlarged liver and spleen as well as debilitating bone disease. Roughly, 90% of patients have the Type I version of the disease. Approximately 3,000 individuals in the United States have this disease. Symptoms will usually emerge in the fifth decade of life. Three drugs are used to treat the disease: imiglucerase, velaglucerase alfa, and taliglucerase alfa. These drugs are described as enzyme replacement therapy. That is, they correct the enzyme deficiency that is the hallmark of the disease, but they do not cure the disease. For symptomatic patients these drugs yield an average gain of 12.8 years free of end organ damage (van Dussen et al., 2014). Each of these drugs costs about $310,000 per patient per year. The lifetime costs for treating a patient with Gaucher's are about €5.7 million or $7.5 million (van Dussen et al., 2014). These are very large numbers. What is clearly ethically relevant is that these drugs are effective; they yield extra years of life of good quality. These patients will not achieve a normal life expectancy, but they will come close. From the perspective of health care justice, is this ethically sufficient to conclude that a just and caring society would be ethically obligated to assure access to these drugs?

---

[8] Up until 2016, 552 "orphan drugs" have received FDA approval subsequent to the 1983 Orphan Drug Act (Silverman, 2016). A drug is eligible for that designation if there are fewer than 200,000 patients alive in a year who could potentially be treated with that drug. Generous financial incentives have encouraged pharmaceutical companies to pursue this research, including the ability to set the price of the drug at whatever level a company believes the market will bear (Herder, 2017). The original rationale was that orphan diseases would never be a profitable market. In fact, most of these drugs are very profitable (Silverman, 2016). There are at least 7,000 diseases identified for which an orphan drug would be an option.

This last question, in complete isolation from all other health care resource allocation needs, would not be wicked. However, imagine metastatic cancer patients in the near future who might gain five extra years of acceptable life at a cost of $1 million from these targeted cancer therapies used sequentially. Ethically speaking, they could ask, "If you (a just and caring society) are committed to spending $7 million for added lifetime for a Gaucher patient, how could you not be committed to spending a fraction of that to provide me with the additional life-years I desperately want?" From a hard-nosed utilitarian perspective, we could justify additional life-years for neither of these groups. If we have made an exception for Gaucher patients, then what would be the justice-relevant considerations that would justify denying the cancer patients their coverage?

Someone could call attention to the sizes of the two populations and the aggregated health care costs associated with each population. However, I can readily imagine a response from within what I have carelessly described as this aggregated cancer population. That response would be: "There is no such thing as *a cancer population*. There are only orphan populations of cancer patients, each of which is identified as a sort of 'genetic tribe' whose distinct genetic features of their cancer require a distinct targeted therapy or succession of targeted therapies. If being an orphan disease group is what justifies special, publicly financed assistance for drug development, then each of us with a genetically distinctive cancer is just as much an orphan disease group as Gaucher or Fabry or Pompe patients."

Implicit in this last line of argument is an egalitarian principle, which ought to ethically resonate with us. But the equally obvious implication would be that as a society we would be ethically obligated to spend unlimited sums on health care interventions that were sufficiently effective. This is an awkward conclusion. Financial limits must be set and respected. Should we be ethically comfortable with letting these patients suffer needlessly and die prematurely? Frigid compassion is not a virtue. Perhaps we ought to make it a problem for individuals or social groups. Individuals can have access to any effective medical interventions they judge to have sufficient value if they spend their own money. Alternatively, private charity could assist with access to these very costly interventions. The clear consequence would be distributional arbitrariness and inadequacy relative to needs. Healthy libertarians might be ethically comfortable with that consequence but virtually everyone else's sense of justice would be offended. A wicked problem is continuing to emerge.

3.2.4. Wickedness and PCSK9 Inhibitors

Let us switch to some other medical problems with a different configuration of medical responses and outcomes, and other forms of wickedness. Consider PCSK9 inhibitors (alirocumab and evolocumab), designed to lower low-density lipoproteins (LDLs), so-called bad cholesterol. The ultimate goal is to reduce the incidence of stroke, heart attacks, and premature death. Statins are currently used to reduce LDL. An LDL level above 100 mg/dL will usually result in a physician recommending a patient start on a statin. About 70 million Americans have LDL above 100 mg/dL. If a patient's LDL is above 130 mg/dL, a physician would very strongly urge the patient to start a statin. Approximately 19 million Americans would fit this latter profile.

Statins reduce LDL on average by about 17%, while PCSK9 inhibitors reduce LDL by 60% or more. The expectation in the major trials of PCSK9 inhibitors (FOURIER; Sabatine et al., 2017) was that the reduction in LDL levels would yield a comparable reduction in major cardiovascular events (heart attacks and strokes). The actual reduction was about 15% in a trial population comprised of individuals with familial hypercholesterolemia or established atherosclerotic cardiovascular disease, which is to say individuals at very high risk for these cardiovascular events. Roughly, 9 million Americans would be in this very high-risk population.

The cost of these PCSK9 inhibitors was $14,500 per person per year, but in 2018 this was reduced to about $6,000. Individuals take these drugs for the remainder of their lives. If all 9 million of these individuals were placed on these drugs, the total additional social cost would be about $50 billion per year. In 2016, the total direct costs of cardiovascular disease were about $320 billion (American Heart Association, 2017). Kazi et al. (2016) estimate that net savings from PCSK9 inhibitors would be about $6 billion per year. This still is a very large overall increase in social costs for one drug. Furthermore, the wicked ethical problem would pertain to the additional 10 million Americans who are at "merely" high risk for these same coronary events, though overall their actual lifetime risk would be somewhat lower. That is, the benefit would be more moderate and less certain than in the case of the very high-risk population, and the additional annual cost would be $55 billion. Would either the very high-risk or high-risk individuals have a just claim to these PCSK9 inhibitors at social expense? In other words, if they were denied these inhibitors at social expense, could they justifiably claim that they had been treated unjustly?

If we had to prioritize access to these inhibitors relative to our targeted metastatic cancer therapies, which would have the stronger justice-relevant claim? Patients with metastatic cancer have a terminal illness and a limited life expectancy. As things were in 2021, most of these cancer patients who received a targeted therapy benefited with extra months of life, not extra years (though there were the super-responder exceptions). One way of making some comparisons would be with ICERs. Three drugs are available to treat metastatic non-small cell lung cancer with the following ICERs: atezolizumab, $219,179/quality-adjusted life-year [QALY]; nivolumab, $415,950/QALY; and pembrolizumab, $236,492/QALY (Institute for Clinical and Economic Review, 2016). PCSK9 inhibitors have ICERs for the very high-risk patient population treated in the FOURIER trial of $503,000/QALY to $414,000/QALY (Sabatine et al., 2017) (roughly half of that after 2018). However, if these inhibitors are provided to the merely high-risk population, ICERs jump to $1.7 million/QALY, primarily because many more patients would have to be treated in order to prevent a cardiovascular event (Kuehn, 2018).[9] Virtually no insurance company will cover the cost of PCSK9 inhibitors for this latter group, given insufficient evidence of benefit.[10] This is also true for the very high-risk category because, even there, 28 patients would have to be on these drugs for a year to prevent one non-fatal heart attack or stroke. We might see this as very selfish behavior by an insurance company (protecting profits), but it also protects the pocketbooks of consumers.

David Eddy, a physician and health economist, notes that we are of a divided mind regarding health care costs. As healthy citizens who must pay for health care through taxes or insurance premiums, we want government or business to do something to control health care costs; as patients (or anxious potential patients), however, we want virtually unlimited funds spent to meet our health care needs, no matter what the likelihood of success might be (Eddy, 1996, chaps. 10, 14, 15). Anxious potential patients might

[9] To be precise, the FOURIER trial showed that approximately 70 patients would need to be treated with evolocumab for two years in order to prevent a single heart attack, stroke, or death. This would be at a cost of $2 million.

[10] Obviously, some number of patients in this high-risk group will have fatal heart attacks and strokes, but from a statistical perspective the number of such events will be roughly the same whether these patients are on statins alone or PCSK9 inhibitors. Equally obvious, we have no way of knowing that *the same individuals* would have had the same fate no matter which group they might have been in. Should this be a source of moral comfort or moral concern? The price of alirocumab was reduced by 50% in mid-2018 to about $6,000 per year. Still, the ICER remains at $997,000 for alirocumab relative to the cost of a statin and ezetimibe (Kazi et al., 2019). To be cost-effective, the price of these drugs must be below $1,138 per year (Hlatky, 2019).

have LDL levels of 125 mg/dL. Statins could bring that level down to 100 mg/dL, still leaving a moderately elevated 10-year risk of heart attack or stroke. PCSK9 inhibitors, however, could take that LDL level down to 40 mg/dL, which would lower that risk only a bit more. This would cost $6,000 per year. Do these patients have a just claim to social resources because these drugs would achieve some (very marginal) risk reduction? The ICER might be as high as $1.7 million/QALY gained. Does cost-effectiveness settle the matter? If so, does cost-effectiveness also settle the matter for very high-risk patients who will have ICERs in the $400,000/QALY to $500,000/QALY range? However, we (as a society) seem comfortable with funding drugs for orphan diseases with ICERs of several hundred thousand dollars per QALY. That would suggest that sometimes other morally relevant considerations override simple cost-effectiveness considerations. If so, what are those overriding justice-relevant considerations? Further, in what range of circumstances do those justice-relevant circumstances have overriding weight relative to cost-effectiveness considerations?

3.2.5. Hepatitis C: Another Warren of Wickedness

Another illustration of our wickedness challenges would be the problems of health care justice raised by the hepatitis C drug sofosbuvir (Sovaldi˚). This drug was priced at $1,000 per pill, or $84,000 for a 12-week course of treatment. Untreated chronic hepatitis C is likely to result in life-threatening liver damage, including liver cancer, though it might require 20 years or more after initial infection for these devastating consequences to ensue. That will be the fate of about 30% of the 3.5 million Americans infected with chronic hepatitis C if untreated. Prior to sofosbuvir, peg-interferon was used to treat chronic hepatitis C. However, the vast majority of patients could not tolerate the treatment regimen (Younossi et al., 2017). However, the cost of that treatment regimen was $19,000 for a 24-week course, which was reasonably effective. By way of contrast, sofosbuvir is extraordinarily effective.

Of the 3.5 million Americans infected with hepatitis C, 750,000 of them have insurance coverage through the Medicaid programs in the various states. Another 500,000 of those individuals are in jail or prison (Liu et al., 2014). If all 750,000 individuals in those Medicaid programs had received sofosbuvir in 2015, the cost to the states would have been $75 billion plus $50 billion for the prisons. Given these taxpayer costs, these are politically impossible numbers. Consequently, most state Medicaid programs have very restrictive policies for accessing this drug (Tumber, 2017; Canary et al., 2015). More specifically, they require a diagnosis of Stage III or Stage IV liver disease before providing these drugs at state expense. This seems harsh. If someone has significantly narrowed coronary arteries, it makes sense to stent those arteries to prevent a heart attack. No one would stent those arteries before a buildup of plaque. However, unlike stents, sofosbuvir can be given within a few years of initial infection to prevent the liver damage and the risk of premature death. No medical consideration would warrant holding off providing the drug at an early stage of infection. What then justifies either Medicaid or prisons in withholding access to the drug from these infected patients? Two answers might be given.

First, 70% of these infected individuals will not develop liver disease during their lifetime. Second, both Medicaid programs and prisons have populations that are constantly turning over. Individuals get jobs and move out of poverty; prisoners serve their time and are released. That means the health care needs of these individuals become someone else's payment problem, perhaps a private insurance company, perhaps the charitable resources of a hospital. However, if this is ethically acceptable (not unjust), then the same logic will apply to insurance programs in the private sector, including employer-sponsored insurance. People change jobs; employers change insurance plans. Consequently, by postponing treatment, those costs are shifted to someone else. However, if treatment is postponed, very high costs associated with treating liver cancer or other forms of liver disease will have to be borne (Rein et al., 2015). Avoiding those costs will economically justify providing sofosbuvir early after infection, and it is the morally decent thing to do. This argument makes economic sense in countries with universal health insurance. The United States, however, has an extremely fragmented system for financing health care, which is what creates the economic incentives and ethical shortcuts I have described and our wicked challenges. Private insurers will ask, "Why should I have to bear the upfront costs when the savings from not treating liver disease accrue to some other insurer?"

Insurers are contractually bound to reimburse the costs of "medically necessary" care. Everyone will agree that an inflamed appendix represents "medically necessary" care. Chronic hepatitis C does not fit this pattern. In 70% of these cases, nothing requiring medical intervention will happen, though we do not know which patients will be in that 70% cohort. Preventing liver cancer or other life-threatening liver problems is a medically and ethically good thing to do. The cost of prevention in this case, however, is $84,000 per patient, and in 7 out of 10 of those cases, nothing will have been prevented. How should we think of this from the perspective of health care justice, whether utilitarian or egalitarian or prioritarian or sufficientarian? Some Medicaid patients will also have metastatic cancer. Some expensive targeted cancer therapies would provide them with some modest (non-curative) benefit. Given limited funding, should priority be given to these targeted cancer therapies (last chance for terminally ill patients) or to earlier provision of sofosbuvir to prevent life-threatening liver cancers? Still more wickedness awaits us.

Roughly half of the 3.5 million Americans with chronic hepatitis C infection are unaware of the fact that they are infected. Should Medicaid and prisons actively screen to identify those individuals? On the one hand, it would be good for these individuals to know their status. On the other hand, it would only make worse the resource allocation problems within the Medicaid program or prisons. The same issue arises for private insurers.

One additional concern needs to be addressed. Approximately 300,000 to 500,000 Americans who have chronic hepatitis C have that status as a result of intravenous drug use. For the time being, we will postpone any extensive critical assessment of responsibility-sensitive conceptions of health care justice. However, we must note that hepatitis C is infectious, and others can be put at risk, including health professionals. How should that factor into a judgment of health care justice. More wickedness.

We need to take seriously both public health considerations and the financial limitations faced by Medicaid programs (Liao and Fischer, 2017). If Medicaid officials followed public health recommendations, intravenous drug users would be treated much sooner for their infection, which would spare them liver damage. Most Medicaid programs have a policy stating that individuals with chronic hepatitis C will only be treated for *one course* of sofosbuvir (given financial constraints). Obviously, this is a policy directed primarily at intravenous drug users. This policy will strike most taxpayers as reasonable and just. However, large numbers of medical problems require costly repeated hospitalizations for the same medical disorder because patients failed to take a reasonable level of responsibility for their own medical care. Type 2 diabetes would be a good example. Neither Medicare nor Medicaid puts a limit on the number of times these patients can be rehospitalized at social expense, costing tens of thousands of dollars per episode. Consequently, it looks arbitrary and unjustly discriminatory that intravenous drug users would alone be faced with such limitations.

3.2.6. Kidney Dialysis: The Headwaters of Wickedness

Consider this historical interlude at the headwaters of our wickedness problems, namely, the invention of kidney dialysis during the 1960s for the benefit of patients with end-stage renal disease (ESRD). At roughly the same time, the surgical ability to do major organ transplants, including kidneys, was also developed. The annual cost of hemodialysis in 2021 was about $90,000 (also the cost of dialysis in 1970 adjusted for inflation to today's values). Few ESRD patients at the time could afford that cost. That meant being condemned to a premature death even though a technology was available that could yield extra years of life. Some patients could pay those costs for a year or two. This would create an ethically and psychologically awkward situation for physicians and hospitals who would have to say to a patient, "We are glad that we have sustained your life for the past 18 months. However, you have run out of money. We could sustain your life for another seven years if you could pay. If that is not possible, this will be your last dialysis session (and you will be dead in two weeks)."

Given uncertain financing for dialysis, hospitals in the late 1960s were reluctant to invest in dialysis facilities, thereby generating a shortage of dialysis facilities. Consequently, at times "social worth" criteria were used to determine who would receive dialysis (Alexander, 1962). For the broad public, however, the most distressing aspect of this situation was that an effective life-prolonging technology was available but was artificially scarce merely because of money. An oft-invoked mantra was that "human life is priceless." There was no absolute scarcity (as with transplantable organs); dialysis units could be constructed until the need was fully satisfied.

Congress was heavily lobbied in 1972. This resulted in passage of the ESRD amendments to the Medicare program. In brief, Congress created what has been described as a national health insurance program for patients with ESRD. Congress believed the program was affordable and that at 20 years out the cost of the program would peak at $500 million (roughly $3 billion in adjusted 2018 dollars). The actual cost of the ESRD program to Medicare in 2018 was about $49 billion to provide either dialysis or a kidney transplant for 786,000 patients (United States Renal Data System, 2020). In 2017,

193,000 Americans were alive with a functioning kidney transplant, the cost of which is about $262,000. These patients also need to be on anti-rejection medications for the rest of their lives costing about $18,000–$30,000 per year (James and Mannon, 2015), initially covered by the federal government. However, Congress later imposed various cost control measures, including a three-year limit on federal funding for those anti-rejection medications (Harris, 2016). The predictable consequence for patients with moderate incomes was going off these drugs followed by transplant failure and a return to dialysis.

Kidney transplantation is moving into the world of precision medicine. Recent research suggests that "precision immunosuppression" is possible (Pineda et al., 2017; DiLoreto et al., 2017; Wiebe et al., 2018). The hope is that future drugs will modulate more finely the functioning of the immune system and the expression of genes related to the transplanted organ. However, if these drugs are as expensive as our targeted cancer therapies, this will be an unsustainable financial burden for both the federal government and transplant patients.

Another point needs to be noted. Patients on these anti-rejection medications have a threefold increased risk of developing cancer relative to the general population. This is obviously because of the suppression of the immune system (Acuna et al., 2016; Sprangers et al., 2017). Some of these patients will only need less expensive standard chemotherapeutic regimens to treat their cancer. Others, however, will need the hyper-expensive targeted cancer therapies. Who is supposed to cover these costs? Should we assume that all these patients have an equally just claim to have these costs socially shared through some insurance mechanism, public or private? This brings us back to our wickedness problem.

The ESRD program has a subtle wicked quality. What will strike some as ethically incoherent, however, is that the ESRD program funds at public expense kidney transplants but no other, more costly, major organ transplants (hearts, lungs, livers, and so on) that are equally effective at prolonging life for years. What explains that apparent ethical incongruity? Do any of the proposed explanations offer sufficient ethical justification?

A bureaucrat might say that the program is just about kidneys, not hearts or lungs or livers. However, the primary rationale for the program was about the pricelessness of human life, not the dignity or moral worth of kidneys. Moreover, kidney transplants achieved the same outcomes as heart or liver or other major organ transplants, that is, roughly 70% survival at five years out and 50% survival at 10 years out. These other transplants are costlier, but fewer can be done, given a limited supply. Heart transplants in 2017 cost about $1.3 million, liver transplants cost about $800,000, heart–lung transplants cost about $2.5 million, and intestinal transplants cost about $1.14 million (Bentley and Phillips, 2017). In 2020 roughly 23,400 kidney transplants were performed, 3,550 heart transplants, 8,900 liver transplants, and 130 intestinal transplants. The total number of major organ transplants was a little under 40,000. In short, nothing morally relevant would distinguish kidney transplants from all other major organ transplants.

Why then would Congress not include coverage for these other major organ transplants? Political reasons could have been a consideration. If Congress had expanded funding, everyone with the relevant need would have roughly equal opportunity to have that need met. From an egalitarian perspective, that would be ideal. From a purely political perspective (satisfying voter preferences), individuals with moderate incomes and modest or no health insurance would be able to compete successfully for these major organ transplants against financially well-off, insured individuals. These latter individuals would raise the self-interested claim that they would be paying taxes to support a transplant program to save "someone else's life" rather than their own, were they to need a major organ transplant. Worse still (from their point of view), they would have ample private insurance coverage, while "these undeserving others" would be using taxpayer funds.

In 1972 Congress believed that dialysis was an utterly unique therapeutic intervention requiring only a trickle of funding. Congress failed to realize that dialysis was at the headwaters of a torrent of expensive life-prolonging technologies that started to emerge in the 1970s. Successful development of the capacity to do organ transplantation was another part of that emerging torrent. By the late 1970s, however, research was going forward to develop a totally implantable artificial heart (TIAH). The ethically and economically significant feature of this device is that an unlimited number can be produced. More than 700,000 Americans died of heart disease in 2021, half of whom (according to computer modeling) could be medically eligible to receive a TIAH if eventually perfected. It would add more than $200 billion annually to US health expenditures if all late-stage heart disease patients became candidates for this device. Congress foresaw and feared this scenario. However, the moral logic behind the ESRD program would require exactly this outcome. The TIAH was projected to yield on average five extra years of life expectancy, mostly, we should add, for elderly patients. This is where wickedness has the potential to become painfully (politically and ethically) evident.

If Congress were unwilling to fund the TIAH as well as other major organ transplants, Medicare would still have to fund these procedures for older patients covered by Medicare, roughly 70% of patients with late-stage heart failure. What would be ethically problematic would be that other non-elderly 30%. For those who were underinsured or uninsured and faced with life-threatening heart failure at age 50, they would be condemned to an unnecessary premature death. Thoughtful individuals would judge it unjust to provide the TIAH at social expense to individuals in their early 80s so that they might achieve age 90 while failing to provide that same technology at social expense to individuals far short of achieving a normal life expectancy. How should that situation be corrected?

The "easy answer" would be to fund the TIAH for everyone with the relevant medical need. Keep in mind our overarching ethical problem, namely, fair health care rationing. If we endorse funding all medically necessary TIAHs because these patients have urgent medical needs which, if unfulfilled, will result in their premature death, then that same moral logic will require assured societal funding (whether public or private) for patients in comparable circumstances, whether those circumstances involve a deadly form of cancer or liver disease or lung disease or pancreatic disease, and so on. That effectively ignores the need for limits or for priority-setting. It also allows health care funding to be ethically hijacked by terminally ill patients, no matter what the social cost, no matter how marginal the benefit.

To see the wickedness of that situation, consider the millions of patients who suffer with osteoarthritis. This is not a life-threatening medical problem. It diminishes substantially the quality of life of individuals. Some relatively expensive drugs might be available to provide significant relief to these patients. However, affordable access to those drugs might be effectively denied to those patients if we are "ethically obligated" to provide unlimited access to any life-prolonging technology no matter how costly for patients judged to be terminally ill. Osteoarthritis is just one example.

Some medical ethicists might argue that the palliative care needs of the terminally ill *must* be addressed, that it would be cruel and inhumane to fail in this regard. Still, wickedness lurks even here regarding health care justice. Specifically, if palliative care physicians are consummate in their care of these terminally ill patients, then many of these patients will be motivated to continue more aggressive efforts at life-prolonging care because the symptoms of their disease or the side effects of the therapy will be effectively managed. This outcome would strike many as both an unjust and unwise use of health care resources, given the unmet health needs of non–terminally ill patients. On the other hand, being stingy with palliative care in order to motivate these patients to choose to die more quickly would clearly be cruel and inhumane.[11] What are the alternatives, given the unmet health needs of non–terminally ill patients?

Among health policy analysts, much discussion today occurs around the notions of "high-value" care and "low-value" care, the thought being (perhaps) that a just and caring society ought to assure access for all to high-value care but leave to individual judgment and willingness to pay access to low-value care (Moriates et al., 2015; Schnipper and Bastian, 2016; Pandya, 2018; Pendleton, 2018; Bassett, 2018). How should this perspective be applied to palliative care?

3.3. Wicked Ragged Edges

Consider again the "ragged edge" problem. From the perspective of health care justice, where should we draw the line when patients presumably "need" a very expensive therapy whose benefits are likely (not certainly) marginal? Again, our paradigm cases will pertain to these cancer therapies. Consider the BRAF V600 mutation, which drives types of cancer. The drug vemurafenib (Zelboraf) is a BRAF inhibitor. In BRAF-positive hairy cell leukemia, vemurafenib has a 98% response rate, which means that the drug causes the cancer to shrink or disappear (which says nothing about a cure). The cost of the drug is about $13,000 per month. In BRAF-positive melanoma, vemurafenib has a response rate of 48%, which would usually imply some gain in survival, mostly measurable in months. In BRAF-positive anaplastic thyroid cancer, vemurafenib has a response rate of 29%. In BRAF-positive cholangiocarcinoma, vemurafenib has a response rate of 12.5% (Prasad et al., 2018). The justice-relevant question is whether all of these patients ought to receive vemurafenib at social expense.

---

[11] Patients on dialysis have had one of the highest "suicide" rates of any type of patient cohort; roughly one in seven patients choose to remove themselves from dialysis. In the past, mood swings and persistent fatigue (associated with red blood cells being "beaten up" in dialysis) precipitated the choice to give up dialysis. But the drug erythropoietin (Epogen) effectively addressed that issue. That drug adds about $3 billion to the cost of the ESRD program each year.

For the sake of argument, let us assume some gain in overall survival for any positive response to the drug. Let us also assume that the gain in overall survival might range from two months to 15 months. From a health care justice perspective, what should be concluded? Must vemurafenib be provided for all the patients in all four of these cancer categories with the BRAF mutation? In the last of those categories, almost 90% of those patients will derive no benefit. In other words, each month of life gained for those patients will cost nine times as much as the cost for a month for patients in the first category. Alternatively, vemurafenib could simply be denied to all the patients in that fourth category, which would mean that 12% of those patients would effectively be denied several extra months of life. If we were inclined to accept this alternative as ethically permissible, would our judgment remain the same if we knew that 1% of these patients would gain several extra years of life if they were to have access to vemurafenib? This is a ragged edge, and it is a wicked challenge.

In our third category, only 29% of those patients will have a positive response to vemurafenib, which means 71% would receive no benefit in terms of survival advantage. In economic terms the real cost for each month gained by the other 29% would be $43,000. Do those patients have a just claim to those social resources? Should a line be drawn at the level of our melanoma patients since 48% of them will have a positive response to vemurafenib? This still means that half the cost of this drug will be wasted or that each month of life gained for the 48% will have a real cost of $26,000. While this is a very high cost, it is what we are currently paying for two-drug combinations of targeted therapies that do yield significant survival gains for many metastatic cancer patients. Should the patients in our third category benignly accept drawing this line at the melanoma patients? Let us assume that the cost for each month of life gained is $43,000, with an average gain of nine months. That would yield a total cost per patient of $400,000. These patients desperately want that additional life. They point out that as a society we are willing to spend $800,000 for an extra year of life for a hemophilia patient with a severe resistance problem. Why, they would ask, are their lower-cost extra months of life of lower priority, ethically speaking, than extra months of life for hemophilia patients? This feels wicked because a simple and ethically compelling response is not obvious.

Ragged edges take many different forms. Some mutations are very specific to one or two types of cancer; others are described as being "cancer-agnostic." They drive many different cancers (Raez and Santos, 2018). TRK fusion-positive mutations are an instance of the latter that can be treated with the drug larotrectinib. However, only 1,500–5,000 patients with metastatic cancer each year would have a TRK-fusion cancer. Because this is a cancer-agnostic mutation, identifying patients with this mutation would require doing next-generation sequencing (NGS) on every metastatic cancer patient at a cost of $5,000 per patient (Regalado, 2016; Mullin, 2017), or an annual sequencing cost of $4 billion, likely for a panel of mutations, not just the TRK fusion. Also, larotrectinib is significantly effective at treating TRK tumors. As reported in the *New England Journal of Medicine* (Drilon et al., 2018), 71% of these patients had ongoing responses at one year, 75% of these patients responded, and 55% had achieved progression-free survival at one year. The monthly cost for this drug is $32,800. Predictably, only about 20% of patients with the TRK fusion could afford this drug (Harrison, 2018). These patients had health insurance, though with high co-pay and deductible requirements.[12]

We need to note that few insurance companies are willing to pay the costs of NGS. Should they be open to justified moral criticism for this reluctance? The argument they make to justify that reluctance is that all that testing (at present) results in only 30% of metastatic cancer patients having a targetable driver mutation. Further, even with insurance only a relatively small percentage of those patients can afford those drugs, which only very rarely achieve a cure.

3.4. Spinal Muscular Atrophy: Wickedness at Birth

Another dimension of wickedness pertains to children born with spinal muscular atrophy (SMA), roughly 400–700 each year in the United States. SMA is a recessive genetic disorder that chiefly affects motor neurons (Prakash, 2017). SMA causes severe muscle weakness that makes walking, sitting, breathing, and swallowing extremely difficult. There are four forms of SMA, the worst of which (SMA1) affects infants at birth. These infants will have a life expectancy of about two years. SMA2 and SMA3 will have onset in very

---

[12] I have provided just one example of a cancer-agnostic drug. There are many others. Pembrolizumab, the anti-PD-1 immune checkpoint inhibitor, has been approved for all solid tumors that are either mismatch repair deficient or microsatellite instability-high when that cancer has advanced or become metastatic (Raez and Santos, 2018).

early childhood with very debilitating results but the potential to achieve something closer to a normal life expectancy.

In 2017 the FDA approved the drug nusinersen (Spinraza*), which is a form of gene therapy. It is given by injection. The first-year cost of the drug is $750,000, and the cost for each year thereafter is $375,000. At this time (2021), no one can say what the effects of this drug are for infants treated near birth. It is believed they will survive more than two years, but no one knows how long survival might be beyond that (Finkel et al., 2017). Children with the less severe (but still severe) version of SMA had what is described as "clinically meaningful improvement in motor function" (Mercuri et al., 2018), roughly 57% of the children in this study.

This form of gene therapy is not curative, and the ameliorative effects are modest. As far as survival is concerned for this latter group, they may come close to a normal life expectancy, despite all the functional limitations. This was true for this group before nusinersen became available, which is where the wickedness issue arises. If these individuals needed to be on this drug for 50 years, the lifetime cost would be $15 million. Do these individuals have a just claim to this level of health resources?

A virtue of the Affordable Care Act is that it did away with lifetime limits regarding medically necessary care. Should we entirely disregard that $15 million number, at least for purposes of making a health care justice judgment? It might be ethically easier to do if this drug dramatically increased survival for these SMA2 and SMA3 children. However, the medical literature says that survival as such might not be affected (Yeo et al., 2022). Instead, the primary effect of the drug will be a modest gain in motor functioning (i.e., quality of life). Consequently, when nusinersen is assessed from a cost-effectiveness perspective, some extraordinarily large numbers are discovered. For SMA1, the cost per QALY is reported as $9.2 million; for SMA2, the cost per QALY is $24.4 million; for SMA3, the cost per QALY is $7.4 million (Michelson et al., 2018). How should we interpret and use numbers such as these as far as health care justice regarding resource allocation is concerned?

No other current health care intervention has ICER numbers this high. If we are willing to underwrite these costs as a just and caring society for very marginal benefits, are there any current health care interventions that we could justly refuse to pay for? The guideline authors from the American Academy of Neurology write regarding nusinsersen: "At societal and clinical levels, there remain unanswered questions about the balance of improving the lives of individual patients vs the societal responsibility to control health care costs and maximize benefits for all" (Michelson et al., 2018, at 930).

Some questions have answers: Babies born with infantile SMA1 will survive longer than the two-year death sentence that would otherwise be their fate. How much longer will they survive and with what level of diminished motor functionality? That is an unanswered question. The same will be true for children with SMA2 and SMA3. Their life expectancy will remain indefinite, and sustained gain in motor functionality will remain uncertain. Would it be ethically acceptable to withhold access to these drugs (given their extraordinary cost) until greater certainty regarding outcomes is achieved for the children who were part of the formal clinical trials? That would strike many as an especially wicked thought. Still, many insurers and some Medicaid programs are unwilling to cover this drug for older children and adults with SMA3 or SMA4 because of the uncertainties regarding functional improvement, quality of life, and value to society provided by nusinersen (Michelson et al., 2018, at 930).

To be specific, what nusinersen would be seeking to preserve would be the ability to manipulate the joystick on a motorized wheelchair. From the perspective of prioritarians, these individuals are clearly among the medically least well off, which implies they have very strong justice claims to the only care that can be at all helpful to them. Insurers would not seem to endorse this perspective, again seeking to protect both their profits and the pocketbooks of the clients in their insurance pool. Still, in the case of SMA1, these children would be condemned to death by the age of two if denied nusinersen. If we knew the drug would only gain an extra year of life for these children, we might judge that outcome tragic and unfortunate, not unjust, given only an extra year of very debilitated life. That would diminish considerably the wickedness of the situation. However, the current (2021) clinical reality is that nusinersen might prolong the lives of these children for some significant period of time, perhaps to early adulthood. No one knows. That intensifies the wickedness of the situation, the unavoidable threat to fundamental ethical and political values.

Imagine a physician saying the following to parents who have just given birth to an infant diagnosed with SMA1: "As I have explained, we have this drug, nusinersen, which *might* prolong your child's life significantly, maybe for two decades, though with profound motor disabilities. Considerable uncertainty exists in this regard. From a societal perspective, I ask you to understand, this is not a wise use of limited social resources. We should be using these same resources to improve the prospects of children with Duchenne muscular dystrophy. Granted, their overall life prospects are limited, but we have more medical confidence in the effectiveness of what we can do for them and at lower cost." It is hard to imagine these parents quietly accepting the implications of this. Put that aside. Consider instead how advocates for persons with disabilities might assess this statement. I would surmise that they would judge it to be especially wicked to play off the needs of one group of persons with disabilities against the needs of other persons with disabilities.

I can imagine advocates for both these groups arguing that it is neither just nor caring that 80-year-old individuals would be feasting on health care resources so that they could achieve a reasonable quality of life into their 90s while brushing a few health care crumbs off the table to these persons with disabilities who would never come close to achieving a normal life expectancy. If it is ethically important to give priority to meeting the health care needs of those who are medically least well off, then surely lavishing health care resources on the elderly while shortchanging much younger individuals with serious disabilities is ethically problematic as a matter of justice. However, this debate overall has an ethically unsavory quality since it appears we are pitting ageists against ableists. That is, which prejudice is more ethically acceptable? Being compelled to ask such a question is itself wicked.

Here is another emerging scenario blossoming with fruits of hope and seeds of wickedness hidden within. Novartis has announced a true gene therapy for SMA, AVXS-101 (Taylor, 2018). This therapy would actually restore the body's ability to manufacture the missing protein responsible for SMA. It would be a true cure. It would be given just one time, presumably very near to birth in an affected baby, at a cost of $4 million. Assume this therapy is a true genetic cure, that these children can achieve a normal life expectancy with no residual muscular deficiencies. It is hard to imagine a just and caring society denying this therapy to any of these children. This is not gene therapy for an 80-year-old with diminishing muscle capacity. These are children at the beginning of life. The aggregated cost for 600 such infants each year multiplied by $4 million would be $2.4 billion.

Note that Novartis does not see AVXS-101 as applying to individuals with SMA2 or SMA3. However, it is working on a version of gene therapy that might be curative in those latter two cases as well. If successful, approximately 4,000 patients would be candidates for that therapy at a one-time aggregated cost of about $16 billion. Again, if the results were that dramatic (full functional restoration), it would be hard to imagine a just and caring society denying individuals that therapy.[13] However, what generates some wicked concerns is that Novartis has several other gene therapies in the pipeline (Taylor, 2018), including ones for hearing loss (linked to a genetic defect), Rett syndrome, and amyotrophic lateral sclerosis (ALS; Lou Gehrig's disease).

Consider the ethical implications of successful gene therapy for ALS. There are about 6,000 new cases of ALS each year in the United States, mostly among middle-aged adults. Currently (2021), about 20,000 ALS patients are alive in the United States. Life expectancy after diagnosis is 2–5 years, though 20% of ALS patients will survive five years, 10% will survive 10 years, and 5% will survive 20 years (ALS Association, 2016). At present, no cure exists for ALS. Consider a possible gene therapy cure for ALS with a cost of $4 million for a single infusion. If all 6,000 ALS individuals were provided with this gene therapy, that would represent an aggregated annual cost in the United States of $24 billion. Again, if this gave individuals several extra decades of good-quality life, ethically speaking, a just and caring society would be obligated to provide that therapy. Still, this will generate some possible wicked problems.

We start with the economic fact that the $4 million front-end costs will not be judged a "good investment" since the cost of caring for most ALS patients for their limited life expectancy would be less than $1 million. By way of contrast, gene therapy for SMA would yield many decades of reasonable quality of life. Does this mean, from a just priority-setting perspective, that we should pay for gene therapy for SMA before we pay for gene therapy for ALS? Or is this question ethically illegitimate because we would be pitting one disability against another when both groups are properly thought of as being among the medically least well off for whom an effective intervention now exists?

The premise for raising these initial questions is that these gene therapies would be curative, completely successful. This might be an excessively optimistic premise. Consequently, consider another scenario. What if the effects of gene therapy gradually wear off, say, over five years? At that point, individuals would need another $4 million infusion to be restored to a normal state of health. Would a just and caring society be ethically obligated to

---

[13] Though I use the phrase "a just and caring society," no such unified entity exists in the United States. We have Medicare, 50 Medicaid programs, and a thousand insurance companies with thousands of insurance plans. That is, we have an extremely fragmented system for financing access to needed health care, and consequently, responsibility is frequently dispersed and uncertain. Consequently, these needs are more likely to go unmet.

provide that second infusion? And a third five years later? And a fourth five years after that? I am raising these questions with regard to both SMA and ALS. As a society we have endorsed through the Affordable Care Act the idea that there should be no lifetime limits regarding health insurance, the background assumption being that we are talking about effective health care interventions that make a significant difference with regard to protecting or restoring length of life and quality of life.

Both of these gene therapies (as imagined) would meet this effectiveness criterion, albeit for five years rather than many decades for each infusion. In addition, it seems cruel if we were simply to allow these individuals to revert to a medical status in which they were among the medically least well off (greatly diminished life expectancy and quality of life) when we had a therapy that would readily prevent that reversion. Further, we are already spending up to $800,000 per year for some hemophilia patients. From an egalitarian perspective, it would seem we would be ethically obligated to provide gene therapy to these patients. Still, we need to take seriously the "just caring" problem. Choices must be made; priorities must be set. The economic math is daunting. If we assume the five-year gene therapy scenario for ALS, then in Year 10 we would have accumulated 60,000 ALS patients who would need a gene therapy infusion for $4 million, or an aggregated cost of $240 billion (constant dollars).

Ethically, we still must do this, but our economic capacity suggests this would be utterly unrealistic. What then would be the right thing to do, all things considered? Among the things to be considered is that a number of other pharmaceutical companies are working just as vigorously as Novartis to develop other gene therapies for other serious single-gene disorders. We might fear a tsunami of gene therapies, but the frightful fact is that a small tidal wave of gene therapies would be sufficient to wreak economic and ethical havoc in our health care system. From an ethical priority-setting perspective, how would we imagine comparing these gene therapies to our targeted cancer therapies or cancer immunotherapies? As advocates for these gene therapies would describe them, they are enormously effective for generally a very young or somewhat younger population compared to a generally significantly older population of cancer patients. Further, for the vast majority of cancer patients, the gains in life expectancy attributable to these targeted therapies are marginal. Alternatively, the number of cancer patients likely to receive some benefit from these targeted therapies is much greater than the number of patients likely to benefit from gene therapy. Further, if the scenario I have laid out regarding gene therapy were to come to fruition, aggregated costs for gene therapy would far exceed likely aggregated costs for targeted cancer therapies and, as noted, for a much smaller population.

3.5. A Wicked Summary

Wicked problems are ethically complex and ethically controversial. No matter what response we choose, we see ourselves in more reflective moments as violating other equally valuable moral norms.[14] Our social sense of health care justice is pluralistic and, consequently, ethically complex. In some circumstances, we emphasize our egalitarian commitments—treat all with equal concern and respect. All who have the same medical problem ought to have assured equal access to the same medical therapy (regardless of ability to pay). No one should be allowed to die if a medical intervention is available that would prevent that death. That will strike many as a worthy moral commitment.

However, utilitarians will beg to differ, especially in cases where patients are faced with a terminal condition, gains in life expectancy are very marginal, and costs to achieve those marginal gains are extremely high, as with metastatic cancer patients who need a costly, targeted therapy. Utilitarians will note that too many other unmet health care needs can be met at a lower cost with more health good achieved than with the targeted cancer drugs. This commitment surely has moral attractiveness (albeit mixed, given the implied sacrifice of some additional life for those cancer patients).

Libertarians will also disagree with egalitarians, claiming it is unjust to use the coercive powers of government to force the healthier to pay for the costly health needs of the less healthy. In addition, some therapeutic interventions are so expensive and so likely to yield only marginal health benefits that it would be both imprudent and unjust to expect that those needs would be met with social resources. Instead, individuals have to decide for themselves whether such interventions are really worth it to them, given their own limited resources and other preferred uses for those resources.

---

[14] Calabresi and Bobbitt (1978) would describe wicked problems as "tragic choices." The choices are "tragic" because all policy options chosen will violate some fundamental social value to protect another equally fundamental social value. Their "solution" to addressing such tragic choices is to choose policy options that effectively hide the violation of that fundamental social value, which violates what Rawls (1971, 1996) refers to as the "publicity condition," which both he and I see as central to any conception of justice.

Next, luck egalitarians will reject the views of moderate non-luck egalitarians, claiming too many individuals have health needs generated by irresponsible health choices. Consequently, luck egalitarians judge that it is unjust that healthy, responsible individuals should have to pay taxes or insurance premiums to assist in meeting the health needs of individuals who made irresponsible health choices. They view a commitment to a non-responsible egalitarianism as being both unreasonable and unjust (Knight and Stemplowska, 2011; Segall, 2010).

Finally, sufficientarians believe that obligations of health care justice have limits. No one has a just claim to anything and everything that might satisfy a health care need. A just and caring society only owes access to health care that is basic or adequate or sufficient (leaving to later discussion "sufficiency"). Their ethical intuition seems reasonable. There are *limits* to the health care a just society owes its members.

When these different conceptions of health care justice are applied to the range of allocation challenges described above, the results are conflicting directives regarding a just enough allocation of resources among these challenges. In the abstract, each of these conceptions of health care justice seems ethically reasonable. In the concrete, however, and while considering the panoply of potential therapeutic interventions, each of these conceptions of health care justice will recommend very different allocation decisions regarding various medical therapies.

Does ethical consistency require that we use the same conception of health care justice for all metastatic cancer patients needing a targeted therapy? However, the predictable result will be specific allocation decisions that are obviously ethically problematic. For example, a strict compassionate egalitarian (Harris, 1985) might wish to provide access to all these targeted therapies for all metastatic cancer patients at social expense. Would that include spending $475,000 for CAR T-cell therapy for a patient we knew with near certainty would not survive 30 days? We might think that a utilitarian perspective would yield a more just outcome in these circumstances, the broader implication being that we would bring to bear different conceptions of justice in different clinical circumstances. However, what then assures us that such decisions are not arbitrary and unfair? Appeal to any one conception of health care justice to justify some specific allocation decision could be plausibly challenged by another conception of health care justice as flawed.

Proposed solutions to wicked problems often lead to unforeseen consequences that are themselves ethically problematic. For example, Congress passed the 1972 Medicare ESRD amendments that paid for dialysis and kidney transplants but not major organ transplants, though all these lives are priceless. Likewise, Congress was unwilling to create a program to pay for factor VIII for hemophiliacs, another extraordinarily expensive intervention that few hemophiliacs could afford. This would have struck many at the time as neither just nor compassionate. One alternative would be to make choices among patients needing very expensive but effective life-prolonging interventions. However, that would have the unsavory political and moral implication that some lives were "worthier" of being saved than others.

Policymakers could "remedy" this situation by closing out the ESRD program. This would be a catastrophic choice, both ethically and politically. Alternatively, policymakers could create a policy of national health insurance for the terminally ill that would pay for any therapeutic intervention that promised any meaningful prolongation of their lives. That would cover all the targeted therapies available for metastatic cancer patients as well as the medical needs of all terminally ill patients. However, that policy option would be equally catastrophic, ethically and economically speaking. Given all the life-prolonging medical technology today, terminally ill patients could hijack the vast majority of current health spending in a year. Wickedness seems to be ubiquitous.

Wicked problems tend to be socially and politically complex and, in the case of health care, medically complex. Health care priorities need to be set. Health care needs, however, are extraordinarily heterogeneous, which makes it extraordinarily difficult to make comparisons that will permit an easy ranking of health care priorities for funding purposes, considering concerns related to efficiency, justice, cost-effectiveness, and compassion. Uncertainty of outcomes contributes to the wickedness of setting health care priorities in medicine. Priorities are typically set with regard to categories of patients and appropriate therapies for those patients in that category. This is relatively easy when virtually all individuals respond either well or poorly to that therapy. However, it is especially difficult to establish the proper ("just enough") priority for a cost-ineffective therapy, such as our targeted cancer therapies, that results in a very broad range of responses in terms of survival gains, quality of life, and costly side effects. Should policymakers just simplify matters by ranking all therapeutic interventions on the basis of cost-effectiveness? However, that would generate some ethically awkward, compassionless outcomes, most especially in the case of children who now can be treated with a very effective and exceedingly costly drug, such as children with enzyme deficiency disorders like Fabry disease.

Wicked problems are *socially complex* when individuals in need of costly care are generally victims of social stigmatization. Recall patients infected with hepatitis C due to intravenous drug use or committing a crime. Also recall HIV-infected individuals, a substantial majority of whom are homosexual. The social complexity is related to the fact that the vast majority of health professionals would feel ethically obligated to treat these patients, given life-threatening health needs and available cost-effective therapies. However, widespread discriminatory attitudes can frustrate the ability of health professionals to meet these obligations because of wicked *political complexity.*

Wicked problems tend to overlap multiple organizational and institutional boundaries. That organizational overlap makes them much more difficult to resolve. Almost half of all health care spending in the United States involves public dollars. However, explicit efforts by any legislative body to reduce public health care budgets has generated the rhetoric of "death panels." Consequently, no legislative body is willing to make visible policy choices to control health care costs perceived as denying individuals costly life-prolonging care. For example, the Affordable Care Act was supposed to create an agency, the Patient-Centered Outcomes Research Institute, that would be responsible for assessing the cost-effectiveness of various new medical technologies. It would generate information used to direct taxpayer dollars to more cost-effective interventions. However, the legislation that brought that agency into existence also eviscerated its ability to do any meaningful sort of cost-effectiveness analysis (Persad, 2015), thereby diminishing any financial threat to many powerful health care stakeholders, such as pharmaceutical companies.

Congress must obviously control health care costs. In 1984, for example, the Diagnosis Related Groupings (DRG) system was put in place for paying hospitals caring for Medicare patients. In brief, a DRG is a mini-budget attached to a Medicare patient admitted to a hospital. There are about 740 DRGs. This is a prospective payment mechanism. The money attached to that DRG is payment in full for that patient's hospitalization. This approach allows Congress to say that it is not practicing medicine or denying any necessary care to Medicare patients. Those judgments are left to hospital administrators and physicians. This creates incentives for discharging patients "sicker and quicker." Bad things can happen to patients discharged early at home (another heart attack). These outcomes are very remote from Congress so far as accountability is concerned. When there are bad outcomes that *might have been averted* if that patient had been in the hospital those extra days, those outcomes will be local, dispersed, and private (invisible to media attention). That sort of ethical obscurity undermines any expectation for institutional accountability.

Consider: How often will some legislative body or hospital or insurer or employer explicitly deny a metastatic cancer patient payment for these drugs (i.e., make an explicit rationing decision)? This will be a rare event. None of these organizations will want to be charged with causing a patient's premature death. Instead, impersonal high co-pays and high deductibles will effectively exclude the vast majority of patients who are financially less well off from accessing these drugs. In effect, it will appear that these patients have freely made these rationing decisions for themselves. That effectively (but wrongly) excuses employers, insurers, and legislators from any responsibility for these rationing decisions, though these organizations all shaped the constraints within these insurance plans that resulted in these patients having to make these choices. This is fairly described as invisible wickedness.

Wicked problems are difficult to define and therefore difficult to solve. Most policy analysts would identify emerging medical technologies since the early 1970s as the most fundamental cause of escalating health care costs. As Callahan (1990) and Kaufman (2015) both point out, those emerging medical technologies create what we would identify as "needs," in the morally valenced sense of that term. The development of effective targeted cancer therapies for metastatic cancer perfectly illustrates the point. These drugs promise some gain in survival and quality of life for patients with metastatic cancer, which is of obvious moral significance. Should we somehow halt or dramatically slow the research that generates these technologies and their dissemination into clinical practice? It is impossible to imagine what political or economic mechanisms would accomplish this, much less compelling moral arguments for such an objective. This is one reason why we are faced with a wicked problem resistant to any resolution.

The wickedness is multifaceted. Another fundamental cause of escalating health care costs in both the United States and the European Union is the expansion of the elderly population, along with a longer life expectancy and a growing burden of chronic illness. Note that 23% of the Medicare population has four or five chronic illnesses (mobility issues, sensory deficits, dementia, cardiac debilitation, cancers, etc.), and another 14% has six or more chronic conditions (Centers for Medicare and Medicaid Services, 2012, figure 1.2a). This is primarily due to the successes associated with the deployment of new medical technologies that have transformed terminal illnesses of relatively brief duration into costly, very long-term chronic conditions. As noted in Chapter 2, a major goal of precision medicine is to transform cancers into manageable chronic illnesses through the use of multiple drug combinations. Again, it is impossible to imagine any political or economic mechanism stifling the need for life-prolonging health care for the elderly. No legislator, no hospital administrator, no insurance executive is going to advocate for an age beyond which the elderly would be denied expensive, life-prolonging health care interventions, lest they be accused of "throwing granny off the cliff." In brief, we are again confronted by a wicked dead end.

The proverbial bottom line, also known as the "warren of wickedness," has been correctly identified by the Princeton economist Uwe Reinhardt (1982). He has proposed the "great equation" in health care: Health Care Costs = Health Care Income. Whatever anyone tries to do by way of controlling health care costs will necessarily involve constraining or reducing someone's (or some institution's) income. Whatever groups of professionals or whatever health care institutions see themselves as being the "victims" of efforts to control health care costs will use whatever political or economic power they have to resist those income reductions. Worse, they will employ any number of pseudo-moral arguments to justify their efforts to resist cost controls aimed at them. Pharmaceutical companies have been the most notorious purveyors of these pseudo-moral arguments (Jones, 2018). Among the worst offenders in this regard are the television and print ads for the drug nivolumab (Opdivo®) for advanced non-small cell lung cancer. The ads show in 30-foot-high letters on either buildings or a cliff "A chance to live longer." In one version of the television ads a voiceover intones, "Who would not want to live longer?" (Bulik, 2017; iSpot.tv 2015; iSpot.tv 2017). What a wicked warren we weave when first we practice to deceive.[15]

We turn next to the challenge of ameliorating some of the wickedness associated with the challenges of allocating health care resources fairly.

---

[15] See also an essay by Liz Szabo (2017), "Cancer Treatment Hype Gives False Hope to Many Cancer Patients," again calling attention to the messages conveyed in television ads regarding these cancer drugs.

4
Precision Medicine, Imprecise Health Care Justice

4.1. Precision Health Reform: What Precisely Should Be Included in a Benefit Package Guaranteed to All?

I assume that a just and caring society ought to guarantee to all its members some level of health care apart from being able to pay for that care. Maybe this is a matter of justice, maybe beneficence. In the ethics and policy literature, this is typically described as a "basic" or "adequate" or "minimally decent" level of care. All of these terms are extraordinarily vague. Even libertarians, unless they have hearts and brains of stone, can accept these modest premises. Our question is this: What medical interventions that come under the rubric of precision medicine ought to be included in a health care benefit package guaranteed to all in our society? Many prominent politicians are advocating that we adopt "Medicare for all." Given the extraordinarily high costs associated with precision medicine and given numerous and persistent demands for health care cost control, how many interventions seen as part of precision medicine ought to be included in Medicare for all?

Let us start by considering a case:

Barbara Kearney was 71 years old in 2017. She was a retired medical technician. She had been diagnosed in 2006 with B-cell lymphoma. In those intervening years, she had gone through four different treatment regimens, including a bone marrow transplant. All of them eventually failed. She was eager to try CAR T-cell therapy, though she knew there was a very high probability of serious side effects. She was one of the first in the country to undergo this therapy outside a clinical trial. (Knox, 2018; see also Bach, 2018, 2019)

Precision Medicine and Distributive Justice. Leonard M. Fleck, Oxford University Press. © Oxford University Press 2022.
DOI: 10.1093/oso/9780197647721.003.0004

We described in Chapter 1 the complexities associated with chimeric antigen receptor (CAR) T-cell therapy. T cells were extracted from Kearney's bloodstream and sent to a lab in California, where they were genetically re-engineered to target the CD19 receptor on cancer cells. Kearney had many of the dramatic side effects associated with this therapy, including cytokine release syndrome, which required three weeks of very intensive care. The entire cost of this episode was approximately $700,000. Unfortunately, Barbara Kearney died three weeks after she received her CAR T-cell infusion.

Barbara Beaudry was diagnosed in 2006 with non-Hodgkin's lymphoma [NHL]. She was in her late 50s. Over the next ten years, her cancer progressed, in spite of the fact that she had tried four different chemotherapeutic regimens. In July of 2015, she took part in the JULIET trial at the University of Pennsylvania Medical Center and received an infusion of CAR T-cells. Three months later, she had achieved a complete response, along with 26 other patients, out of 81 in the trial. Of those 26 patients, 19 were still cancer free at six months. Barbara "graduated" from the trial in June of 2017 "cancer free." Approximately 75,000 patients per year in the United States are diagnosed with NHL. (Abramson Cancer Center, 2018)

Ms. Beaudry was alive and doing well in the middle of 2018. No one can say with confidence what her prospects for long-term survival might be.

Doug Olson was diagnosed with chronic lymphocytic leukemia [CLL] in 1996 at the age of 49. He did not require treatment for a number of years. Then he needed chemotherapy, which yielded a 5-year remission, followed by more chemotherapy, which yielded a 2-year remission, followed by more chemotherapy, which failed to yield any remission. He was offered the option of a bone marrow transplant but turned that down because of a 50% chance of dying from the transplant itself. Instead, he entered a trial for CAR T-cell therapy in 2010. He was the second patient in that trial. He experienced some of the more serious side effects, which required a brief hospitalization. He has been cancer-free since then. (Olson, 2018)

Doug Olson is correctly described as a super-responder, since he is alive and doing well in early 2022 (Kolata, 2022). I have no statistics on the fate of others who were in that trial. However, in the JULIET trial, the 19 patients (25%) who achieved durable remissions at six months still had durable remissions at 29 months, which says nothing about seven-year survival.[1] Should CAR T-cell therapy be included as part of a minimally decent (or basic or adequate) health care benefit package guaranteed to all in our society?

Behind our fundamental question is an equality premise: Everyone in our society is entitled to equal concern and respect. This is about both fairness and beneficence. If any patient with a specific medical condition is treated with a reasonably successful therapy at social expense, then all with that condition should have access to that therapy at social expense. Think of an appendectomy. A society with the sophisticated medical technology we have in the United States would be open to serious, justified moral criticism if it allowed such patients to die for lack of ability to pay. Consequently, this *sort of care* (however we might define that) would have to be included in a minimally decent health care package guaranteed to all in our society.

Perhaps we should say that no one should be allowed to die "prematurely" if we have the medical ability to prolong their lives. This would be a starting point for defining a minimally decent health care package for all. However, this rule has at least two disadvantages: (1) It is too inclusive and diffuse and (2) potential costs could inappropriately skew other health care resource allocations within a limited social budget. What is characteristic of our appendectomy example is that this patient is at imminent risk of dying *and* we have the effective ability to prevent that death from occurring. Precision medicine, in contrast, is about patients with metastatic cancer and a terminal prognosis. None of these drugs can promise a cure. Rare super-responders may gain extra years of life. However, to save those extra years of life, we would have to fund all these cancer drugs in a basic benefit package, even though in the vast majority of cases only a few extra months of life would be gained. This would seem to be neither economically nor ethically reasonable. If we include these targeted cancer therapies in the basic benefit package, then what would be the justice-relevant considerations that would justify excluding any other costly medical intervention that promised any degree of likely life-prolonging benefit? The short answer, I believe, is that no such justice-relevant considerations exist.

We have no way of identifying before the fact which few metastatic cancer patients might be super-responders. Suppose, however, that we were able to

---

[1] The CAR T-cell research we have been reporting involves having the CD19 antigen as its target (June and Sadelain, 2018). However, other versions of CAR T-cell therapy have other targets and other approaches to engineering those T cells. There are at least 21 CAR T-cell therapies in development (National Cancer Institute, 2022).

identify biomarkers that could identify with greater than 90% confidence the super-responders. Would that make such patients more ethically akin to our patients with life-threatening appendicitis? If so, does their treatment become part of the basic benefit package? These patients may have a just claim to these drugs at social expense, but the justification for that claim is not to be found in the language of "basic health care." The language of basic benefits fits most readily the sufficientarian conception of health care justice. This view is ethically insufficient for addressing the justice challenges raised by the dissemination of precision medicine, and this is also true for all the major theories of health care justice.

4.2. Key Challenges to Health Care Justice

Our broad question is this: Can any conception of health care justice fairly and adequately address the complex challenges to health care justice posed by precision medicine? I will offer a negative answer. Let's do a quick recap of those challenges.

(1) *The ragged edge challenge*: How can a bright line be drawn that distinguishes just social payment for metastatic cancer patients who need a targeted cancer therapy and who are most likely to gain substantial medical benefit above that line from patients whose likely benefit is below that line? If we refuse to draw that line, we are in effect refusing to control these social health care costs.

(2) *The super-responder challenge*: Super-responders clearly gain the most medical benefit from these targeted therapies. Does that imply that we must fund a specific targeted therapy for a specific cancer for everyone with that cancer to avoid condemning potential super-responders to a premature death? If so, we surrender cost control and risk cancer therapies making unjust claims on social resources. On the other hand, if future biomarkers permit identifying super-responders before the fact, what should that imply for moderate and marginal responders who might be in their 20s or 50s or 80s?

(3) *The very high cost-effectiveness challenge*: Many targeted cancer therapies have high cost-effectiveness ratios, such as $200,000 per quality-adjusted life-year (QALY), for the majority of cancer patients needing that specific drug. However, very high cost-effectiveness

ratios exist for some range of non-cancer drugs, such as nusinersen (Spinraza®) to treat spinal muscular atrophy (SMA), at $400,000 per QALY. These orphan drugs are often approved for social funding. Is that unjust to the cancer patients whose targeted therapies might not be funded due to high cost-effectiveness numbers? More broadly, how can cost-effectiveness numbers be used to make just allocations of health care resources?

(4) *The very high front-end cost challenge*: We have called attention to CAR T-cell therapy for treating various blood cancers (and future research aimed at attacking solid tumors).[2] The front-end cost can be $475,000, with several hundreds of thousands of dollars in additional costs for 30%–50% of patients needing intensive care unit care for cytokine release syndrome. If these high costs yield extra years of reasonable-quality life, then the costs are worth it (I would argue), so far as health care justice is concerned from multiple justice perspectives. However, if 30% of these patients fail to gain a year of life, and we can identify them before the fact, would it be unjust to deny them that therapy? Another example would be onasemnogene abeparvovec-xioi (Zolgensma®), a form of gene therapy used to treat SMA with a front-end cost of $2.2 million and with unknown long-term effectiveness.

(5) *The medically least well off/terminally ill challenge*: The terminally ill can fairly be regarded as being among the medically least well off. Metastatic cancer patients are among the terminally ill. Patients with factor VIII resistant hemophilia would be among the medically least well off, enduring considerable lifelong suffering at very great expense to the health care system. Many patients in this latter category have open-ended life expectancies, certainly if they have assured access to extraordinarily expensive (but non-curative) treatments. The health care justice challenge is whether social resources should be preferentially directed to patients in this latter category as opposed to funding somewhat open-endedly targeted cancer therapies for these metastatic cancer patients.

(6) *The fair treatment of the very old challenge*: Are the elderly (over 65) and hyper-elderly (over 85) hijacking the health care system

---

[2] Solid tumors are much more of a challenge for CAR T-cell therapy because the microenvironment of the tumor has many strategies for evading the immune system (see Titov et al., 2020; DeRosier, 2019).

and health care resources to the potential disadvantage of the non-elderly? Elderly patients have many more health needs (generally) than the non-elderly, both needs related to quality of life and needs seen as being life-threatening. The non-elderly have those needs as well, for which expensive and effective medical technologies are available. Few would doubt the just claims to these technologies by the non-elderly, but often these interventions will be less effective in the elderly and hyper-elderly. This *may* be true for many of the targeted cancer therapies. However, if these targeted cancer therapies were often 50% less effective in treating individuals over age 75 with metastatic cancer, would that justify withholding such drugs from these individuals so that those dollars could be reallocated to more promising therapies that would be more effective at earlier stages of a cancer?

(7) *The very high aggregated cost challenge*: Very expensive interventions, say, $100,000 for every metastatic cancer patient, are economically tolerable and might be required as a matter of justice. However, we introduced the scenario in which metastatic cancer becomes a managed chronic care condition for at least five years through the sequential use of these drugs with each of those years costing $100,000 for the 610,000 cancer patients who would otherwise die that year. Those aggregated costs would quickly become unsustainable and represent a threat to the just allocation of health care resources to non-cancer health care needs. What considerations of health care justice would justify limits on such multi-year aggregative therapies?

(8) *The comparative cost challenge*: In the case of end-stage renal disease (ESRD), we already use public resources of $90,000 per patient per year for dialysis, for 7–10 years. If we sought to control the costs of providing life-prolonging targeted cancer therapies for multiple years at $100,000 each, as in challenge 7, would cancer patients who saw themselves as the "victims" of such cost-control efforts have just cause for complaining that this was unfair, given societal willingness to pay $90,000 per year for ESRD patients? Alternatively, society will spend $1 million to sustain the life of a patient with HIV for 30 years with quadruple drug therapy or several million dollars for a hemophilia patient. Can the metastatic cancer patient justly complain that society must be willing to spend equal sums to prolong their life with

whatever targeted therapies or immunotherapies might be available and effective?[3]

(9) *The ibrutinib/CLL/CAR T-cell challenge*: For most CLL patients ibrutinib is very effective in yielding many extra years of life (7–10) at a cost of $156,000 each, or $1.5 million at 10 years, often at an advanced age. Recall that 71 was the median age at diagnosis with CLL. Some patients will develop resistance to ibrutinib within a year or two. Their one other treatment option will be CAR T-cell therapy with those very high front-end costs. For those who respond well, that might mean an extra three to four extra years of life. At that point we raise again the question of whether with reliable biomarkers we could again deny CAR T-cell therapy to those predicted to gain less than a year of life. However, others will fail ibrutinib after 4, 6, 8, or 10 years. Should all of these individuals have an equally just claim to CAR T-cell therapy as those who failed ibrutinib after one or two years?

(10) *The fair treatment for persons with disabilities challenge*: All persons with disabilities should be treated with equal concern and respect. However, the heterogeneity of disabilities can have consequences so far as effectiveness is concerned. Under what circumstances should that likely effectiveness affect the just claims to that treatment for a person with some specific disability? Imagine an individual with a cardiac condition and a three-year life expectancy. They have a leukemic cancer that would require CAR T-cell treatment. However, the CAR T-cell therapy is very unlikely to result in a gain of one year. If we had agreed to a societal rule requiring one-year survival for CAR T-cell therapy, then would there be anything discriminatory and unjust in denying this individual with the cardiac disability access to that therapy? More problematic is the use of quality-of-life judgments in allocating health care resources, as many critics of QALYs have noted (Pettitt et al., 2016; Harris, 1987). However, even there, distinctions in making allocation decisions might be just and justified. For example, should an individual in advanced stages of dementia with a metastatic cancer have as strong a just claim to a

---

[3] The number of these ultra-expensive multi-year, multi-decade therapies is steadily increasing and challenging our sense of justice.

$150,000 checkpoint inhibitor as a quadriplegic with an open-ended life expectancy?

(11) *The personal responsibility challenge*: Luck egalitarians defend a version of responsibility-sensitive justice. In brief, one of their central claims would be that individuals whose costly health problems are the result of choices they have made should have to pay all or most of the costs associated with that health condition by themselves. Consequently, should individuals with metastatic lung cancer be denied access to targeted therapies at social expense, at least as a matter of justice (as opposed to some degree of social compassion)?

Before assessing various conceptions of health care justice in relation to the challenges posed by precision medicine, let me make one very large point: *No conception of health care justice can yield anything remotely acceptable as even "rough justice" within the context of the US health care system as it is now, and this will be even more true with regard to the challenges posed by precision medicine.* The primary reason for this judgment pertains to the fragmentation associated with health care financing in the United States: thousands of private health plans, 50 Medicaid programs, Medicare fragmented by Medicare Advantage plans. In addition, individuals have been denied insurance coverage for "preexisting conditions." Typically, these are individuals who are at greatly elevated risk for various cancers or heart disease or other life-threatening disorders, often for genetic reasons outside the control of that individual. We have to accept as a fact of nature our vulnerability to various life-threatening diseases, but lack of secure access to needed and effective therapies for those disorders is not a fact of nature. That is a fact of social choice and/or indifference.

In Chapter 3 we introduced the notion of "wicked problems." The complexity and heterogeneity of health care needs, along with the complexity, uncertainty, heterogeneity, and cost of therapeutic interventions for those needs, along with the complexity and heterogeneity of policy and administrative options for financing access to meeting and managing those needs, along with competing understandings of health care justice, compassion, and responsibility for meeting those needs, result in the creation of fertile ground for multiple wicked problems. As noted already, the defining feature of wicked problems is that they are not solvable. In the right circumstances such social problems may be manageable and ameliorable. However, this is precisely what is impossible in the present US health care system. We need a health care system that is universal with a fair system for health care financing. A universal health care system (e.g., those of Canada, the United Kingdom, and Germany) will not necessarily be "ideal." However, all of them are more just than the US health care system.[4] They too will have to struggle with the wicked health care justice problems identified in Chapter 3, though with a better chance of realizing "rough justice" in managing these problems.

None of the prevailing conceptions of health care justice can adequately address the ethical challenges described above in connection with metastatic cancer and precision medicine. In part, this has to do with the heterogeneity of medical needs; the complexity of therapeutic options for meeting those needs; the uncertainty of the health outcomes associated with those therapies, both globally and at the level of the individual patient; the socially unsustainable costs of these therapies, especially when the therapeutic benefits are marginal and uncertain; and the conflicting social values necessary to inform any policy options. These are the circumstances that generate what Rawls (1996) has dubbed the "burdens of judgment." No hard numbers or elegant economic equations or insightful and astute ethical analyses will yield what all rational minds would agree are the best policy options for addressing the challenges posed by advancing precision medicine. This is the realm of reasonable disagreement (McMahon, 2009; Gutmann and Thompson, 1996). This is the realm where multiple policy options in a specific context might be "reasonable enough" and "just enough" and "affordable enough." Still, in the real world of public policy one option will have to be chosen and implemented. This, I argue, should be through a fair, inclusive process of rational democratic deliberation. Recall that the core of the problem of health care justice in this context is setting limits, making rationing decisions, identifying just trade-offs. Such choices should come about through the exercise of social autonomy, which is what the deliberative democratic process offers. Such choices then are collectively self-imposed upon all along with a rationale that fair-minded individuals could not reasonably reject. If the deliberative process is fair, then no social group will be able to justifiably claim

[4] Ezekiel Emanuel reaches this same conclusion in his book *Which Country Has the World's Best Health Care?* (2020). He provides a very detailed picture of 10 health care systems (Canada, United Kingdom, Germany, the Netherlands, Norway, Switzerland, France, Australia, Taiwan, China). No one will be surprised to learn that no system is best in all respects; all make trade-offs regarding cost, access, quality, and financing. Still, the United States would be among the least just of these health care systems.

that they were exploited by the process. The healthy, wealthy, and politically powerful will not be able to impose their will on the sick, the poor, and the politically and socially vulnerable.

4.3. The Insufficiency of a Sufficientarian Conception of Health Care Justice

Harry Frankfurt (1987) was an early proponent of the sufficientarian conception of justice. He wrote: "What is important from the point of view of morality is not that everyone should have the *same* but that each should have *enough*. If everyone had enough, then it would be of no moral consequence whether some had more than others" (at 21). Frankfurt is not writing specifically about health care. If we were to use Rawlsian language, we would say that he had *primary goods* in mind, that is, adequate food, shelter, clothing, and money to have a decent life. Social welfare policies in Europe and the United States represent a reasonable practical interpretation of what "enough" is. The poor receive a *fixed amount* of Food Stamps to purchase food for the month. The assumption is that every family will have roughly the same nutritional needs. This assumption is irrelevant with regard to health care.

Health care needs vary from one person to another, from one point in time to another, and are extremely heterogeneous. Likewise, health care interventions for more complex health needs often have high degrees of uncertainty with regard to therapeutic efficacy for individuals who technically have the "same" health problem. That might be related to the unique physiology of each individual, their unique genetic endowment, consequences of past health care interventions, or challenges associated with intolerable side effects of particular interventions, not to mention a host of social determinants of health. Further, the vulnerability of individuals to accident and disease will vary enormously from one person to another across the life span, including the complexity of the bodily assaults effected by disease or accident (or violence and war). Finally, the costs associated with being responsive to these complex health needs will vary from modest to exorbitantly expensive. Unlike the need for food, the costs and complexity and uncertainty associated with health care and health care needs make identifying a standard of "enoughness" for health care a practically impossible task. Still, the sufficientarian must address this task in order to claim to have a useful theory of health care justice.

Virtually everyone will agree that a just and caring society should fix broken bones as part of basic health care. That will remain true even if an individual suffers broken bones 50 times over the course of a decade.[5] The same will hold true for repeated bouts of pneumonia or urinary tract infections or childbirth or lacerations or precancerous mole removal or chronic pain or rashes or high blood pressure, and so on. We can move up a step to somewhat more complex health problems, still part of basic health care, that would include managing heart disease at various stages; treating early cancers; managing diabetes; treating various sorts of lung, liver, kidney, and gut disorders that tend to be responsive to well-established medical interventions; and so on. We can add some of the more common and effective surgical interventions, as well as a long list of common, relatively inexpensive, effective drugs and related diagnostic procedures. My guess is that some fairly complex, somewhat expensive surgeries would also be included in this basic benefit package, though some sufficientarians might balk at 85-year-old patients with early dementia.

Two claims seem to be at the core of the sufficientarian view: (1) Everyone should have the opportunity to lead a decent life, in our case, a healthy enough life. If someone has a health deficiency that leaves them below some threshold of a "healthy enough" life, then they have a just claim to be brought above that threshold if that is medically possible (or at least as close as possible to that threshold). (2) There are no issues of health care justice above that threshold (assuming the threshold is set sufficiently high). Both these claims are intuitively plausible. With respect to (1), a just and caring society ought not allow individuals to suffer the consequences of disease or accident when we can remedy those problems. However, with respect to (2), no one has a just claim against society for unlimited resources to achieve superior states of health. For example, if some future medical anti-aging technology offered individuals the opportunity to live 20 extra years beyond a normal life expectancy in excellent health, no one would have a just claim to have access to that technology at social expense because that would be "more than enough." In a liberal society, individuals would be free to use their own resources to purchase those gains in life expectancy. Their use of personal resources to achieve this goal does not threaten the just claims of less fortunate others to social health care resources.

---

[5] Some readers will recall Evel Knievel, the daredevil motorcyclist, who earned his living jumping over a progressively longer string of cars. He would likely be a real-world example of someone who had broken bones 50 times in a decade.

However, this enhancement scenario poses a puzzle. If this enhanced individual (who has paid for this with their own funds) is 90 years old and develops a treatable cancer, would that individual have a just claim to the social resources needed to treat that cancer? Imagine this is a curable cancer costing $40,000. On the one hand, it would seem to be indecent and unkind to simply allow this individual to die "prematurely" from a treatable cancer (assuming 10 life-years at risk). On the other hand, this individual has no *just claim* to the social resources they need (given that they are well above the assumed sufficiency threshold). Perhaps obligations of social beneficence are relevant (to be discussed in Chapter 7).

Consider, however, our imagining this alternate scenario in which this 90-year-old individual has an advanced version of CLL, not curable but potentially treatable with ibrutinib at a cost of $156,000 per year. Given that this individual has this medically engineered enhanced life expectancy, ibrutinib could yield eight extra years of life for them at a social cost of more than $1.2 million. In addition, assuming ibrutinib failed at some point, the CAR T-cell option would be available. This individual could not be cured, but the potential for a substantial number of extra years of life (congruent with their enhanced status) would be there. Why would this not require another act of social beneficence (albeit a more expensive act) if that first act of social beneficence was seen as being obligatory? Or has this individual already had "more than enough" as a result of their purchase of this anti-aging therapy?

Here is yet another challenge to the sufficientarian perspective. Imagine another 90-year-old in very good health who achieved that status as a result of healthy choices, good luck, and an excellent genetic endowment. That individual could either have the $40,000 curable cancer or CLL with the potential for many extra years of life if they have access to ibrutinib at social expense. If they were refused the necessary social resources in either or both cases, the justification for that denial could not be that they had purchased privately this anti-aging therapy. Instead, the argument would have to be that they already had had "more than enough" good-quality life. This does not appear to be a judgment that most non-sufficientarians would accept as just or reasonable.

If a hard age limit cannot establish a sufficiency threshold, what other criteria might be invoked? Perhaps individuals are entitled to a "reasonable quality of life" so far as health status is concerned or, as one author put it, basic functional human capabilities (Ram-Tiktin, 2017). If individuals are functionally impaired as a result of disease or accident and if some thera-peutic intervention can repair that deficiency, then individuals would have a just claim to that intervention. That avoids the health enhancement issue. Still, that implies that our 90-year-old (excellent genetic endowment) with the $40,000 treatable cancer would have a just claim to have that treatment at social expense. Perhaps that is the ethically correct conclusion.

This brings us back to metastatic cancer, precision medicine, and our targeted therapies or immunotherapies. As noted, cancer is largely a disease of older individuals. It can easily be viewed as a natural part of aging, just like sarcopenia. But some younger individuals will be afflicted with a potentially fatal cancer. In both cases (young and old) treatment of an advanced cancer will be extraordinarily expensive. In some cases (childhood leukemias) the therapeutic benefits will be substantial. These children will be able to achieve a normal life expectancy. In older patients with chronic myelogenous leu-kemia (CML) the benefits of the drug imatinib will also be substantial (years of a reasonable quality of life gained). But the large majority of targeted ther-apies for metastatic cancer will yield only costly marginal gains in life expec-tancy (Prasad, 2020). How should a sufficientarian respond to the just claims of these patients?

More problematic for the sufficientarian is the future scenario I sketched above where a number of targeted therapies or immunotherapies are used in combination with five-year survival rates for a majority of those patients at a cost of more than $500,000 per patient. Some will be in their 40s or 50s, others in their 70s or 80s. Projected benefits would be roughly the same for all. Again, invoking some sort of age limit would be ethically awkward, even for the sufficientarian. One of the hallmarks of the sufficientarian position is some commitment to a prioritarian view. That is, they see those who are worst off health-wise, far from the threshold of sufficiency, as having the strongest just claims to social resources to meet their needs so long as the therapies available are effective enough. However, those patients cannot make unlim-ited claims on social resources for very marginal benefits. Recall our some-what futuristic scenario where sequential use of multiple targeted therapies yielded five or more extra years of life at substantial social cost. That would seem to represent a just claim on social resources for our sufficientarian be-cause this represented a very effective therapy (recall our HIV patients re-ceiving quadruple combination therapies). That seems to be part of the logic of their position, though integral to the sufficiency view is the notion of "limits."

How should the "threshold problem" be addressed? If the threshold is set too low (society is very stingy), the consequences for patients will be ethically unacceptable (i.e., letting patients die prematurely or suffer unnecessarily even though we have a costly but effective technology for preventing that because they are just above that threshold). On the other hand, if the threshold is set too high (society is imprudently generous), then too much health care will be purchased at too high a price for too little benefit. Anywhere we try to set a threshold will be arbitrary (Axelsen and Nielsen, 2017; Casal, 2007). This is a matter of great moral consequence that should not be haphazardly set if negative allocation decisions are going to be fairly justified to individuals adversely affected by those threshold decisions.

Fourie (2017) imagines some number of individuals (we will say 20,000) who are in severe pain, very far from wherever the sufficiency threshold is set, and a much larger number of individuals (we will say 500,000) who are just a bit below the sufficiency threshold. I will concretize her abstract example. The 20,000 individuals have sickle cell disease; their suffering is intense. Two new drugs, crizanlizumab-tmca (Adakveo®) and voxelotor (Oxbryta®), were approved in late 2019 by the US Food and Drug Administration (FDA) to treat the severe quality of life–diminishing symptoms of sickle cell disease, the pain and anemia (Kolata, 2019; Vichinsky et al., 2019). They are believed to be about 70% effective, thereby lifting these individuals much closer to the sufficiency threshold. However, these drugs cost on average $100,000 per patient per year for the rest of their lives. The 500,000 patients are patients with treatable cancers at an average cost of $40,000 per patient treated and cured (i.e., brought up to the sufficiency level). From a justice-based sufficiency perspective, is it more important to maximize the number of individuals who can be brought to the sufficiency level at a lower cost per person or to dedicate more resources to caring for those far below the sufficiency threshold at very substantial cost who will never achieve the sufficiency threshold but whose quality of life would be substantially improved, as in our example? If our two drugs improved the quality of life of these patients by 10% or even 20%, an answer would be easy. However, the improvement in quality of life is very significant for the sickle cell patients, though for the 500,000 individuals the cancer therapy is life-saving. Which of these allocations should have higher priority from the perspective of a sufficientarian conception of health care justice?

The correct answer to this last question is not obvious because the various proposed thresholds for sufficiency are either arbitrary or ambiguous or both. In brief, the sufficientarian perspective fails to address most of the wicked problems described in Chapter 3.

4.4. Luck Egalitarianism and Health Care Justice: Should Responsibility Count?

We turn next to the luck egalitarian or responsibility-sensitive conception of health care justice.[6] The defining feature of luck egalitarianism is that everyone deserves equal concern for their health care needs, unless their health care needs are a product of bad health choices. This applies to everyone, which is why it is egalitarian. Health needs related to option luck (bad personal choices) cannot make a just claim on social resources for resolving those needs. Individuals are free to use their own resources. However, if they are lacking sufficient personal resources to obtain some very expensive intervention, they cannot claim they have been treated unjustly so far as the luck egalitarian is concerned, even if the result is a very premature death. This is what generates both the abandonment and the harshness criticisms of this view.

A provocative illustration of the sort of behavior that luck egalitarians find most objectionable would be that of drug addicts who use "dirty needles" that will repeatedly result in infected heart valves, thereby creating a life-threatening problem for themselves. Many surgeons object to doing more than one valvuloplasty on these individuals. This is unjustly harsh. It is cruel to allow these patients to die when an intervention is readily available that would save their life, even if those individuals seem indifferent to whether they lived or died. To my mind, this is a decisive criticism. However, Segall (2010) offers a complex, pluralistic version of luck egalitarianism that deserves more careful assessment.[7]

Segall contends that his version of luck egalitarianism can bypass the harshness and abandonment objections. His basic contention is that "individuals should be compensated for losses for which they are not responsible" (2010, at 63). He further explains that individuals are not "responsible" for

---

[6] An excellent overview of luck egalitarianism as a responsibility-sensitive conception of justice would be Arneson's (2011) essay in *Responsibility and Distributive Justice* (Knight and Stemplowska, 2011).

[7] I will focus on Segall's version of luck egalitarianism because of its sophistication and complexity and because Segall does explicitly address health care issues.

bad health outcomes when it would be *unreasonable to expect individuals to avoid* the behavior that resulted in those bad health outcomes. A coal miner in West Virginia must risk a life-threatening lung disease to feed his family. The same reasoning would hold for police, firefighters, soldiers, and construction workers. Still, Segall realizes many imprudent individuals will do things that result in serious health needs. Consequently, Segall endorses the claim that we (a just and caring society) are ethically obligated to meet the health care needs of these individuals at social expense. His version of luck egalitarianism is *pluralistic* because multiple ethical values may justifiably override the otherwise strict requirements of a luck egalitarian conception of health care justice. Thus, when it comes to "basic health care needs," a society (with sufficient resources) is ethically obligated *as a matter of compassion* to meet the basic health needs of both the prudent and the imprudent. The imprudent do not have a *just claim* to have those needs met with social resources. Nevertheless, society is ethically obligated for reasons of compassion to meet those needs according to Segall.

Segall is an egalitarian who contends that the basic health needs of *everyone* ought to be met, for reasons of either justice or compassion. However, Segall's egalitarian commitments are limited above that sufficiency threshold because it will be fair (not unjust) to treat differently the health care needs of the prudent and the imprudent. He writes, "Luck egalitarianism is compatible with the view that equality (or egalitarian distributive justice) does not trump all other considerations of justice, let alone all moral considerations" (2010, at 66).[8] Still, Segall would not endorse providing unlimited access to needed health care for the prudent above that sufficiency threshold, especially for high-cost, marginally beneficial interventions. What then are the non-arbitrary, justice-relevant considerations that would determine for the luck egalitarian above the sufficiency level the just distribution of limited health care resources?

Recall all the targeted cancer therapies and immunotherapies reviewed above. What Segall does say is that considerations of utility or self-respect or publicity or autonomy or compassion or cultural diversity might all trump or constrain commitments to egalitarian health care justice in various circumstances.[9] Also, prioritarian or libertarian considerations of justice

---

[8] Segall (2010) writes elsewhere, "Egalitarian distributive justice is but a narrow slice of morality and thus allows for a plurality of other moral considerations to be coupled and traded off with it" (at 74).
   [9] Segall cites other philosophers who would endorse an egalitarian perspective that is constrained by other justice-relevant or morally relevant considerations, including Temkin (1993, 2003),

might constrain or override a strong egalitarian commitment when consid-erations of fairness are indeterminate. However, when we reflect on all our wickedness problems, they are all indeterminately fair. What then? How do we know, when we invoke these other considerations, we will get a result that is "just enough" from an egalitarian perspective?

Segall is most concerned to refute the abandonment objection. Segall opposes dumping seriously ill imprudent patients into the hospital parking lot to die. Those patients have serious health care needs to which compas-sionate egalitarians must be responsive. Still, Segall also believes it would be unfair for the prudent members of society to be required to bear the health costs of the imprudent. The imprudent must bear those costs, though this is a practical impossibility in a health crisis, such as needing a targeted therapy for metastatic cancer. Consequently, he would mandate the purchase of health insurance by everyone, and he would heavily tax products that would increase substantially the health risks of those who used those products, such as cigarettes or alcohol or high-calorie, sugar-laden foods. This would seem to protect sufficiently Segall's *egalitarian* health care commitments since the health needs of the prudent and imprudent would be paid for and somewhat in proportion to individual degrees of imprudence. However, some critical comments are in order.

Though libertarians will object to the mandated purchase of health in-surance, Segall effectively addresses their objections. The more challenging question (as a matter of justice) would be how premiums would be adjusted for that mandated insurance. Determining a fair premium for various kinds and degrees of imprudence (which would have to be self-confessed, maybe easy enough for Roman Catholics) would be a very fuzzy affair, in effect, being penalized for what *might be* a very costly bad health outcome that can be properly attributed to consistently bad health choices. If we consider the Affordable Care Act and uninsured individuals who must purchase in-surance through the exchanges, then those individuals within 400% of the poverty level would have their actual purchase costs reduced by the federal subsidies. Consequently, they would pay only a small portion of the "impru-dence premium" for which they were responsible. Prudent taxpayers would

McKerlie (1996), and Scanlon (1976). Scanlon (1976) is quoted by Segall as saying, "we temper the demands of equality with other considerations. Equality is not our only concern" (at 10). Again, what is the scope of egalitarian health care justice in the context of marginally beneficial, extraordinarily expensive targeted cancer therapies and immunotherapies?

have to bear those costs instead. This is not the result Segall intended to achieve.

Another Segall proposal would be to tax heavily products associated with costly health consequences. This idea will work well for smokers and lung diseases. However, what would be taxed in the case of melanoma? What would a sunshine tax look like? Segall's egalitarianism would seem to require that the metastatic melanoma of these patients would still be treated, presumably with very expensive targeted cancer therapies. The same problem occurs with regard to substance abuse with illegal drugs or casual sexual encounters or high-performance competitive sports, and so on. Again, the prudent would pay the health care costs of the imprudent, contrary to Segall's intent.

Sorting out the complex factors that might be used to distinguish responsible from irresponsible health outcomes will be more difficult than Segall imagines. Consider someone with a moderate smoking habit, maybe 10 cigarettes per day. This person does have a risk for lung cancer, though less than that of a 40 cigarettes per day smoker. Unbeknown to them, they are genetically susceptible to lung cancer. This is brute luck. They are mindful of their lung cancer risk and have tried quitting on several occasions. They have deliberately (responsibly?) restricted their smoking to 10 cigarettes per day. Nevertheless, they have lung cancer at age 60. From the perspective of Segall's luck egalitarianism, how should we judge whether this individual is responsible for their lung cancer? Alternatively, if this individual had whole genome sequencing performed and knew about genetic vulnerability to lung cancer but continued their moderate smoking habit, occasionally trying to quit, should we make a different judgment regarding their responsibility for their lung cancer? Translating these expectations for responsible behavior into social practice would require enormous violations of privacy (Arneson, 2000),[10] not to mention the professional integrity of physicians who would have knowledge of these behavioral transgressions (Fleck, 2012).

Segall asks what it is "reasonable to expect" of individuals regarding behavior that can result in bad health outcomes. Many will say that the person "chose" to smoke, likely at age 13 at the behest of smoking friends. This hardly represents a *deliberate* mature choice, but neither is it correctly described as

---

[10] Arneson (2000) writes: "In a luck egalitarian society all members will find their privacy violated by intrusive and offensive investigative procedures that aim to classify them according to the level of badness of their lives and the degree of responsibility of their life choices" (at 342).

brute luck. Moreover, smoking is addictive. We might imagine that these fine-grained judgments would be irrelevant if we simply tax cigarettes. But these taxes vary from state to state, depending upon lobbyists. In the states where the lobbying is successful, prudent non-smokers will pay a large portion of the health costs incurred by the imprudent smokers, contrary to what Segall would intend.

To reiterate, Segall would not endorse denying expensive, life-prolonging care to smokers for their lung disease. That would be abandonment and contrary to his egalitarian commitments. However, this egalitarian commitment must address at least two other ethical challenges: the "same disease" challenge and the "cost control" challenge.

What precisely counts as the "same disease" in the era of precision medicine? In ordinary conversation, we simply talk about cancer. In the era of precision medicine, a cancer will be identified by the genetic mutation that drives that cancer. A particular cancer might be driven by a mutation in VEGF or KRAS or NRAS or ALK or HER2, and so on. Different targeted therapies will be used to attack each of these cancers. Given this way of categorizing cancers, more than 200 cancers could be listed. Further, cancers are typically staged from I to IV, which determines how aggressively the cancer will be treated and whether a cure is possible. How is this related to Segall's egalitarianism? If a woman is diagnosed with a Stage IV, HER2$^+$ breast cancer to be treated with trastuzumab, then for Segall's egalitarian, every woman with that same breast cancer would have an equal just claim to that same treatment.

That brings us to the "cost control" challenge. How is health care cost control to be accomplished fairly? The generic luck egalitarian has an easy answer. It is unfair that individuals who have costly health problems that are a product of brute luck should have to assist through taxes or insurance premiums in paying the costs of health care for the imprudent and irresponsible. Those are "excess costs," due to irresponsible choices. This is where cost control can be justly imposed. If these imprudent individuals cannot bear those costs, then it is not unjust to deny them needed but undeserved care. If this results in unnecessary suffering or debility or premature death, this is unfortunate but not unjust. However, this is precisely the abandonment outcome Segall rejects. Segall still needs to tell us what he would accept as being a "just enough" approach to controlling health costs that would be consistent with his egalitarian commitments, most especially with regard to metastatic cancer patients and these targeted cancer therapies.

Recall our earlier discussion of imatinib and CML. Roughly, 70% of patients with CML taking imatinib will survive 10 years. The cost of this drug peaked at $146,000 per year. It is hard to imagine Segall not endorsing funding this drug for patients with CML, given its effectiveness and given that CML appears to be the product of brute bad luck.

We turn next to metastatic non-small cell lung cancer. If your cancer is ALK$^+$ (primary driver of the cancer), you might get the drug crizotinib. If your cancer is driven by an EGFR mutation, you might receive erlotinib or gefitinib. If no such genetic driver can be identified but you have high PD-L1 expression, you would be started on a checkpoint inhibitor, such as pembrolizumab. All of these interventions would have costs of about $150,000 per year. More recently (Hellmann et al., 2018), non-small lung cancer with high tumor mutational burden has been treated with nivolumab and ipilimumab. This combination would have costs of $250,000 with a one-year progression-free survival rate of 42% compared to 13% for chemotherapy. Median progression-free survival for the combination was 7.2 months (range 5.5–13.2) compared to chemotherapy with median progression-free survival of 5.5 months (range 4.5–5.8). These are smokers treated at social expense. This preserves both elements of Segall's luck egalitarianism, though obviously these drugs are nowhere near as effective as imatinib for CML.

Consider again our metastatic melanoma situation. Some melanoma patients will be undocumented immigrants harvesting fruits and vegetables; others will be just plain sun-worshippers (seeking greater social acceptance with the perfect tan).[11] Traditional chemotherapy has provided only marginal gains in life expectancy for these individuals: median survival of 6–9 months, less than 10% surviving five years. Precision medicine has promised significantly more for patients with certain genetic markers. Almost 60% of the patients with metastatic melanoma will have a BRAF-mutated version. The best treatment option for them will be a combination first-line anti-PD-1 plus an anti-CTLA-4 (nivolumab + ipilimumab), which might be effective for six years or longer. A second-line treatment would be a combination of a BRAF inhibitor with a MEK inhibitor (dabrafenib + trametinib). For patients for whom this treatment regimen works very well (30%–40% of these patients), the gain in life expectancy would be 8.4 years at a lifetime cost

[11] Roughly 1.2 million Americans are living with melanoma; about 92,000 new cases were diagnosed in 2019; 9,320 individuals died of melanoma in 2018, approximately 2.4% of all cancer deaths.

of $656,692 (Tarhini et al., 2019). A less expensive lifetime regimen would start with a combination of a BRAF inhibitor and a MEK inhibitor, which would yield a gain of 3.2 life-years at a cost of $345,693.

Would Segall endorse the following proposal: Melanoma patients would need to accept the less expensive treatment for metastatic melanoma (i.e., the treatment that yielded a gain of 3.2 life-years for a cost of $345,000), as opposed to the regimen that would yield more than eight extra life-years for a substantial portion of patients at roughly twice the lifetime cost? This might seem harsh since it would feel like punishment, which Segall would not endorse. Also, it would not be congruent with his egalitarianism. Further, if this were an ethically acceptable way of controlling health care costs, generalizing this rule would mean that costs would be controlled by providing less effective and less costly treatment for patients whose expensive health needs were judged to be a product of their imprudent behavior. Such patients would not have been "abandoned," completely denied needed and effective health care. Still, receiving second-rate care would mean being treated like a health sinner, while health saints received top-tier care. That would not be congruent with the version of egalitarianism Segall endorses.

Segall is a welfare egalitarian, not a resource egalitarian. If it is medically possible for individuals to achieve an average or normal level of health, including a normal life expectancy, then this is what a just and compassionate society must provide. In the case of metastatic melanoma for patients below age 70 (at least), this would imply that all these patients should be provided with access to the more expensive life-prolonging combination cancer therapies. However, this generates other justice-relevant problems. Would this imply, for example, that all metastatic cancer patients ought to be provided with the most effective cancer therapy available for their cancer, no matter what the cost might be? If so, the Segall egalitarian could hardly say that this commitment was for cancer patients only. This would suggest that cancer was somehow ethically special. Segall would have to be committed to providing the best care available for somewhat younger end-stage heart patients, lung patients, liver patients, and so on. Implicitly, this would represent an affirmation of the belief that human life is priceless. This would be congruent with a very strict understanding of egalitarianism (Harris, 1985), but it would not be congruent with the "luck" aspect of his egalitarianism. More importantly, such a view would represent a rejection of the need for health care cost control. That conclusion would be neither reasonable nor just. That conclusion would bypass our wickedness issues. However, that would require taking social resources from many other areas of social need requiring social expenditures, which means our wicked problems would be transferred or displaced rather than resolved.

I assume that Segall does accept limits on health care spending because he is committed to some version of sufficientarianism. In other words, he is clearly committed to the idea that a just and compassionate society will meet the *basic health care needs of all.* However, non-basic health needs, health needs above some justice-relevant threshold, will be viewed by most sufficientarians as being "beyond justice." That does not seem to be Segall's view. For Segall, *some* justice-relevant considerations will determine access to needed health care above that threshold. This is where Segall would suggest that a commitment to fairness may be indeterminate, which is to say that non–luck egalitarian considerations of justice will determine an acceptable distribution of health care resources. However, which values are supposed to determine that?

Segall does not recognize any hierarchy among many possible values; he is a pluralist. How then are we supposed to avoid an entirely arbitrary outcome? How can we be ethically confident that any specific allocation outcome is either "fair enough" or "just enough" or "compassionate enough"? Is his egalitarianism limited to distributional health care needs and concerns below that sufficiency threshold level? Or are there some egalitarian considerations that would apply above the threshold as well? How should we imagine Segall would address all the wickedness issues we raised earlier?

Consider the following questions. If we are going to use CAR T-cell therapy to treat some form of leukemia at a cost of $475,000 at the front end and if we are able to identify biomarkers that tell us with 90% confidence that patient will be among the 30% who will not gain more than an extra year of life expectancy with that therapy, would it be ethically acceptable to deny access to that therapy at social expense for patients like that? It would be easy to see that a utilitarian would give an affirmative answer to this question. It is not at all obvious that either a prioritarian or an egalitarian would also endorse that answer.

An egalitarian could endorse the view that either every leukemia patient has access at social expense to CAR T-cell therapy or none do. This seems intuitively fair. On further thought, however, consider all the possible life-years that would be lost, especially for individuals who might have gained five or seven extra years of life. These would be life-years of reasonable quality, certainly better than the life-years we currently save for ESRD patients on dialysis.

Consider the age distribution of this hypothetical cluster of leukemia patients. Some patients might be in their 30s or 60s or early 80s. Assume that all these patients are reasonably likely to gain five to seven extra life years with access to this CAR T-cell therapy. Do they all have an equal just claim to this resource at social expense? Segall, the egalitarian, might have to give an affirmative answer. However, we must control health care costs. Numerous unmet serious health needs exist among the non-elderly. As a welfare egalitarian, Segall ought to be committed to doing everything medically possible to maximize the likelihood of achieving a normal life expectancy. That perspective would suggest that our leukemia patients in their 30s and 60s ought to have assured access to CAR T-cell therapy but not our patients in their 80s, which looks like ageism.

Would a cost-effectiveness perspective clarify matters? However, by hypothesis, all these patients will gain five to seven extra years of life, which is to say the cost per life-year saved would be the same for all of them, roughly $90,000 or less, which is what we currently pay to sustain the lives of patients on renal dialysis at social expense.

Here is another wrinkle. Suppose those in their 80s were in the early stages of some form of dementia, still pretty much capable of managing their own lives with some minimal social assistance. If they live those extra years, they will end up with the very advanced stages of their dementia (and some substantial additional social expenses for long-term care). Would that represent a sufficient, ethically relevant consideration that would justify denying access to CAR T-cell therapy for those individuals with early-stage dementia? Or is this a choice that must be offered to these individuals as a matter of respect for patient autonomy, as opposed to regarding it as a matter requiring the wise use of social resources? How should a luck egalitarian, such as Segall, respond to this last question?

Recall that luck egalitarians are concerned with individuals who make poor health choices and impose unjust health costs upon the rest of society. Our leukemia patients in their 80s have gotten there (in all likelihood) as a result of both brute luck and good health choices. It would clearly be wrong to prevent these individuals from living longer. However, would it be equally wrong to fail to provide them with the substantial costly social resources they would need to gain seven extra years of life with CAR T-cell therapy? Those patients in their 80s have clearly benefited from brute good luck. Should that be ethically relevant in determining whether those patients had a just claim to health care social resources to further extend that brute good luck? I am certain Segall would argue (and I would argue) that these individuals would have strong just claims to basic health care. But CAR T-cell therapy must be outside anything reasonably described as basic health care.

Recall our ibrutinib discussion in Chapter 3. Ibrutinib is used to treat CLL. This was one of our wicked problems. The median age of patients at diagnosis is 71. Ibrutinib costs $156,000 per year. Treatment-naïve patients have a five-year progression-free survival probability of 92%. If the entire cost were socialized, the annual social cost would be $21 billion. Virtually all patients will develop resistance to the drug at some point, maybe after a year or two, maybe 10 years out. Median survival with CLL after ibrutinib failure will be only three months. However, CAR T-cell therapy is a follow-up option. Again, half these patients will be more than 70 years old.

Consider patients who fail ibrutinib after one or two years. CAR T-cell therapy offers the promise of several extra years of life (at least for the 70% who get beyond the first year). Do these patients have a strong just claim to be provided CAR T-cell therapy? How should a Segall-like egalitarian respond? Though half the patients will be over 70, the other half will be below 70. Should that difference be ignored?

A 10-year survivor with ibrutinib would have accumulated health care expenses for society of $1.56 million and is now requesting $475,000 more for CAR T-cell therapy, or a total CLL expenditure of $2 million. Some of those individuals might be beyond age 80. For one version of an egalitarian perspective, all of these patients have an equal just claim to CAR T-cell therapy, though the social costs would be many additional billions of dollars more per year. More ethically interesting would be ibrutinib patients who only gained two years on the drug. They could make the claim that they nevertheless ought to get CAR T-cell therapy because society was willing to spend $2 million for individuals who had already gained 10 extra years of life. Segall does not seem to have an ethically persuasive response to any of these questions.

Segall would see this as an "indeterminate justice" situation. Does this mean that all those choices would be ethically acceptable? That is, none of these CLL patients would be treated unjustly. All would get what they wanted or needed. If these CLL patients get everything they want or need in the way of social resources, then someone else somewhere else in the health care system will not have available the social resources they need.[12] Segall's ethical pluralism above the sufficiency threshold is not unreasonable in itself, though this way of addressing the indeterminacy of justice above sufficiency would likely have determinately unjust consequences elsewhere in the health care system. The alternative is to make rationing decisions among these CLL patients (or some other cluster of metastatic cancer patients) in accord with some of these other relevant ethical values. However, how are these alternate, competing values to be non-arbitrarily weighed and assessed so that the result can be recognized by all as "just enough"? Consider again all of our wicked scenarios. Luck egalitarianism does not provide the resources needed to answer all those questions.

4.5. Prioritarianism and Health Care Justice: Are Precise Priorities Possible?

We next consider prioritarian conceptions of health care justice in relation to our wicked scenario challenges. Derek Parfit (1991) is regarded as the godfather of prioritarianism.[13] Parfit defines his priority view as follows: "Benefiting people more matters more the worse off these people are" (at 19). His view is not that of egalitarians. Consequently, he says that it is neither bad nor unjust that some people are worse off than others. He then clarifies by saying that "what is bad is not that these people are worse off than *others*. It is rather that they are worse off than *they* might have been" (at 22, his italics). In other words, they are at a lower *absolute* level. That is what matters, not their welfare or health status relative to anyone else. The other key claim in Parfit's view is that benefits to the worse off have greater weight than those same benefits for those who are much better off. This would be one justification for some degree of redistribution from the better off to the worse off. Such a redistribution, from a prioritarian perspective, represents a net gain in social benefit. What does it mean for Parfit to be "worse off"? People can be worse off because "they may be poorer, or less happy, or have fewer opportunities, or worse health, or shorter lives" (at 2). Parfit concludes that distribution according to need is essentially a reflection of a commitment

[12] This would certainly be true in the United Kingdom, where the National Health Service must remain within a fixed budget every year.
[13] As always, variations of prioritarianism have emerged over the intervening decades. I will call attention to some that are distinctive if useful in our discussion of precision medicine.

to prioritarianism. One final point: For the prioritarian, nothing will justify making the well off even better off if it causes the worse off to become even more worse off.

Next: How should prioritarians address problems of health care justice that arise in connection with precision medicine and the needs of metastatic cancer patients for these ultra-expensive targeted cancer therapies and immunotherapies? Certainly, patients with metastatic cancer facing a terminal outcome are among the worse off. In general, prioritarians have said little about health needs. They mostly address garden variety needs: malnourishment, homelessness, poverty, unemployment. As Parfit would point out, these are all individuals whose lives are significantly deficient in *absolute* terms.

Now imagine individuals in the top 10% of the income spectrum who have very nice homes, enjoyable vacations, very satisfying culinary experiences, lots of respect, and cultural opportunities; but many of them are now faced with metastatic cancer. Would a prioritarian say that such individuals were among the worse off? We can imagine that these individuals had very good health insurance as well as access to very good cancer care. I have not seen a case such as this discussed by a prioritarian, though this is a real-world type of situation. It is puzzling. On the one hand, such individuals are getting very good care for their cancer. Relative to other individuals with metastatic cancer who are uninsured or underinsured, doomed to die prematurely, our financially well-off individuals with metastatic cancer do not belong among the worse off. On the other hand, relative to individuals in very good health with an indefinite life expectancy ahead of them, our financially well-off individuals would be in *absolute health terms* among the worse off. This is an unfortunate but not an unjust situation, unlike uninsured patients with metastatic cancer for whom more could be done if given the financial means. This is a matter of prioritarian justice. What would justify *not* regarding this as a matter of prioritarian justice?

Parfit would counsel against the comparative reference to the fully insured, financially well-off patient with metastatic cancer. That would be an egalitarian commitment. What matters for the prioritarian is the absolute diminished health status of our uninsured cancer patient. But then we need to notice something else. A health state can be diminished or greatly diminished only relative to some standard of good health or adequate health. That sounds like the sort of perspective that the sufficientarian would endorse (Benbaji, 2006). This is not intrinsically objectionable. However, that does mean the prioritarian must have some objective, rational basis for establishing the location of that health threshold. This is not something explicitly addressed by Parfit or most other prioritarians. Perhaps they think it is just obvious to everyone what that threshold is. Moreover, the prioritarian would agree with the sufficientarian that no one had a just claim to social resources that would be used for health enhancement, such as a future anti-aging technology. Let's just accept this as a reasonable enough threshold. What then?

The challenge I see at this point for prioritarians is the "Callahan problem." Callahan (1990) calls attention to how the domain of what we regard as health care needs is directly related to novel medical technologies and treatments. No one needed targeted cancer therapies before targeted cancer therapies were invented. No one needed etanercept (Enbrel®) for their rheumatoid arthritis until etanercept was invented. No one needed PCSK9s to lower their low-density lipoprotein (LDL) cholesterol until PCSK9s were invented. The result of all this technological creativity is a profusion of health care needs, very expensive health care needs. This is the primary reason why we have a health care cost containment crisis and our problems of health care justice. No society can afford to pay for every such medical intervention. Choices have to be made fairly. What does the prioritarian say to address that challenge?

The prioritarian might say that we need to give first priority to urgent and serious health care needs. This has an intuitive appeal. We think of the heart attack patient. We will save them, but they will have heart failure, though it would be better if we could prevent that heart attack in the first place. The drugs known as PCSK9s can help to accomplish that objective, though they are expensive in the aggregate. Do patients with significantly elevated LDL levels have a serious and urgent health care need? How would a prioritarian answer this question for determining the just allocation of health care resources? The annual cost of providing those PCSK9s could be about $133 billion. Would the prioritarian say that is something that a just and caring society ought to fund? Consider this hypothetical scenario: We spend $133 billion for these PCSK9s for the at-risk population, and we reduce annual heart attacks by 30% and related hospitalization and treatment costs by $40 billion. Is this a trade-off that a prioritarian ought to endorse as representing a more just allocation of health care resources?

This is the "prevention challenge." The worse off are identified by the prioritarian as the *absolute* distance of an individual's health status from a state of good health. However, the 19 million Americans with substantially elevated LDL at risk for either a heart attack or stroke actually feel quite well on any given day. In addition, over a 10-year period of time, the risk of a heart attack or stroke for these individuals would be less than 20%. Consequently, they do not have "urgent" health needs. Everyone agrees with the prioritarian intuition that we are obligated as a matter of justice to treat heart attacks, and they might endorse a vague intuition about prevention. However, virtually no one will endorse spending that $133 billion for the PCSK9s. Economists have pointed out that these drugs are simply not cost-effective, typically having cost-effectiveness numbers in the hundreds of thousands of dollars per QALY. Also, statins are available at greatly reduced cost (less than $200 per year), though they are not nearly as effective at reducing heart attacks and strokes as the PCSK9s. How should the prioritarian respond to this trade-off?

Prioritarians rarely talk about the cost-effectiveness of health care. This would make them sound too much like utilitarians. Prioritarians have in mind only garden variety health care needs that are relatively inexpensive, either at the individual patient level or at the aggregated social level. I imagine prioritarians would endorse this statement as a core element of their position: Whatever can be done medically to cure a disease state or repair damage to one's health (thereby restoring an individual to good health) and whatever can be done medically to manage a chronic condition (thereby keeping an individual as close as medically possible to a state of good health) ought to be done as a matter of justice. These patients with well-managed chronic illness could have been among the medically worse off, except they have now been restored to something close to good health, though they need costly ongoing medical support to remain there for years. That brings us to our metastatic cancer patients and our precision medicine challenges.

How do we imagine the prioritarian would respond to our ibrutinib scenario for CLL patients? Recall that these are mostly older patients, that ibrutinib costs $156,000 per year, that these patients might gain anywhere from 1 to 10 years from this drug. This part of the scenario looks indistinguishable from our ESRD, HIV, or totally implantable artificial heart (TIAH) scenarios. I conclude that a prioritarian would have to endorse funding this drug as a matter of justice. The harder part of the scenario is what the prioritarian would be required to endorse after a CLL patient fails ibrutinib. Would they then be logically obligated to endorse CAR T-cell therapy? This therapy might yield one to four extra years of life expectancy for these patients, very like our ESRD, HIV, and TIAH scenarios. However, 30% of these patients offered CAR T-cell therapy would not survive a year. Future research might discover biomarkers that would identify those patients with 90% confidence. Would the prioritarian then deny CAR T-cell therapy to those patients, given the very high front-end cost and limited benefit? These patients are certainly among the least well off, which would seem to require the prioritarian to ignore that limited life expectancy. These patients cannot be restored to good health, but they might be able to get a few extra months of acceptable health. Also, if the prioritarian balked at funding the CAR T-cell therapy, then it would appear that the prioritarian would be making a cost-effectiveness judgment, just like a utilitarian. What would be unclear would be the justice-relevant considerations that would justify such a limitation from within a prioritarian perspective.

Let us assume instead that the prioritarian would endorse funding CAR T-cell therapy for these CLL patients, whatever their future survival prospects. This creates a different sort of problem for the prioritarian, that is, limits on health care spending. Must all health care needs which represent a deficiency from good health be socially funded as a matter of justice from a prioritarian perspective? Consider again all the targeted therapies and immunotherapies that we have discussed. The prioritarian would have to endorse funding all of these interventions as a matter of justice, even though the benefits were marginal for *most* patients. Recall our strong responders. What is the appropriate justice-relevant response for the prioritarian? All of these patients are among the worse off. What criteria would the prioritarian endorse to control health care costs?

What about quality-of-life considerations for the prioritarian? Are there quality-of-life considerations that would justify limits on access to care? Are patients in a persistent vegetative state (PVS) among the medically least well off? With aggressive medical care such patients could be sustained in that state for many years. If such patients develop a life-threatening but treatable cardiac or cancer problem, would the prioritarian say we were ethically obligated to treat them? If so, that would only reinforce my main criticism of the prioritarian perspective, namely, that they fail to take seriously the need for health care limits.

Priorities have to be established among health care needs. However, prioritarians seem to resist making such comparative judgments. Parfit (2012) seems to reaffirm this last point. Parfit writes: "We have a stronger reason to give people benefits, or expectable benefits, the worse off these people are, or expectably are" (at 436). Holtug (2006) writes: "Prioritarianism is the view that, roughly, a benefit has greater moral value the worse the situation of the individual to whom it accrues" (at 125). Two points in these quoted passages speak to our PVS example. First, we cannot compare the needs of cardiac patients with the needs of cancer patients with the needs of renal patients. All that matters for a prioritarian conception of health care justice is how far patients in specific disease states might be from a state of good health. Second, patients who are worse off have stronger claims to have their health needs met than patients closer to a state of good health. If a cancer patient can be given an extra year of life of reasonable quality with some therapy and if someone with asthma (not life-threatening) can be given an additional year of life through some therapy with the same quality as our cancer patient, then from a moral point of view (justice-relevant) the value of that year for the cancer patient is much greater. Health gains have differential moral value depending upon how far from a good health state those gains are achieved. This would seem to imply for the prioritarian that effectiveness matters. However, nothing in medicine today will improve the welfare status of PVS patients.

Here is another challenge for the prioritarian. Consider the drug aducanumab, which is used to treat mild Alzheimer's-type dementia. This drug only received FDA approval in early 2021. At present there are about 3.1 million Americans with mild dementia. This drug is given by monthly injection at a cost of $56,000 per year for the drug and another $15,000 for the injections.[14] If 3.1 million patients were on this drug for a year, the cost would be $220 billion per year.[15] This would not result in any long-term care savings because the disease process would simply be slowed. Does the prioritarian conception of justice require social funding for this drug? Are these patients among the medically least well off?

This last question might seem odd. These individuals are just below good health status. They have minor memory lapses; they struggle occasionally to find the "right word." They certainly are not suffering in the way numerous end-stage terminally ill patients might be suffering, struggling to breathe, enduring excruciating pain from cancer that has invaded bone, and so on. Still,

[14] Roughly 600,000 Americans will be newly diagnosed with Alzheimer's each year over the coming decade. Further, it is estimated that by 2050 the number of Americans with Alzheimer's will grow to about 13.8 million (Alzheimer's Association Report, 2020). Total payments from all sources for the care of Alzheimer's patients in the United States in 2019 were estimated to be $305 billion.

[15] In the real world of health insurance and financial limits this figure represents a gross exaggeration. All manner of financial constraints (co-pays, deductibles, non-coverage) would serve as a barrier such that only a relatively small fraction of patients with early Alzheimer's would be able to afford this drug. However, I assume that prioritarians would regard all such barriers as being essentially unjust. Consequently, they would have to address my critical challenges in the text.

they will become among the medically least well off in several years. Recall that we do not wait until patients are in the end stages of cancer or heart disease or lung disease before initiating treatment. We are ethically obligated to provide effective treatments that slow the disease process. The cost of doing this is not usually judged to be exorbitant.

However, all of these chronic degenerative disease processes eventually get to late stages. At some point we run out of medical options. But before that happens, we have, in the case of various cancers, all manner of targeted therapies and immunotherapies, which both prolong life and improve quality of life (to some degree). The same will be true for many chronic degenerative conditions, though these are extraordinarily expensive interventions that are a major contributor to escalating health care costs. It is understandable why we (prioritarian citizens wanting to sustain a just and caring society) would believe that justice required funding these end-stage interventions. These patients are faced with a relatively imminent terminal prognosis and no other therapeutic alternatives. It would seem cruel to just "allow them to die."

At this point a critic might say to the prioritarian, "Surely you should establish some priorities among all the patients you regard as being among the medically least well off. Consider the children with various leukemias now capable of being cured in a large majority of cases at a cost of several hundred thousand dollars. Consider the children with cystic fibrosis who could benefit from this $300,000 per year drug or children with hemophilia who need these very expensive drugs or children with sickle cell disease or children with Gaucher's disease or Pompe disease, or SMA that might benefit from a $2.2 million gene therapy or Duchenne's muscular dystrophy, and so on. Surely individuals in the earliest stages of life must have a stronger just claim to limited societal resources than individuals faced with a terminal prognosis who have already lived a very full life." Is this where the prioritarian reiterates their commitment to a non-comparative assessment of the justice of meeting health care needs?

A certain moral virtue may be attached to this non-comparative perspective. The suffering attached to a late-stage metastatic cancer is of no greater or lesser moral value than the suffering attached to end-stage heart disease or end-stage chronic obstructive pulmonary disease or advanced sickle cell disease, and so on. Consequently, no priorities should be established among these disease states. Recall one of our wicked problems, cancer patients who might need a $200,000 therapy for only four extra months of life. That is a bad buy, given limited resources. But that patient complains about the million dollars we will spend to sustain the life of an ESRD patient or a cystic fibrosis patient or a hemophiliac. The prioritarian (it seems) will agree with that complaint, thereby bypassing that wicked problem. All those patients, no matter the overall cost of meeting their health care needs, are equally entitled to have those needs met. Dodging wicked problem seems commendable, but overall health care costs must be controlled. The prioritarian can also dodge the personal responsibility challenge, that is, the smoker with lung cancer because all that matters for reasons of justice is that the smoker is among the medically least well off.

In summary, prioritarians seem to dodge the "just caring" problem, assuming (it seems) that health care budgets have no limits. To be fair, the prioritarian perspective does have real-world moral and political utility, especially in the US health care system. Consider individuals with preexisting conditions (i.e., very costly health problems) who are denied health insurance. These individuals are clearly among the medically less well off and at risk of dying prematurely. The prioritarian perspective rightly calls attention to this injustice. Likewise, the relatively poor, very often people of color, who have been victims of long-standing social discrimination, would also be among the overall least well off who would be faced with economic barriers to accessing needed and effective health care. These are injustices that must be remedied; this is the right and reasonable message delivered by prioritarians. However, remedying those injustices will require rationing decisions (i.e., not meeting some genuine health care needs). The prioritarian fails to provide us with the intellectual tools needed to address that challenge.

4.6. Egalitarianism and Health Care Justice: What Is Inequitable?

We turn next to egalitarian perspectives regarding health care justice. There are many varieties of egalitarianism. Consider the broad distinction between strict and moderate egalitarians. The strict egalitarian emphasizes that all in our society are entitled to equal concern and respect, equal fundamental moral and political rights (also fully endorsed by the moderate egalitarian). Welfare rights distinguish these views. The strict egalitarian wants welfare for all equalized as much as possible. The moderate egalitarian is satisfied if all are guaranteed a reasonable or adequate package of welfare-sustaining social goods, what Rawls (1971) refers to as "primary goods," the "social bases of self-respect."

With regard to health care, the language sometimes invoked is that of everyone having a "right to health care." Those with the same health needs have a right to the same socially funded therapy. This has an obvious moral attractiveness that reflects equal concern and respect for all, especially preventing premature death and unnecessary suffering. However, there is the heterogeneity of health care needs problem: How are we supposed to figure out which health care needs make a just claim to social resources when they are so incomparable? The strict egalitarian can bypass this problem by paying for all health care needs. The strict egalitarian then faces the same problem as the prioritarian: The noble sentiment captured by this commitment is not affordable unless some just rationing decisions can be identified and justified. The strict egalitarian does not provide us with the resources to accomplish that.

The moderate egalitarian, in contrast to the strict egalitarian, will accept as "just enough" some inequalities in accessing needed health care. But then the moderate egalitarian is faced with the same challenges as the sufficientarian: What justice-relevant criteria determine the threshold of sufficiency or the content of an adequate health care benefit package? Most people for most of their lives are reasonably healthy, but a substantial number of others have extremely complicated and costly health care needs at various points in their lives for which that basic benefit package would be entirely inadequate. In the United States, in any given year 5% of the patient population will account for 50% of health care costs (Weissmann, 2012; Cohen and Yu, 2012).[16] These individuals are of primary concern for prioritarians. They make strong claims on health care resources for reasons of both justice and compassion. Egalitarians would verbalize a commitment to equal concern and respect for all. However, given the enormous heterogeneity of health care needs, the uncertainty of significant health benefit from various therapies (our targeted cancer therapies), and the extraordinary costs of these therapies, translating into health care policy and practice "equal concern and respect for all" will be a challenge, especially for the moderate egalitarian who needs to control overall health care costs in the face of endless (and legitimate) health care needs.

---

[16] The composition of that 5% of the population will vary from year to year. Some patients will have had a very costly terminal illness and die. Others, however, will have had a very costly illness, but they have gotten beyond that health crisis and again have an indefinite life expectancy.

Given the complexity and heterogeneity of health needs, what precisely does the moderate egalitarian believe should be equalized? Some will argue for equality of resources. However, resources have no relationship to the satisfaction of health care needs. Imagine guaranteeing to all in our society $1 million to purchase needed health care for a lifetime. That could be exhausted in the first year of life for an extremely premature infant. Others will live to age 90 and use only several thousand dollars in health care. In general, health needs are unpredictable. This is why health insurance exists as a prudent social response to the heterogeneity and unpredictability of health needs.

Dworkin (2000) defends the "prudent insurer" perspective. For Dworkin, "a just distribution is one that well-informed individuals create for themselves by individual choices, provided that the economic system and the distribution of wealth in the community in which these choices are made is just" (at 313). Dworkin is a critic of the "rescue principle" for defining what a just universal health care system ought to look like.[17] Instead, he imagines that individuals with a reasonably just, adequate income would make more constrained choices. Thus, he does not see prudent individuals wanting expensive life-prolonging interventions if they were in a persistent vegetative state or an advanced state of dementia or faced with a terminal illness and only a few months of additional life at great expense (as in, I surmise on behalf of Dworkin, our targeted cancer therapies for metastatic cancer). Consequently, he concludes that a universal health insurance scheme would be "a disservice to justice" (at 315) if everyone were forced to have such comprehensive rescue-like health insurance through a mandatory scheme. He adds, "we would therefore accept certain limits on universal coverage, and we would accept these not as compromises with justice but as required by it" (at 315). Dworkin does concede that "some of these decisions would be particularly difficult" (at 316). He mentions specifically some very expensive diagnostic procedures. He also mentions the case I brought up of an extremely premature infant who might require $1 million in health care. However, the more challenging scenarios would involve children with cystic fibrosis or hemophilia or any of the lysosomal storage disorders where life-sustaining costs of $300,000 per year might be required for years or decades. What

---

[17] As the term "rescue principle" suggests, it is about spending unlimited sums in an attempt to rescue individuals faced with a serious or life-threatening health crisis. Dworkin regards this as being both imprudent and unjust.

sort of decision should the prudent egalitarian make in those situations for Dworkin? These are rare cases, but the therapies are very effective, often yielding many years of an acceptable quality of life. However, as a prudent purchaser of health insurance (with a just but limited income), would I include coverage for the above disorders (and numerous others like that)?[18]

When a country offers universal health insurance, and this includes a fairly comprehensive set of health care benefits, we have something that approximates the egalitarian ideal. Still, no society can afford to cover every health care need. Consequently, the moderate egalitarian must be able to justify limitations and exclusions from that health plan. One option would be to use cost-effectiveness criteria. Such criteria, however, would result in justifying significant inequalities in access to needed and effective health care. Examples would include patients with hemophilia, Gaucher, Pompe, Duchenne muscular dystrophy, or SMA. The care needed by these patients would often cost several hundred thousand dollars per year, far outside any accepted understanding of cost-effective care.

Equalizing overall health welfare is another goal that an egalitarian might see as reasonable for a more egalitarian society. That might mean doing everything medically possible to give everyone an opportunity to achieve a normal life expectancy, say, age 75. This view has a certain ethical attractiveness. We, an egalitarian society, will spend whatever it takes to provide as long a life as possible of reasonable quality for children with sickle cell disease or hemophilia or cystic fibrosis or various lysosomal storage diseases or cancer. And we will do the same for anyone with heart disease or renal disease or HIV or Alzheimer's, and so on.

Recall that the moderate egalitarian must control overall health care costs to society. Dworkin endorses this. If their view is as open-ended and unqualified as I have presented it, then no limits exist regarding health spending for genuine health needs below age 75. Extraordinary sums would be paid to achieve merely marginal benefits. Recall the vast sums that could be commandeered by the PCSK9s to reduce LDL to achieve a marginal reduction in heart attacks and strokes. Recall the vast sums that could be commandeered by aducanumab (Mintun, 2021) to achieve a *possible* moderate slowing of Alzheimer's dementia. The same will be true for all

---

[18] Clackson (2008) regards Dworkin's prudent purchaser as a rationally self-interested individual who is making trade-offs between possible health benefits and other consumer goods. He does not see how this perspective is supposed to yield a just outcome. Clackson suggests that Dworkin's prudent purchaser ought to adopt the perspective of a prudent citizen capable of transcending self-interest.

the targeted cancer therapies and immunotherapies. The egalitarian could deny everyone therapeutic interventions likely to yield only a marginal benefit, which is congruent with a moderate egalitarianism. That still leaves the ragged edge problem.

What would be the relevant egalitarian criteria that would determine where that marginal benefit line will be drawn? Is this a line drawn at the level of individual patients, as opposed to some clinical classification of patients? Recall the circumstances of metastatic cancer patients offered some targeted therapy or immunotherapy. We know that the majority of those patients will receive only a very marginal benefit (Prasad, 2020). But we only know that about a specific type of cancer patient whose cancer is defined by a specific genetic mutation. Some of those patients will gain an extra year or two, and a very small number will be super-responders. If we cannot sort out likely outcomes, should the moderate egalitarian aim to save social resources by denying the therapy to everyone in the cohort? That means we sacrifice the opportunity for more substantial gains in life expectancy by the strong responders. This outcome might be congruent with egalitarian commitments, but it would likely not be regarded as being just or caring from the perspective of relatively younger patients in their 40s or 50s without other options for a somewhat improved life expectancy.

Perhaps the moderate egalitarian would only deny this marginally beneficial care to those over age 75. This proposal has a sufficientarian character to it with all the related problems, such as ageism. However, let us put that aside for the moment. Other ethically awkward problems need to be addressed. Consider our scenario with metastatic cancer patients where we have the ability to use several targeted cancer drugs in succession, thereby gaining for these patients on average five extra years in life expectancy. Such a patient initiates therapy at age 73. They now have a real possibility of at least reaching age 78. Would the egalitarian conception of health care justice permit social funding to exceed that age 75 threshold? It would feel unconscionable to withdraw therapy when that patient reached age 75, knowing that the therapy would be effective for several more years. But it would also be ethically problematic for this egalitarian to withhold initiating the cancer therapy at age 73 knowing that this patient could then reach age 78.

Perhaps the egalitarian would think of age 75 as a soft threshold. If so, what would that softness mean so far as the just allocation of health resources was concerned beyond age 75. If someone developed metastatic cancer at age 76, would they be entirely responsible for covering the cost of the needed care from their own funds or have to accept an earlier death without treatment? It would be hard to imagine (for reasons of compassion) not providing any socially funded health care beyond age 75. This is why a soft threshold would be desirable. That only raises the question of what criteria would be used by the egalitarian to determine what care would be provided at social expense beyond age 75 (i.e., the sufficientarian arbitrariness problem).

The egalitarian might have in mind that "basic" health care would be socially funded. What precisely does that mean? Everyone would agree on lots of examples of basic care. What about examples right at the edge of basic care or just slightly beyond that edge? Consider a patient diagnosed at age 80 with an early cancer that could likely be effectively treated. Is that basic treatment? Alternatively, if that same patient had instead a very aggressive version of that same cancer with an unalterable terminal outcome, and treatment would provide an extra year of life for $50,000, would that treatment be regarded as "basic"? If we did think about the example this way, then "basic" would be about therapeutic effectiveness. The latter example represents "low-value" care.

Presumably, prudent egalitarians would endorse denying low-value care to those over the age of 75. Of course, that just generates the additional question: Why would a prudent egalitarian not agree to forgo low-value care below age 75 as well? This seems perfectly reasonable. However, this commitment would generate some ethically awkward situations. Consider the care of somewhat younger cancer patients. Imagine a 50-year-old with metastatic cancer. He could be given a $150,000 combination of immunotherapies that we would know before the fact would yield only three extra months of life. That would be low-value care. But the moderate egalitarian wants to maximize the opportunity for an individual to come as close as possible to age 75. This looks like an internal conflict for the egalitarian. Perhaps it is resolved by invoking Dworkin's prudent egalitarian, who would have chosen at an earlier point in life an insurance plan that would not cover this intervention under these circumstances.

Consider our 80-year-old with a refractory B-cell lymphoma. He has the option of CAR T-cell therapy with a front-end cost of $475,000. Imagine that we have successfully found biomarkers that identify patients who will be strong responders to the therapy and gain several extra years of life. This is high-value care, costly but very effective (though not curative). This is care that ought to be socially funded for the egalitarian, especially if the egalitarian has endorsed continued funding for cancer care initiated prior to age

75 that now sustains the life of that patient for many years beyond that age. This would not be an uncommon situation if we were talking about CLL and treatment with ibrutinib. Again, this has the appearance of an internal conflict for the egalitarian. Some of these patients will be given access to CAR T-cell therapy at social expense, while others unlikely to survive a year with CAR T-cell therapy would be denied it as low-value care. What about patients who might gain one or two extra years of life for whom this might be labeled "mid-value care"? How should the prudent egalitarian think about those patients?

4.7. Utilitarianism and Health Care Justice: What Care Is "Worth It"?

We next consider utilitarian theories of health care justice. The basic goal of utilitarianism in a health care context is to maximize total health benefits, given a fixed budget. Efficiency in using limited resources is a critical part of economic life. The virtue of utilitarian justice is that it is impartial. In effect, the utilitarian says before the fact, "I have no idea who the beneficiaries will be of our commitment to deliver health care services in the most efficient and cost-effective manner possible. It is just a matter of luck. Some individuals will have extremely costly health problems that are chronic and will benefit to only a small degree from current therapies. Given limited budgets, we cannot afford to pay for those health care needs. This is unfortunate, but it is not unjust."[19]

Recall our wicked challenges: all patients with metastatic cancer who need some targeted cancer drug costing $100,000 for only three extra months of life. We rarely know before the fact who those patients or the super-responders might be. In either case, this would provide a strong motivation for funding research to discover biomarkers that would identify either of these patients with a high level of probability. Economists are concerned about cost-effectiveness. Economists are not in agreement regarding the maximum cost per QALY. A rough consensus in the United States would put that figure at $100,000 per QALY, roughly $80,000 per QALY in the European

---

[19] I discuss more critically the "impartiality" of a utilitarian theory of health care justice below in this section. In brief, the utilitarian focus on outcomes fails to consider how outcomes are affected (often adversely) by a variety of social determinants of health "upstream." This has justice-relevant consequences.

Union. If it cost $100,000 to gain three extra months of life for a metastatic cancer patient, then that represents a cost of $400,000 per QALY.[20]

No utilitarian wants to be a health care Scrooge. A utilitarian could propose funding much more cancer research aimed at improving less costly cancer therapies that were more effective at earlier stages. Funding could come from not funding marginally beneficial efforts to prolong life with metastatic disease. This would seem both reasonable and economically and morally rational, especially for those patients who would benefit from this change of perspective. However, some patients are first diagnosed with metastatic disease (i.e., lung and pancreatic cancers). They would derive no advantage from this proposal. On the contrary, they would be worse off relative to the prior state of affairs. For egalitarians and prioritarians this would be ethically problematic. Many ordinary folks would see such an outcome as being heartless.

The utilitarian is going to run into this same problem elsewhere. Recall the children with cystic fibrosis or sickle cell disease or SMA or various lysosomal storage disorders. Treating all of these disorders can have costs of $300,000 or more per year for years or decades. These are effective interventions, but they are not curative; and they are clearly far outside the normal cost-effectiveness limitations. It seems unconscionable that we (a just and caring society) would simply allow these children to die, given these therapeutic options.

An alternative to denying all these children costly but effective life-sustaining care would be to claim that other values were relevant, not simply cost-effectiveness. The obvious value would be compassion. These are children. They are entirely dependent upon the care of others. What should be the scope and limits of this compassionate response? Hemophiliacs with more severe forms of the disease, for example, would start out as children but need this costly and intense level of care for their adult life as well. We could not be ethically justified in cutting off life-sustaining care once an individual reached age 18. However, other adults faced with a very costly life-threatening disorder, something far outside cost-effectiveness limits, would expect to be recipients of comparable societal compassion. This looks like a matter of ethical consistency, justice as fairness. Again, we are dealing with a fixed social budget.[21]

[20] Many individuals will find this whole discussion about cost-effectiveness and rationing to be abhorrent. They will often mutter something about human life being priceless. At the same time, they will resist raising taxes or insurance premiums to pay for the real costs of their moral commitments.

[21] Very recently, a new form of gene therapy for hemophilia was announced (Stein, 2020b). It has a cost of $3 million. It is a one-time therapy that, in theory, would be a cure for an individual's

The more that compassion motivates us to provide life-prolonging care that is not cost-effective, the more we would have to give up any form of care that was cost-effective.[22] What criteria would the utilitarian use for making these trade-offs that were congruent with a utilitarian conception of health care justice? The utilitarian could lower the cost-effectiveness threshold from, say, $100,000 to $80,000. The funds saved would pay for compassionate care above the threshold. However, tens of thousands of metastatic cancer patients whose care would cost $100,000 per year would no longer have their care covered at social cost. They would have the right to ask for compassionate support not warranted on grounds of cost-effectiveness. What would justify not responding positively to these requests? Some of these cancer patients would be in their 70s or 80s, quite a distance from our children. However, if these patients are getting an extra year of life for each $100,000 expenditure (as opposed to three months), that represents a significant benefit. What would justify not extending our compassion to these individuals? A brutally honest answer would be that these individuals were simply too old to elicit compassion; they were expendable. This would represent the worst sort of ageism, reasonable grounds for rejecting as "just enough" a utilitarian conception of health care justice.

Another challenge for utilitarians, given fixed budgets, is aggregated medical success of expensive medical interventions. If everything should be socially funded that has a cost-effectiveness value of less than $100,000 per QALY, then the number of life-years funded at that level may increase to unsustainable levels with ongoing medical success. Recall the goal of some was to make cancer a manageable disease through a succession of targeted

hemophilia because it would introduce into an individual the healthy gene necessary to produce the protein that would cure them. From a utilitarian cost-effectiveness perspective, the manufacturer claims the therapy is worth that high price. Still, the front-end cost of $3 million must come from a current hard budget while the savings would only accrue over 10–20 years. That can have justice-relevant consequences that require assessment today.

[22] A real-world example may be found in the United Kingdom in the form of the National Institute for Clinical Excellence (NICE). NICE assesses all new medical technologies that might be incorporated into the National Health Service (NHS). Its assessment relies heavily on cost-effectiveness data as well as social value considerations. NICE has ultimately rejected for NHS funding a number of cancer drugs that were too expensive and yielded too little clinical benefit. This was creating problems for the British government because angry patients were demanding these drugs. The government could not overrule NICE. Instead, the government set up the Cancer Drug Fund to which patients could appeal, generally on grounds that the drugs represented "last chance" therapies. No doubt the government saw this as a justified compassionate response. However, the obvious criticism is that the government did not create a Cardiac Drug Fund or Renal Drug Fund or Rheumatoid Arthritis Drug Fund. What would justify such selective compassion? Apart from that, the Cancer Drug Fund delivered very little real benefit to patients (Aggarwal et al., 2017; Cohen, 2017).

therapies. Five-year survival at $100,000 each for three million cancer patients would be $300 billion on top of whatever other funds were expended on non-metastatic cancer patients. Also recall our artificial heart example. The aggregation of these very expensive gains in life-years would require painful, justice-relevant trade-offs within constrained health care budgets. What trade-offs would the utilitarian endorse? Would the utilitarian endorse reducing the ultra-expensive compassionate expenditures discussed above, many of which are associated with meeting the life-prolonging needs of children. Allowing those children to die when an effective life-prolonging therapy was available to them is not a trade-off most people would embrace with equanimity, especially if such trade-offs seemed necessary due to our extending the lives of much older individuals, even with cost-effective precision cancer care.

Utilitarians are not friends with prioritarians. Utilitarians are certainly committed to meeting at least some of the claims of the medically least well, if cost-effective. Otherwise, those individuals will have no just claim to social resources. Stein (2012) states with absolute clarity the view of a strict utilitarian: "Finally, there are examples in which it is indeed clear that the worse-off candidate would benefit less from scarce resources than the better-off candidate. In these examples, it seems to me that the scarce resources go to the candidate who can benefit most, even if she is better off" (at 51). Stein goes on to say, "Prioritarianism gives extra weight to the welfare of those who are worse off. From a utilitarian perspective, this is like placing a thumb on the scale of justice; it violates the principle of equal respect" (at 52). The problem with this utilitarian conclusion is that the ethical focus is entirely on the quantity and quality of outcomes, ignoring altogether justice-relevant considerations regarding the larger causal history behind those outcomes, such as the social determinants of health. Individuals raised in an impoverished environment may be predictably less responsive to specific therapies than more advantaged individuals with the same diagnosis. Those background conditions may reflect deep and sustained social injustices, which should not be perpetuated through the health care system; Stein would simply ignore those background conditions.[23] To summarize, a utilitarian theory of health care justice will have too many ethically unsavory consequences relative to

---

[23] A clear real-world example of this ethical challenge is what is occurring as I write in the middle of the COVID-19 crisis. A disproportionate number of individuals from impoverished backgrounds are infected with COVID-19, have more serious symptoms, require more frequent and intense hospitalization, and end up with higher fatality rates (Abrams and Szefler, 2020; Yancy, 2020).

our 11 health care rationing challenges. Still, the core idea at the heart of utilitarian justice is not without merit. In making health care rationing and allocation decisions, effectiveness matters and cost-effectiveness matters. But that mattering needs to be constrained and balanced by other justice-relevant considerations, ultimately, as I argue, through fair processes of rational democratic deliberation.

4.8. Libertarianism and Health Care Justice: Only Getting What You Can Pay For

The preeminent value in political life for libertarians is respect for individual liberty. Numerous social values are worthy of political acceptance and respect. How those values are organized into the life of any individual must be left entirely to that individual. The state must protect the right of individuals to make those choices. These are the rights of non-interference. There are no welfare rights (i.e., state-supported assistance with accessing societal goods). There is no such thing as a right to health care, nor does the state have responsibility for distributional justice related to health care.

Tristram Engelhardt (1996) has been the most vocal proponent of a libertarian point of view in health care: "The imposition of a single-tier, all-encompassing health care system is morally unjustifiable. It is a coercive act of totalitarian ideological zeal, which fails to recognize the diversity of moral visions that frame interests in health care, the secular moral limits of state authority, and the authority of individuals over themselves and their own property. It is an act of secular immorality" (at 375). Nothing wishy-washy is in this passage, no subtle qualifications, no carefully crafted exceptions, no thoughtful balancing of competing values. Here are some of the practical implications of this passage.

(1) Employers are free to offer health insurance to their employees if they wish. This is a product of a free contractual agreement. If this benefit becomes too expensive, an employer may cease offering this benefit or pay more for that benefit. Employers are free to include or exclude whatever health care services they wish. If targeted cancer therapies or CAR T-cell immunotherapies or major organ transplants are seen as being too costly, employers are free to delete these services from their contracts.

(2) Private health insurers have exactly the same rights as private employers. If an individual has or is likely to have a costly preexisting medical condition, then that insurance company is free either to deny that individual health insurance or to exclude from that contract health care related to that preexisting condition or to charge an exorbitant premium that an individual is "free" to accept or reject.

(3) If individuals cannot afford private health insurance, they will have to rely upon the private charitable impulses of hospitals or physicians or churches or charitable organizations. If some uninsured individuals are faced with a life-threatening illness for which some costly life-prolonging intervention is available (dialysis or a left ventricular assist device) and there is no charitable response, these individuals will die prematurely. For Engelhardt (and other libertarians) such an outcome would be unfortunate but not unjust. Engelhardt (1996) writes: "Loose talk about justice and fairness in health care is therefore morally misleading, because it suggests there is a particular canonical vision of justice or fairness that all have grounds to endorse" (at 375). If there is no society-wide shared understanding of health care justice, then society at large cannot be rightly accused of being unjust when uninsured individuals are denied life-prolonging care they cannot afford.

(4) Of course, the prior unfortunate state of affairs can be avoided if a society such as Canada or Germany mandates health insurance for all. However, libertarians absolutely reject taxpayer-funded health care because coercively collected taxes are required to support such a system. Likewise, they reject all mandated health insurance as a violation of liberty rights. Some individuals may prefer not to have health insurance at all and accept the consequences of such a decision.

(5) The worst of all possible worlds (according to the libertarian) would be a world with government-funded universal health care, the same health coverage for everyone. Individuals would see themselves as having to pay for health care services they would never purchase for themselves. This would be regarded as a violation of basic liberty rights. Likewise, numerous health care interventions are the object of religious or ethical controversy. No one would be compelled to use these services, but if they are included in universal health care, then those who conscientiously objected would be legally obligated to pay taxes to provide these services. For the libertarian, that represents

unwarranted and unjustified state-authorized interference in the lives of individuals.

(6) Engelhardt is aware of the need to control health care costs; many individuals would prefer to spend their money on other things they might value more than health care. Engelhardt writes: "One cannot provide the best possible health care for all and contain health care costs" (at 376). That implies that rationing would be inescapable in a universal health care system. But it would be extremely unlikely that there would be broad societal agreement regarding rationing decisions acceptable to everyone. Some people would want very limited life-sustaining care provided to patients in advanced stages of dementia or strict limits on costly care provided to individuals whose health needs were the result of poor behavioral choices. Others would want all metastatic cancer therapies protected from rationing because of the ubiquity of cancer and the lack of therapeutic alternatives. Again, these challenges represent violations of the liberty rights of individuals in a universal health care system. Engelhardt concludes: "That few openly address these foundational moral tensions at the roots of contemporary health care policy suggests that the problems are shrouded in a collective illusion, a false consciousness, an established ideology within which certain facts are politically unacceptable" (at 377).

Ultimately, Engelhardt endorses inequality in access to needed health care as unavoidable because of private resources and human freedom. In brief, individuals have a right to the health care that they need if they can pay for it themselves or through health insurance. For Engelhardt, these are inescapable "facts" about the real world, though these are really tragic and unjust "facts" related to health care financing in the United States. In concluding, however, I must concede that Engelhardt (and other libertarians, such as Lomasky [1980]) have identified issues that cannot be easily dismissed with an insightful philosophic quip. Libertarian concerns represent legitimate justice-relevant considerations that need to be part of rational democratic deliberative efforts to forge a more just approach to the wicked problems associated with the need for health care rationing. If a just health care system cannot cover every therapeutic possibility, would there be anything unjust about permitting wealthier individuals to purchase supplemental insurance that would pay for those services denied to everyone else under the social insurance package?

4.9. Fair Equality of Opportunity and Health Care Justice

Norman Daniels (1985) defends the moderate egalitarian fair opportunity account of health care justice. Daniels emphasizes the "normal opportunity range" of a society, all the possible activities in a specific society for a typical member. If an individual is prevented from fully participating in that normal opportunity range as a result of disease or accident or disability and if effective medical or rehabilitative interventions are available that would allow an individual to regain access to that normal opportunity range, then a just society would be obligated to provide assured access to those interventions.

Two broad consequences of this view should be noted. First, it is the "normal" opportunity range that matters. Some individuals might have developed extraordinary talents as musicians or artists or financial analysts or woodworkers or engineers or physicians, and so on. Those individuals might be afflicted with some disease that severely compromises their ability to continue to do their work with a very high level of expertise. Those individuals would have a just claim to whatever medical interventions were available that were effective enough that they could do their work again, though not necessarily with that very high level of expertise. In other words, if it were medically possible to restore that very high level of expertise but at great expense with uncertain likelihood of success, that individual would not have a just claim to that intervention at social expense. This would be the analogue of the "expensive taste" objection that Dworkin (1981) introduced into the literature.

A second consequence of the normal opportunity range is that it is about "opportunity" that can be *protected or restored*. In some cases, disease or accident has had such tragic results that medicine cannot restore that individual to the normal opportunity range (i.e., a persistent vegetative state, maybe very advanced dementia, and very late stages of many other terminal disorders). Such patients clearly have a just claim to hospice care. However, such patients would not have a just claim to some extraordinarily expensive intervention with a very low probability of success in supporting only a very debilitated state of existence. In other words, they could not meaningfully engage any portion of the opportunity range.

One of the virtues of Daniels' view is that it does establish limits on access to social resources to meet health care needs. There is nothing unjustly discriminatory in those limits. One of the common criticisms of the US health care system is that it contains hundreds of billions of dollars of waste: millions of unnecessary tests and procedures, low-value care, low rates of preventive care, and so on (Shrank et al., 2019).[24] No one has a just claim to wasteful care. One way of defining wasteful care is to say, with Daniels, that it does virtually nothing to improve access to concrete opportunities for a patient.

On a more positive note, a clear implication of Daniels' commitment to equality of opportunity is that those who are least well off health-wise but capable of significant benefit from costly but effective life-prolonging medical interventions will have a just claim to those interventions. Children with cystic fibrosis or sickle cell disease or Duchenne muscular dystrophy or various leukemias or lymphomas or lysosomal storage diseases would all have a just claim to the social resources needed to pay for the relevant life-prolonging interventions, even if these interventions cost several hundred thousand dollars per year. I take it the same would be true for older patients requiring renal dialysis or metastatic cancer patients who might gain several extra years of life from a succession of targeted cancer drugs or immuno-therapies, including CAR T-cell therapy. Likewise, patients who were HIV$^+$ would have a just claim to the drug combinations that would manage their HIV for decades, and patients with end-stage heart disease would have a just claim to the $250,000 left ventricular assist device that might yield one to four extra years of life for them. Having said all of this, several problems re-main for Daniels.

Daniels' account will have to struggle with ragged edge challenges. The PCSK9 drugs will yield significant medical benefit in the form of reduced heart attacks and strokes for patients with extremely high LDL levels, most often the result of familial hypercholesterolemia. Patients with LDL levels above 130 mg/dl are also at elevated risk, though the likelihood of benefit will diminish substantially. To be clear, the benefits are not negligible. All along that continuum patients will continue to have strokes and heart attacks that might have been prevented, some of which will be fatal, others of which will result in diminished life opportunities. Where should Daniels' moderate egalitarian draw a line? It is easy to draw a bright line at familial hypercholes-terolemia. What happens to those below that line? They will be told to engage in a substantial exercise program and dramatically alter their diet. Relatively few patients will have the psychological motivation to act on those directives. Is this outcome congruent with Daniels' opportunity egalitarianism? The

---

[24] I will mention, with the authors, that the most expensive sort of waste in the US health care system is excess administrative costs associated with private health insurance.

basic problem is that the aggregated social cost of funding 19 million lives per year for PCSK9s is imprudent, unsustainable, and a likely misallocation of resources, given a fixed health care budget. In addition, unlike the HIV drugs which produce a substantial medical benefit for *each and every* patient taking them, the PCSK9s prevent a stroke or heart attack only in a relatively small proportion of the population taking them (even though they will reduce LDL in all of these patients). Some of these patients might complain that this denial is not congruent with an egalitarian commitment to equal concern and respect for all. They will argue that they are asking for $6,000 per year, while HIV⁺ patients get $35,000 worth of care per year. In the case of the HIV⁺ patients, these drug combinations effectively prevent the premature deaths of all these individuals. It is not as if only a small fraction of HIV⁺ patients are helped by these drugs. In the case of patients with elevated LDL levels, the PCSK9s do reduce LDL levels in all these patients, but only a relatively small percentage will be spared a premature death from either a stroke or heart attack. This is a difference that makes a difference, so far as health care justice is concerned.

Clinical testing is now occurring on a TIAH, with a projected cost for surgery and hospitalization of about $500,000. Average gain in life expectancy for such patients would be five years. In the United States, projected need for the device would be about 350,000 patients per year at a social cost of $175 billion. From the perspective of Daniels' opportunity egalitarianism, this is something society would be ethically obligated to pay for as a matter of egalitarian justice. These are patients with advanced heart failure losing access to the normal opportunity range. The TIAH would restore normal access to that opportunity range. This is precisely the rationale requiring egalitarians to pay for the sickle cell drugs that cost $100,000 per year or the cystic fibrosis drugs that cost $300,000 per year. Still, the need for limits is inescapable. How high a priority ought the TIAH have, all things considered?

The vast majority of these devices would be allocated to patients over the age of 70. Many of these patients will achieve something more than a normal life expectancy. An 80-year-old would live to age 85 or beyond, thanks to this device and its social financing, instead of dying a "premature" natural death at 80. Daniels would certainly endorse as ethically necessary providing this device to relatively younger individuals in their 40s or 50s who were unfortunately afflicted with a life-threatening bacterial endocarditis as well as individuals in their 60s with advanced heart failure, whether due to bad luck or bad health habits. But maybe something is ethically amiss in providing this device to individuals in their late 70s or 80s. Moderate egalitarians are ethically comfortable with various degrees of health inequalities that are not a product of unjust social policies or practices. In this case, however, if TIAHs are available at social expense to individuals already well above normal life expectancy, it would feel like the inequality is being generated and sustained by a commitment to opportunity egalitarianism. In other words, this could be an inequity.

This potential inequity could be corrected by denying the TIAH to anyone over age 70. However, Daniels' egalitarianism would endorse social funding for a series of targeted cancer drugs for five years or more that in some cases would carry patients far beyond age 70. The same would be true for the CLL patients needing ibrutinib, potentially followed by CAR T-cell therapy. A TIAH limitation of age 70 would not be ethically congruent with these other commitments. Again, a patient in heart failure at age 69 gets the TIAH and the opportunity to live to age 74 or beyond. A patient in the same situation at age 71 would have to accept dying at that age, having been denied the TIAH at social expense. What does ethical consistency require?

Daniels did not have to consider explicitly any of the wicked problems that represent serious challenges to some aspects of his account of health care justice when he wrote his first book (1985). However, his second book (1988) addressed resource allocation issues related to aging. Emerging life-prolonging technologies at the time made clear that the major beneficiaries of these technologies would be older individuals who would live longer with more costly chronic degenerative conditions that would only worsen the problem of health care cost escalation as well as the just allocation of resources across the life span.

The elderly had the benefit of Medicare, while the non-elderly were entirely at the mercy of the financial concerns of employers regarding health care benefits. Of course, the non-elderly were helping to pay for Medicare through the payroll tax, hoping they would not die prematurely from an unaffordable illness. Daniels believed there was something essentially unjust about the non-elderly helping to pay for medical care that would permit the elderly to become hyper-elderly while they themselves were at risk for dying prematurely. However, constraining access to expensive life-prolonging care for the elderly to improve access to care for the non-elderly would be ageism.

Daniels consequently proposed his "prudential life span account" of health care justice. In brief, he asked individuals to imagine themselves as young people, very healthy, knowing statistically the health risks all faced over the course of a lifetime, also knowing the costly effective medical interventions that could allow those individuals to reach old age without serious but preventable disabilities if they were afflicted with a life-threatening but curable medical disorder. In addition, these individuals would be mindful of the random events that could threaten their insurance coverage in the United States as things were then. Moreover, despite these concerns, these individuals wanted to see their health care costs controlled. What Daniels imagined is that such prudent individuals, if given the opportunity, would deny their future possible elderly selves certain very expensive but marginally beneficial life-prolonging interventions if the money saved could be transferred to their younger selves in order to maximize their opportunity to achieve an average life expectancy. This would be rationing health care to the elderly, but it would be autonomously self-imposed rationing for my own future possible elderly self, as opposed to someone else's elderly self. This would not represent some discriminatory form of ageism. This would be a prudent choice that rational individuals would make for themselves. In addition, the outcome would be just, or at least more just than the current state of affairs with Medicare and unstable employer-based health insurance.

Daniels offered this model in 1988. How would this model hold up if Daniels' prudent individuals had to address any of our wicked problems, such as ibrutinib, CAR T-cell immunotherapies, or our targeted cancer drug scenarios? The short answer, as Daniels himself would attest, is that his account would not fare well against these challenges. He believes, as I do, that this would be true for every other philosophic theory of health care justice. The basic problem is that all these theories are too abstract to address the complexities associated with health care needs and therapies today, though each of these competing theories has as its defining core a social value that is reasonable and legitimate.

For Daniels, the outcome of this state of affairs is what Rawls (1996) refers to as "reasonable disagreement." Such disagreement cannot be allowed to simply stand because, in the real world of money and public policy and limited resources, decisions will have to be made that are judged to be reasonable and legitimate. For Daniels, that means we must have a process for resolving concrete disagreements (as opposed to resolving philosophic disagreements about a correct theory of health care justice). Daniels and Sabin (2008) write, "We must rely on fair process because acceptable general principles of justice fail to give us determinate answers about fair allocation and because we have no consensus on more fine-grained principles" (at 30). Daniels refers to this approach as "accountability for reasonableness."

First, the entire process of deliberating about some specific rationing protocol must be public and transparent, nothing hidden from those who could potentially be affected by this rationing protocol. This is what Rawls (1971) refers to as the "publicity condition." It is absolutely essential to our understanding of justice.[25] Second, the process that leads to legitimating some specific rationing protocol must be deliberative. That is, it is about giving reasons, providing evidence, critically assessing arguments for and against some specific rationing protocol. It is the opposite of gathering opinions through a survey or taking a vote and aggregating the preferences. The deliberation itself is a social process. Daniels, following Rawls, contends that participants in the deliberation must be *reasonable*. That is, they must be seeking "fair terms of cooperation" in an enterprise (the health care system) of which all are a part.

In the United States and the European Union, for example, virtually all members of those societies have helped to create the health care system through their payment of taxes and health insurance premiums. Those funds subsidized the cost of medical education as well as the medical research that has generated numerous powerful therapies. Consequently, all should have the opportunity to benefit from their contributions to that system. Still, given resource constraints, not every health care need can be met. The purpose of the deliberative process is to determine fairly which health care needs will not be met. Those unmet needs will belong to individuals who can be accepting of those denials if the deliberative process has been careful to lay out fully and explicitly the reasons and reasoning that resulted in a specific rationing protocol. Daniels and Sabin (2008) write, "Specifically, a rationale will be reasonable if it appeals to reasons, evidence and principles that are accepted as relevant by fair-minded people who are disposed to finding mutually justifiable terms of cooperation" (at 45). In other words, individuals may not agree with the outcome, but they understand the reasons and reasoning

---

[25] In several of my earlier articles (1987, 1990) I called attention to the practices of "invisible rationing" that have been integral to the US health care system. Much invisible rationing is done by ability to pay through the use of co-pays and very high front-end deductibles. Mechanisms like that do not require any identifiable individual to be the denier of access to some needed health care. Hence, no one can be held accountable for clear injustices. Several writers defend the social utility of such practices on the grounds that this minimizes social divisiveness (Calabresi and Bobbitt, 1978). I vigorously disagree with that rationale.

that justified that outcome, which they see as relevant and reasonable. Consequently, they accept that they cannot reasonably reject that outcome.

Who is supposed to be accountable for being reasonable? Daniels and Sabin mention managed care plans and private health insurance, which they believe ought to include some form of broader rational democratic engagement. The primary source of justice and legitimacy in the making of rationing decisions should be the autonomous self-imposing of these rationing protocols. Having specific rationing protocols "come down" from the board of a managed care plan will not reflect the autonomous choices of those who will be affected by those protocols. Options, concerns, relevant values beyond justice, weighting of justice-relevant considerations pertinent to a specific rationing problem—all that needs to emerge from a broader democratic deliberative process for some rationing protocol to be genuinely autonomous.

What should that deliberative process look like? What conditions must be met for that process to be just and legitimate? How might our "wicked challenges" be addressed through such a process? How is it possible to achieve "sufficient agreement" regarding these wicked challenges when such diverse understandings of justice, as well as many other fundamental social values, are prevalent in our society, not to mention the complexity of our health care system and its therapeutic options? We turn next to address these challenges.

5

Rational Democratic Deliberation

Seeking Justice Together

5.1. Rational Democratic Deliberation: Taking Seriously the Tragedy of the Commons

Why do we need rational democratic deliberation to address the problems of health care rationing? We are faced with a "tragedy of the commons" problem. Health insurance, whether public or private, represents a shared pool of financial resources. Contributors to the pool share financial risk for meeting health care needs and have the right to withdraw funds from the pool. What health care needs justify taking resources from that pool to meet those needs? One short answer would be "whatever is medically necessary." Professional medical judgment determines what is medically necessary.

Most of us will accept these judgments of need based upon expertise. However, imagine a physician informing a patient that they are terminally ill but that there is an intervention for $100,000 that will yield an extra week of life. Other members of the insurance pool would be reluctant to allow that individual to withdraw that $100,000. What would justify that reluctance? The patient would insist they had a right to that payout because of the pain they are in. Others in the pool would object: "What if everyone in the pool wanted to draw out $100,000 for an extra week of life?" For insurance to be affordable, limits must be identified and agreed to for taking resources from the pool. Otherwise, we have a "tragedy of the commons" situation, which would result in the destruction of the commons.

To prevent that tragedy and have reasonable agreement, rational democratic deliberation would be necessary. Multiple basic values will be integral to this conversation. Everyone will want to limit the cost of health insurance. Everyone will also want to assure sufficient concern for the well-being of others afflicted with various disorders. Compassion is essential. However, not every legitimate health care need can command resources from that pool.

Precision Medicine and Distributive Justice. Leonard M. Fleck, Oxford University Press. © Oxford University Press 2022.
DOI: 10.1093/oso/9780197647721.003.0005

A fair process is needed for determining which needs rightfully commanded those resources.

We all would want to fund effective therapies that are reasonably priced. If we want effective cost containment/rationing in health care (no cost shifting), then we have to find a way to link cost and value through patients. And if we want a fair approach to health care cost containment and rationing, then rationing protocols will have to be public or explicit, reasonable, rationally justifiable, autonomously imposed, and impartially generated and applied (as opposed to being a product of interest group politics and power). These are conditions that can best be met through processes of rational democratic deliberation (I shall argue).

David Eddy (1996, chap. 12) and Norman Daniels and James Sabin (1997) have identified the essential moral insight that makes rational democratic deliberation fair and feasible. Any fair approach to health care rationing must be a product of patient choice, freely and rationally self-imposed, and from the point of view of an indefinitely large number of possible healthy/unhealthy selves I (and others) might become. The distinction Eddy makes is between patients with a small "p" (who have health problems at the moment) and "Patients" in that all-inclusive sense that embraces both the currently well (who will be ill) and the currently ill. When we are engaged in deliberative efforts aimed at articulating fair and cost-effective rationing protocols, we must occupy both those perspectives simultaneously. We must have the capacity to empathize both with the sick and anxious in our midst (patients with a small "p" who really represent future possible versions of myself) as well as the mostly healthy (Patients) who are presently responsible for covering those health care costs through taxes or insurance premiums. In this latter frame of mind, the thought will intrude that perhaps some of these very expensive health interventions might not be worth it.

Our key question: Do we have good reason to believe that a fair and inclusive process of rational democratic deliberation would be able to manage all of the "wicked" problems of health care justice that we identified in Chapters 3 and 4? What are the alternatives? We could control societal health care costs by rationing by ability to pay. This works. The consequence of this arrangement might be perfect economic efficiency but enormous deficiencies of justice and compassion. A child born into a poor family with a curable life-threatening condition will die prematurely and unnecessarily. No one could accept such an outcome with equanimity unless they had a heart and brain made of stone. Still, if this same child needed a life-prolonging therapy for only an extra week of life for $100,000, it would be reasonable and just to deny that request. Such an outcome would be tragic.

We could imagine Obamacare-lite. Such a proposal would require everyone to have insurance; but no subsidies would be available, and insurers could refuse to cover patients with preexisting conditions. Individuals who were among the medically least well off would both suffer unnecessarily and die prematurely. This would be neither just nor compassionate, especially since all would have contributed to creating this health care system. Consequently, all ought to be able to benefit. Still, no one has the right to make unlimited claims on social resources. Some mechanism is needed to determine limits on access to needed health care that reflects our collective sense of what a just and caring society ought to be.

Employer-based health insurance is not a solution because it is unstable, unfair, and often inadequate for the specific health needs of employees. The instability is related to the economic strength or weakness of the company itself, not to mention the larger economic climate, as we saw with COVID-19 in early 2020. In the space of months, 10 million workers were added to the ranks of the uninsured, and this was in the midst of a pandemic! The unfairness is related to both the scope of benefits and the cost-control measures embedded in those plans, all of which affect more adversely lower-wage workers. The co-pays are supposed to incentivize workers (as patients) to make more cost-conscious choices. Unfortunately, half the time the choices of workers to forgo some intervention are the wrong choices with potentially disastrous consequences.[1] It is ethically disingenuous to minimize these consequences.

5.2. Medicare: An Impending Tragedy of the Commons

The Medicaid and Medicare programs are also flawed from the perspective of health care justice. Medicaid can vary enormously from state to state. Medicaid is typically the most expensive item in state budgets. Consequently, given pressures to control state budgets, Medicaid is a target. Medicaid can control its costs by limiting the eligibility of individuals for coverage. Many

---

[1] Chernew (2020) writes: "Specifically, blunt cost-sharing approaches, such as high-deductible plans, have failed to encourage price-shopping, and though they have reduced utilization, these reductions have affected higher- and lower-value care simultaneously" (at 1403).

southern states will limit Medicaid coverage to the lowest 25% of those below the poverty level. Those above that line are uninsured and entirely dependent upon the instability of private charity. Likewise, physicians are not legally required to accept Medicaid patients. This is especially problematic for medical specialists, such as oncologists.

Medicare was initiated in 1965 to bring about a more just health care system. As a group, the elderly population has three times the number of health problems of the non-elderly. To be retired at the time meant the loss of health insurance. Medicare was universal access to a comprehensive set of health care benefits for the elderly at the same price for everyone. The technology revolution in health care started in 1960, which rapidly drove the cost of the Medicare program higher than anyone had forecast. However, Congress was not going to engage in any explicit rationing. Consequently, the Diagnosis-Related Groupings (DRG) system was put in place to control hospital costs in 1984 (as discussed at section 3.5 above). This did constrain costs, with ethical risks. Physicians remained motivated to provide the best care possible for their patients, but hospital administrators saw such compassionate behavior as a threat to their bottom line. Prior to the DRG system hospital administrators wanted to keep their beds filled. Under DRGs the incentive was to empty those beds as quickly as possible. The ethical risk was that patients would be discharged "sicker and quicker." Is this an unjust outcome? Does it matter that the injustice would be randomly distributed?

Would the elderly themselves have embraced the DRG system as a fair and reasonable way to control health care costs? More recently, Medicare has relied upon privatization through the development of Medicare Advantage plans. Medicare Advantage plans are less expensive in terms of monthly premium costs compared to traditional Medicare. Medicare Advantage plans "save money" by limiting the range of discounted providers that plan members can use. They also tend to rely upon substantial front-end deductibles. Medicare Advantage plans are attractive to the healthy elderly. The elderly with more costly chronic conditions stay with the traditional Medicare program and supplement it with a Medigap policy. That means that the traditional Medicare program is perceived as being more costly, thereby creating the illusion that these Advantage plans are really more efficient.

The justice-relevant policy question is this: What would happen if Congress suddenly dissolved the traditional Medicare program and declared that everyone had to find a Medicare Advantage program willing to accept them. What would the cost of those programs then become? Would Medicare raise the premium paid to these programs to reflect that most of these individuals had more health problems and much greater health care costs? This sounds like a speculative academic question. However, in 2017, Speaker of the House Paul Ryan was pushing legislation that would convert all of Medicare into a "defined contribution" program (Sprung, 2016). The goal was to reduce the cost of the Medicare program by $1 trillion over a 10-year period.

Recall that in a strict sense Medicare has no annual budget. However, with a defined contribution approach, Medicare would have a fixed budget. Medicare would divide up some fixed sum of federal funds into "vouchers" for each Medicare recipient. Recipients would then go into the marketplace to purchase a private insurance plan that met the core benefit requirements established by Medicare. Each year Medicare would determine a medical inflation number for the coming year but then reduce that number by 1%, the announced goal being to motivate insurance companies and health care providers to find more efficient ways to deliver health care services. However, after a number of years, the actual effect of this process would be to reduce the "purchasing power" of that voucher, thereby requiring Medicare recipients to supplement with their own funds the value of the voucher in order to pay for a private Medicare plan (Komisar, 2017). This actually represents cost-shifting to the Medicare population. This would mean access to needed health care would be increasingly determined by individual ability to pay. This would be especially problematic regarding the targeted cancer therapies and immunotherapies that define precision medicine as well as many other very expensive, life-prolonging therapies. In effect, Medicare would reflect the ethical flaws characteristic of employer-based private health insurance.

Could the vouchers be risk-adjusted to reflect the likely health care needs of elderly individuals with preexisting chronic degenerative medical conditions? Without risk adjustment, these individuals would have vouchers that no insurance company would accept. Consequently, insurance companies would build in care limits for those chronically ill individuals, thereby either forcing individuals to pay more for their care or to deny themselves that care, as would likely be the case for these costly targeted cancer therapies. This would again be a form of invisible rationing. Neither Congress nor insurers were explicitly denying access to needed health care for anyone.

Instead, individuals would be denying themselves needed health care because of their limited ability to pay.

How would the risk-adjusted value of a voucher for an individual be determined? This would be an annual event for every Medicare patient to reflect their changing health circumstances. Imagine, for example, a patient in late-stage heart failure who could easily be predicted to need a left ventricular assist device (LVAD) in the coming year at a cost of $250,000. What would be the risk-adjusted value of that voucher? It certainly would not be $250,000. Would an insurer agree to accept a $25,000 voucher to insure that individual, with the understanding that that individual would be responsible for half the costs of the LVAD, should they choose that option?

In earlier chapters, we noted the outrageously high prices attached to the targeted cancer therapies. Most European countries pay substantially less for prescription drugs than we do in the United States. They bargain as a country with the pharmaceutical companies. Germany, for example, has 80 million covered lives, which gives them considerable bargaining power. Medicare represents 47 million covered lives, which represents considerable bargaining power as well. However, Congress passed a law in 2003, the Medicare Modernization Act, that forbade Medicare from bargaining as a unit, thereby protecting the profit margins of those companies at Medicare expense. Likewise, that same law forbade Medicare from using the cost-effectiveness of a drug as a basis for excluding it from the Medicare formulary. As long as a drug was safe and marginally effective, Medicare would have to cover it. Pharmaceutical companies, consequently, have enormous latitude to price their drugs as they wish. The Congressional Budget Office estimates that if House Resolution 3 had been passed by Congress in 2019, Medicare would have saved $345 billion in prescription drug costs for the period 2023–2029 (Cubanski et al., 2019). Over 10 years we would get half that trillion dollars in savings that Paul Ryan was seeking without engaging in the ethically problematic forms of invisible rationing integral to the Ryan plan.

What conclusions should we draw from this review of cost-control efforts?

(1) Fragmented financing of health care means fragmented, insecure, inequitable access to needed health care. Is it fair that access to needed and effective health care should depend upon the whims of workplace chief executive officers (CEOs), insurance executives, Medicaid directors, or legislative bodies?

(2) Fragmented financing means fragmented, invisible, unaccountable, inequitable efforts to control health care costs. Fragmented financing permits all manner of cost-shifting, most often to those who are medically and financially among the less well off.

(3) Fragmented financing will often mean that those with the greatest health needs will have the least secure access to needed health care since such patients represent a threat to the profitability and/or financial solvency of the companies responsible for financing health care access. Fragmented financing also has the untoward effect of pitting relatively healthy patients against patients with persistent costly health care needs. The question many relatively healthy individuals will pose to themselves is, "Why should I, in very good health (as a result of good fortune as opposed to assiduous efforts to make good health choices), have to pay for the costly health needs of others by being in the same health plan as them when I am certain their poor health status is the result of their own irresponsible health choices?"

A Canadian-style single-payer system has the moral advantage of affirming that "we are all in this together." That does mean addressing the "tragedy of the commons." Participants can collectively discuss rationally what they would regard as a reasonable (just and affordable) health care benefit package guaranteed to all, both their currently healthy selves and their future possible selves afflicted with many possible costly chronic degenerative conditions. This is impossible in our current highly fragmented system for financing health care and controlling health care costs. In our current system individuals must simply accept whatever is offered as a health benefit package by an employer or a state Medicaid program. Medicare does offer choices in the form of Medicare Advantage options, but those are options for the relatively healthy elderly. However, this does nothing to encourage conversation among the elderly as a whole regarding whether this represents the fairest way of meeting the health care needs of the elderly *and* controlling health care costs. On the contrary, what is created are self-interested silos of health care financing intended to exclude those with the most serious and costly health needs. This is an ethically problematic outcome because all of our wicked problems of health care justice are left to fester, mostly at the expense of those with the greatest health needs who will be the victims of various forms of invisible rationing.

5.3. The Just Caring Problem: A Quick Review

Let me summarize the argument of the book so far. We are faced with the "just caring" problem. We have limited resources (money) and unlimited health care needs. We ought to be meeting genuine health care needs for whoever has those needs because otherwise those individuals suffer unnecessarily and are at risk of dying prematurely. This is a matter of equal concern and respect. However, meeting those needs has become increasingly costly, in part because the volume of needs has grown dramatically with constant medical innovation.

If these costly medical innovations were curative, we would have a strong moral obligation to find the money needed. However, the vast majority of these medical innovations are "halfway technologies," representing limited medical success (i.e., prolonging life of diminished quality for a number of years that require costly and constant medical attention). More problematic are those medical innovations that are successful for a small number of patients but that are extraordinarily costly and yield only relatively small benefits for the vast majority of patients.

These last few sentences characterize perfectly precision medicine. For the most part, precision medicine involves targeted cancer therapies and immunotherapies for patients with a terminal prognosis and no other life-prolonging options. These patients are among the medically least well off and most deserving of a compassionate response. However, in the current fragmented system for financing health care in the United States access to these targeted therapies will be arbitrary and uncertain. Is that fair? Is that just?

Cancer is not our only costly life-threatening medical problem; literally hundreds of other diseases make similar claims on social resources, which is why we are faced with a tragedy of the commons. Not all of those claims can be met, which is the problem of health care rationing. How can we adjudicate justly among all these claims when we are faced with a number of wicked problems of health care justice?

To further complicate matters, the various conceptions of health care justice discussed above are all reasonable but nevertheless inadequate to address the very complex problems of health care justice generated by precision medicine. To put my position briefly, there is no "most just" resolution of these problems, only competing, reasonable, morally relevant considerations that must be considered. Trade-offs among these considerations need to be thoughtfully assessed. What we seek is a reasonable balance among these competing considerations, something "roughly just." More than one reasonable balancing of these considerations is possible, which also implies that other balancings will be flawed, as a matter of justice.

In the real world (as opposed to a world of philosophic hypotheticals), choices have to be made within a limited period of time. These are social choices, policy choices. Given the nature of health care, these choices can affect anyone and everyone. Consequently, such choices ought to be a product of fair and inclusive processes of rational democratic deliberation so that the results are "just enough," legitimate enough, reasonable enough, stable enough, and autonomously imposed. We turn now to a fuller explication of what that must mean in practice.

5.4. Public Reason: The Core of Rational Democratic Deliberation

At the core of our conception of rational democratic deliberation should be the notion of *public reason* as articulated by John Rawls (1996). For Rawls this notion applies to controversies regarding constitutional essentials and the basic structure of society. However, I will argue that the "just caring" problem should be thought of as being part of the basic structure of society. The need for effective health care is more fundamental than the need for food or economic support.

Rawls has three parts to his two fundamental principles of justice: equal basic rights and liberties for all, fair equality of opportunity, and the difference principle. Daniels (1985) has (in my judgment) correctly built a general argument for the just claims to needed health care that all have on the basis of Rawls' fair equality of opportunity aspect of justice as fairness, as discussed in section 4.9 above. One of the virtues of Daniels' account is that it does connect with Rawls' difference principle. In other words, some inequalities in access to needed health care are not unjust. Which inequalities might those be? We need rational democratic deliberation to address that question. Likewise, the first principle of justice for Rawls states that "each person has an equal claim to a fully adequate scheme of equal basic rights and liberties" (Rawls, 1996, at 5). Again, what does that mean with respect to needed health care? This too needs to be worked out, defined, and legitimated, through our fair and inclusive process of rational democratic deliberation.

Next, we consider Rawls' notion of political liberalism. "How is it possible that there may exist over time a stable and just society of free and equal citizens profoundly divided by reasonable religious, philosophical and moral doctrines" (Rawls, 1996, at xxvii)? Given this description, how is it possible to have a process of rational democratic deliberation that can effectively address the "just caring" problem in general or in relation to the complexities associated with precision medicine and our wicked problems? Would we have nothing but unending contentiousness? How does one work around that contentiousness?

Rawls' most fundamental insight in response to this last question is that we need a *political* conception of justice. Such a conception is *free-standing*, which is to say that it is not attached to any comprehensive religious, philosophic, or moral doctrine. Consequently, Rawls admits that "justice as fairness," as presented in *A Theory of Justice* (1971), was attached to a comprehensive doctrine, Kantian constructivism. In *Political Liberalism* Rawls (1996) seeks to redescribe "justice as fairness" as a free-standing *political* conception of justice. I believe the same can be accomplished with respect to health care justice. It can be articulated and justified as a free-standing *political* conception of justice.

Public reason is the stance all of us are capable of adopting when we think of ourselves as *citizens as such* who need to solve fundamental political problems with our fellow citizens. When we think of ourselves simply as citizens, we are not thinking of ourselves as Catholics or utilitarians or Kantians or as committed to any other reasonable comprehensive doctrine. There is nothing intrinsically illegitimate or objectionable about any reasonable comprehensive doctrine. One of the defining features of a liberal society is that it embraces a reasonable pluralism with respect to how individuals choose to live, what they choose to believe, and what they choose to value.[2] Liberalism takes the view that there is no one ordering of values or way of living that is superior to every other possible ordering of values or way of living. This requires an understanding of toleration that allows for mutual respect, in spite of these differing orderings of values and ways of living. This is primarily accomplished through a mutual commitment to a political conception of justice which, in effect, establishes the boundaries for what can be regarded as reasonable orderings of values and reasonable ways of life.

---

[2] Rawls credits Joshua Cohen (1993) with introducing him to the notion of a "reasonable pluralism" as opposed to a simple pluralism of comprehensive doctrines. Fanatics of whatever stripe tend to place themselves "beyond reason" and "beyond being reasonable."

How do we imagine achieving that mutual commitment to a political conception of health care justice? We must be willing to be *reasonable* citizens. Rawls writes: "Citizens are reasonable when, viewing one another as free and equal in a system of social cooperation over generations, they are prepared to offer one another fair terms of cooperation (defined by principles and ideals) and they agree to act on those terms, even at the cost of their own interests in particular situations, provided others also accept those terms" (1996, at xliv). Rawls refers to this as "reciprocity." Reciprocity is about mutual respect, not seeking to take advantage of another. No one, as a citizen, has superior rights or liberties relative to any other citizen. We are engaged in a system of social cooperation that will span generations, namely, our political system. This is not a short-term contract, and everyone is included.

Our political system is what Rawls describes as a "social union of social unions" (Rawls, 1971, at 527). Quite literally, in the United States today there are hundreds of thousands of social groups that interact in complex ways to form this social union of social unions. Though these groups are often enough both cooperative and in conflict with one another, the social union as a whole is stable and reasonably peaceful. This is because relations among all these groups are governed by a shared political conception of justice as well as some range of public interests and public values that are also divorced from any particular comprehensive doctrine but nevertheless capable of being endorsed as reasonable by virtually all reasonable comprehensive doctrines.

What binds this social union together is a commitment to fair terms of cooperation. We have to start by imagining ourselves as free and equal citizens *and nothing more*. That is the common role we all share. This is what Rawls represents with his thought experiment of everyone behind the veil of ignorance. Behind that veil of ignorance, we are not Catholics or Protestants or Buddhists or atheists. We are not Democrats or Republicans. We are not liberals or conservatives. We are neither men nor women. We are not heterosexual or homosexual or asexual or bisexual. We have no idea how long we might live. We have no idea what our health status might be at various points in a whole life. We have no idea what diseases or disabilities we might be afflicted with. We do not know whether we might have to struggle with psychiatric disorders of one sort or another. We have no idea what our level of educational attainment might be or what sort of work life we might have. We have no idea what our level of wealth or income might be at various points in our life. We do not know whether we will marry and have children.

In spite of all this ignorance, we also have an enormous amount of knowledge. We know (collectively) everything known today in all of medicine, in all of the different areas of science (physical, biological, social), including all the possible options for designing political and economic systems. We know the full diversity of religious and philosophic perspectives. We know the full range of life opportunities, accessible by skill, constrained by chance. We know we want to live in a liberal society. Consequently, we want to define a specific list of rights and liberties assured to all.

There are all sorts of beliefs and life choices that I believe are ridiculous or embarrassing or clearly false. I am certain Hinduism is not a true religion; the same is true for Zoroastrianism. People waste an enormous amount of time on Facebook and Twitter. Those platforms really need to be very heavily regulated; they are cesspools of stupidity. Of course, if I take more seriously my role as a liberal citizen, I quickly realize that numerous fellow citizens have similar feelings of disgust regarding some of my beliefs and practices. I would clearly resent their using the political process to constrain my ability to engage in practices I enjoyed but that they found worthless or disgusting. I enjoy a very good steak, but I can see how vegetarians would have serious objections to this bit of indulgence. Consequently, I realize it would be wrong to use the policymaking process to outlaw Hinduism or atheism or pantheism or meat-eating or any other reasonable social practice or reasonable comprehensive doctrine. Such efforts would be contrary to my being a liberal citizen.

This is a political conception of justice because it is free-standing; it is not connected to any particular comprehensive doctrine, but it would be supported by all reasonable comprehensive doctrines because, in effect, it protects those comprehensive doctrines and their adherents from being discriminated against with respect to any of their basic rights and liberties. Justice as fairness protects equally all of these comprehensive doctrines that accept those same protections for what we might regard as their rivals. Likewise, what everyone behind the veil of ignorance would realize is that effective life opportunities will require substantive rights or welfare rights that would remove or minimize obstacles to fair competition for desirable social positions. In contemporary American society, this will require access to quality educational opportunities as well as quality health care for those whose opportunities would otherwise be severely constrained by an untreated health problem for which there were effective therapeutic interventions.

Rawls' difference principle allows differences in income, wealth, social status, and so on, as long as the basic structure of society is organized in such a way that those who are least well off are made as well off as possible, given efforts to enhance the well-being of society as a whole. More specifically, if some form of capitalism can maximize the wealth of a society by motivating and releasing the creative energies of entrepreneurs and if those creative energies bring about the economic destruction of some enterprises, then we need to have in place welfare policies that will assure an adequate standard of living for all who are adversely affected by this sort of social and economic dynamism. It would clearly be unjust to permit economic activity that left those already less well off even worse off while allowing those very well off financially to become extraordinarily well off. It would be equally unjust if individuals did have jobs but were reduced to being "wage slaves" (as Marx uses that term). That too would represent a diminishment of their status as free and equal citizens. Again, the values that are represented by the difference principle are free-standing political values, not attached as such to any comprehensive doctrine. They are values that can be endorsed by any reasonable comprehensive doctrine. These are the values that provide substantive content to public reason.

At the end of this discussion behind the veil of ignorance, what motivates all the participants to endorse Rawls' conception of justice as fairness? This was a reasonable and a *rational* choice to make. To say it was a *rational* choice is to say that it was a matter of self-interest. This might at first sound odd because everyone is behind a veil of ignorance. However, they do have self-interests that are attached to being citizens as such, liberal self-interests. These exist at a high level of abstraction. To illustrate, one liberal self-interest would be my right to change my life goals or to change my allegiances to particular associations or to change my fundamental beliefs (i.e., give up being a Catholic to become a Buddhist). I would also be mindful of the frequent role of chance in determining how my life might go. I could be in a horrible accident that left me largely paralyzed and unable to earn money through work. I would still want to live; I could still imagine ways in which I could enjoy life. But I would want to know that my most basic needs for food and shelter and health care would be securely met. Hence, I would want a conception of justice that assured the creation of the basic structure of society that would provide for my welfare needs. If additional motivation were needed for embracing justice as fairness, then imagine all 330 million Americans behind the veil of ignorance being randomly allocated to the 330 million vacant "life slots" at the conclusion of deliberations. This is how the difference principle gets endorsed.

How does this Rawlsian perspective apply to the justice-relevant challenges raised by precision medicine and the targeted cancer therapies? One of the standard criticisms made of Rawls' veil of ignorance experiment is that it has no application to the real world. No one can literally put themselves behind a veil of ignorance. However, the vast majority of us are behind a health care veil of ignorance at most points in our life. We have no idea what particular diseases or disorders or accidents might befall us. Certainly, as I write, no one imagined in mid-2019 that we might be facing the COVID-19 pandemic in early 2020, including the disruption to our economy, the disruption to our health care system, and the disruption to the health of millions of Americans. Hence, we can ask from behind a health care veil of ignorance what principles of health care justice would we collectively agree to as representing fair access to needed and effective health care, given our overall commitment to mutual respect as free and equal citizens/ patients (vulnerable to an indefinite array of life-threatening or quality of life–diminishing health problems).

Rawls initiates his thought experiment with the empirical truth that as citizens we are part of a political society for generations as we seek to work out fair terms of cooperation. This creates a certain kind of stability of expectations. We are all in this together. I will respect your rights and liberties because I trust that you will respect my rights and liberties. However, in the United States, very few people will literally be part of the same system for financing their access to needed health care over the entire course of their lives. One further point: Public reason is about public interests, public goods. In the United States, however, health care is treated as a private commodity. Justice-relevant decisions are made by executives and management teams in these various institutions without any significant input from patients. Moreover, given the huge variety of institutions and insurance products, there is no consistency across all these institutions with regard to justice-relevant considerations that would affect patients.

The rhetoric of a right to health care is a staple at many political rallies. However, that is *just rhetoric* because no practical way exists to make that rhetoric a reality in the current fragmented US health care system. The health care systems in which such democratic deliberation (as I envision it) could meaningfully occur today would be in Canada, the United Kingdom, and many European countries. Our wicked problems remain.

5.5. Public Reason, Precision Medicine, and Wicked Problems

What we want is a political conception of health care justice. How can public reason address the wicked problems related to precision medicine? Public reason includes everything that is medically and scientifically known today. Facts do matter when making many normative judgments. Scientific facts are not embedded in any religious or philosophic doctrine, which is why they are part of public reason.[3] We can say with certainty that an eight-cell embryo has human DNA and is, therefore, a human life form. We cannot say on the basis of scientific evidence that an eight-cell embryo is a person or has a soul. For the same sort of reason, a political conception of health care justice will not be utilitarian or egalitarian or libertarian, and so on.

However, the values that are at the core of those theories can be separated from those theories and are capable of universal agreement by all reasonable persons. Hence, all can agree that all deserve equal concern and respect. That is clearly a defining value in egalitarian theories of justice, but it is a value that can be reasonably embraced by non-egalitarians. Likewise, doing more good for more people can be embraced by any reasonable person as a worthy social value, though it is at the core of a utilitarian conception of health care justice. Embracing that value is not embracing utilitarianism. Understanding the value of individual liberty as a fundamental social value in a liberal society is another value all reasonable persons in a liberal democratic society can embrace without any commitment to libertarianism. These are freestanding social values. Again, everyone ought to be able to enjoy a basic level of well-being, barring irresolvable health challenges. This is why the "least well off," whether for health or financial reasons, are especially deserving of social assistance.

All of these fundamental social values are part of public reason, which is what allows us to talk reasonably with one another about controversial social policies. Two points to note. First, we need democratic deliberation to determine a reasonable balance among these values when there is a conflict among these values in specific circumstances. This occurs because there is a plurality of reasonable values *and no one of these values is intrinsically superior to all*

---

[3] Many people deny various scientific facts, such as plate tectonic theory or the origin of the universe as we know it 13.7 billion years ago or the evolution of species. If their views are rooted in biblical passages or other religious doctrines, then their views deserve only a respectful dismissal from the domain of science and public reason.

these other values. At one point, Rawls observes that the most fundamental conflict of values, given the political history of the United States, is the conflict between liberty and equality. However, this is not a conflict that we can imagine being settled once and for all time, certainly not by philosophers. It needs to be settled in hundreds of very specific contexts that will reflect a complex balancing of liberty-relevant considerations and equality-relevant considerations. This is the fundamental task of public reason and rational democratic deliberation.

Second, public reason has a critical role to play in our public life, but it is not an all-encompassing dominant role. Its scope is limited to addressing conflicts related to our common interests as citizens (i.e., public interests). What counts as a public interest? The integrity of our judicial system is a public interest. In testifying in a court of law, truthfulness is absolutely essential to protecting the integrity of our judicial system. This is an interest that everyone has but that we as individuals are unable to protect on our own. We rely upon all the machinery that defines our judicial system to ensure that value is protected in practice. The judicial system can affect the lives of everyone in fundamental ways, which is why this is a public interest. In contrast, individuals may lie to one another in their personal lives for any number of less than admirable reasons. Such conduct will be unethical but not subject matter for public reason. We always have the right to "un-friend" people who lie to us through Facebook. (I think this is one of those rights constitutional scholars would say is in the "penumbra" of the Constitution.)

Health care and our health care system are also public interests. Again, a public interest is an interest that each and every one of us has that we are unable to protect or manage as individuals. Instead, we need government and public policy to put in place the protections and institutional structures necessary to maintain and enhance that public interest. I have no ability to assess the competence or trustworthiness of physicians and surgeons in whom I might have to place my life. Instead, I have to rely upon all sorts of government or quasi-government agencies to establish standards for the training and licensing of physicians and all other health professionals. Likewise, I have no ability to assess the quality of thousands of drugs available for treating numerous health disorders. I have to rely upon the Food and Drug Administration (FDA) to protect my interest in using only safe and effective drugs. Recall that our health care system is a product of massive public investment in medical research and the training of health professionals. All of this is the result of enormously complex forms of social cooperation. This is what makes the health care system a public good to which all in our society will have presumptive (limited) just claims.

Many will argue that there are inefficiencies in how we are using our health care resources, that we are not spending wisely. Failing to spend wisely is one problem requiring democratic deliberation. More problematic is that we are also failing to spend justly, as our account of wicked problems in our health care system demonstrates. We should emphasize that those two problems, spending wisely and spending justly, are linked with one another. The more we spend unwisely through public programs, such as Medicare and Medicaid, the more disinclined legislators are to expand public health insurance coverage for the currently uninsured and underinsured.

What should the deliberative process look like in practice? Do we imagine it as an adversarial process? That would not have a constructive outcome. How can it not be an adversarial process? I have done large-scale deliberative projects with two National Institutes of Health grants exploring ethics and policy issues related to emerging genetic technologies. I posed to each deliberative group scenarios that were very realistic and that were designed to elicit in the mind of each participant significant internal conflict. If I was successful in doing that, then it did not matter whether an individual would describe themselves as liberal or conservative, Democrat or Republican, religious or non-religious, right-to-life or non-right-to-life. Instead, what emerged through the initial discussion was a shared sense that "this" was a real problem that required a social solution.

I imagined this thought in the mind of each individual: "I am really puzzled by this situation. I know it requires an answer. I do not feel good about any answer that occurs to me off the top of my head. Can anyone suggest how we might think about this problem?" In other words, each individual was open to hearing what others might have to say that might prove constructive. Further, it was clear in the minds of all that a specific problem was not one that individuals could address as individuals; some sort of social resolution was going to be necessary. To illustrate with an example that I actually used in that project, I started with the case of a 26-year-old individual whose father had died of Huntington's. I made sure everyone understood what that disorder was. I explained that this individual knew there was a 50% chance that he would have the disorder as well, that a likely onset would be in his early 40s with a decline toward dementia over 10 to 15 years. I noted that at the time there was a genetic test that would tell this individual whether or not he had the genetic mutation that would result in his being afflicted with Huntington's.

I posed to the audience this statement: "This individual has the right to decide whether or not he wants to take this test, especially if he believes his life would be miserable, were he to receive a positive result. In other words, he has the right to be genetically ignorant about his own genetic fate." I used audience response devices to elicit responses from everyone on a five-point scale. Virtually everyone agreed with the statement: He had a right not to know. Then I asked them whether he had a right to privacy so that he had no moral obligation to reveal to anyone this possible genetic fact about himself. Again, virtual unanimous agreement. Then I said that he did intend to marry and have children. Did he have a moral right to withhold from a future possible marriage partner his possible genetic status? I suggested to participants that the "future possible marriage partner" could be their daughter or sister or good friend, and so on. That created the genuinely confused state of mind in virtually every member of that deliberative group. They had already affirmed his right to not know as well as his right to privacy. But failing to reveal this fact about himself to a potential marriage partner with whom he hoped to have children seemed wrong; it seemed like it was a serious harm.

A whole series of questions emerged in the discussion. How strong was his right to privacy relative to the rights of a future possible marriage partner? Would we say that he *ought* to reveal this fact about himself in this situation, meaning that it would be a good and decent and ethically honorable choice to make? What if she were positive for the BRCA1 gene with the lifetime risk of breast cancer entailed by that genetic fact? There are more than 700 variants of the BRCA1 gene with a lifetime risk of breast cancer in the 40%–85% range. Would she be obligated to reveal that to a future possible marriage partner? How comparable is that to the risks associated with a 50% chance of being positive for Huntington's? If we think of this as an "ethical" matter, would that mean it was up to each individual to decide the right thing to do? That conclusion did not feel right to a substantial majority of these deliberative groups. Where does public policy fit regarding this matter?

I asked each deliberative group whether we should have a law requiring the divulging of some range of genetic information by potential marriage partners to one another. That proposal was very strongly rejected within all the deliberative groups. I would press them on this issue. Was this a serious public health matter, given that future possible children might be adversely affected if individuals were unaware of the risks they posed to future possible children and, consequently, not motivated to consider alternative reproductive options that would protect their reproductive rights as well as the genetic health of future possible children. These considerations did not alter the views of very many. Such a proposed law was too intrusive, too much a threat to individual liberty. I softened the proposal a bit. I reminded them of the law passed in the late 1980s in some number of states that required AIDS counseling/education prior to marriage. This law did not require anyone to do anything other than participate in this counseling session.

I am not trying to recount how all those conversations evolved. Some options elicited strong support, while others elicited strong rejection. No enlightened consensus emerged from these deliberations. That last sentence might be a little misleading. We did not achieve agreement on our Huntington case. Keep in mind this was just one case of many that were discussed. There were seven deliberative groups in seven cities in Michigan. Each group met 12 times for two hours with a different discussion agenda each evening, so there was only limited time for considering each scenario. However, what is important is that the deliberative process was mutually educational and constructive.

There was not a single instance of yelling, screaming, or disrespect at any of the deliberative sites, though all the issues we discussed were controversial. I should mention that we deliberately sought to recruit individuals beforehand who might hold strong opinions on some of these genetic issues, such as right-to-life individuals or individuals with various disabilities. In spite of the diversity of perspectives represented in each group, civility prevailed. Public reason proved to be possible. Public reason proved to be more than just a philosopher's chimera.

No one's life was going to be altered for better or worse in these deliberative sessions. However, sometimes decisions need to be made with life-altering consequences. Consider the allocation of intensive care unit (ICU) beds or vents or vaccines during a pandemic when demand exceeds a limited supply. A fair policy is absolutely essential; it would be unconscionable and irresponsible to try to make up something "on the fly" as patients are admitted to the hospital. It would be equally unconscionable and irresponsible to simply allow each attending to admit or remove patients from the ICU on the basis of their personal medical and moral judgment. The ICU is a shared, public resource; some shared sense of health care justice is necessary to make these allocation decisions. Rawls is correct; just policies and procedures must be public. Nothing needs to be hidden. Still, politicians generally fear such public decisions. Could such conflicts be better managed if deliberative practices were an integral part of our political system?[4]

What should we expect if we were to have broad-based public deliberation regarding our wicked rationing problems? I will argue that we need to have these public conversations, no matter how politically and socially painful they might be. Some politicians might wish to deny that the rationing problem is real. However, it is real but mostly hidden from public view, which is why politicians can easily choose to ignore it.

In the United States, rationing is mostly accomplished through individual ability to pay. Insured individuals faced with very high co-pays or deductibles deny themselves needed and effective health care. A treatable cancer may go undiagnosed and untreated until it has become metastatic, resulting in an unnecessary and unjust premature death (Wharam et al., 2018). What public interest is satisfied by allowing such outcomes to occur, as if they were not preventable? Alternatively, what public interests are violated by allowing such outcomes to occur? Is such an outcome congruent with the equal concern and respect that we owe to all members of our society?

It is disingenuous to contend that individuals in these circumstances have made these autonomous choices themselves. These individuals had no actual choice to make. This example helps to make clear the value of rational democratic deliberation as a mechanism for determining the just claims to needed health care in a world with limited resources. More precisely, a fair, inclusive, well-structured process of rational democratic deliberation will yield more just judgments of health care justice than judgments made by private insurers (seeking to maximize profits) or legislators (seeking to not incur the wrath of taxpayers).

5.6. An Outline of a Fair Deliberative Process

The basic elements of a *fair* deliberative process will include everything we have said so far regarding public reason.

---

[4] In the pandemic of 2020–21 extracorporeal membrane oxygenation [ECMO] was in extreme shortage at many major medical centers, though there was little public awareness of this fact (Fink, 2021).

(1) Participants need to see themselves simply as *citizens*, as opposed to seeing themselves as liberals or conservatives, as CEOs or professors, as religious or irreligious, and so on.

(2) Participants need to be mindful of the fact that they are deliberating behind a health care veil of ignorance.

(3) Participants need to be reminded that they care about the well-being of many others in their lives (i.e., family members, friends, co-workers, acquaintances in a variety of social groups, and so on), all vulnerable to future health crises.

(4) Participants need to be reminded that all citizens as citizens are entitled to equal concern and respect. The health care needs of any citizen in our society are just as important as the health care needs of any member of my family or of my dearest friends.

(5) The process itself must be *inclusive*. We must assure fair representation of racial and ethnic minorities. That is *one* important sense of being inclusive. The more important sense, however, for purposes of a fair deliberative process is that it includes a diversity of reasonable political, economic, ethical, religious, and sociocultural perspectives. The deliberative process needs to address that complex mix of issues that represent the "just caring" problem. The goal of this deliberative project is to identify fair and reasonable health care rationing protocols justified by considered judgments of health care justice that reasonable citizens *as citizens* can accept. Those rationing protocols could apply to any of the deliberators depending upon their future health status and the future health status of those they care about. Again, the deliberative process is intended to yield freely self-imposed rationing protocols. If the deliberative process is not sufficiently inclusive, then non-included sorts of individuals can justly complain that these rationing protocols will be imposed upon them without their rational consent. Still, ardent racists or other fanatics who are incapable of endorsing the idea that all in our society are entitled to equal concern and respect are justifiably excluded.

(6) Participants need to be reminded that health care is a public good and a public interest created through shared investment. Still, it is a limited resource, while health care needs are expansive and enormously heterogeneous. This is what generates an extraordinarily complex problem of health care justice that needs to be addressed through this public, democratic, deliberative process.

(7) A fair approach to health care cost containment and rationing will have to be public or explicit, rationally justifiable, autonomously imposed, and impartially generated and applied (as opposed to being a product of interest group politics and power). The publicity condition is what Rawls sees as the core of any conception of justice. When public interests are at stake, nothing should be hidden. The avoidable, premature death of individuals is a public interest whether that death is a result of opioid addiction or an unaffordable co-pay or deductible which prevents access to effective life-saving care.

For both insurers and politicians, it is socially convenient that individuals unable to pay for effective cancer care die what looks like an unfortunate natural death, a private event that will merit an obituary but no problematic public attention. The political/psychological advantage of this approach to health care rationing is that the outcomes of these mechanisms are widely dispersed, uncertain of application to any individual patient, and invisible to any form of public scrutiny. In addition, any bad outcome is directly attributable to a choice made by an individual. This is a matter of personal responsibility, or at least that is the preferred view of insurers and politicians. However, I argue this is fundamentally unjust. Such outcomes ought to be public and explicit so that they can be thoughtfully and fairly assessed through a democratic deliberative process.

Among academics, philosophers, and political scientists, there has been considerable discussion regarding the virtues of democratic deliberation (Bachtiger et al., 2018; Gutmann and Thompson, 1996, 2003, 2004; Bohman and Rehg, 1997; Cohen, 1997; Estlund, 2008; Christiano, 1997; Richardson, 2002; Goodin, 2003; Gaus, 1997). However, no broad political movement has been ignited that would make such broad deliberation an integral part of the political landscape. This is worth some comment. The likelihood is that many of us will be rescued from death several times by contemporary medicine, and these rescues will be very costly. We will be rescued from both our first and second heart attacks, from two or more bouts of cancer, from a significant stroke, and from kidney failure. Of course, in medicine the word "rescue" is highly relativized; it is not like being rescued from a mountaintop, after which I go on to live a full and normal life. Each of these life-threatening events leaves an individual somewhat more debilitated. Most often, the first event is the beginning of a chronic downhill course that might be extraordinarily prolonged. Are all of us entitled to every rescue effort that is medically possible, no matter the costs or probability of success? We want choices to be made that are just and compassionate and cost-effective.

We have handed off responsibility for making these hard choices to insurance companies or to Medicare. These institutions are the managers of the health care commons. However, when they deny us health care interventions which we desperately want for ourselves or our loved ones, we are outraged. We are certain that we are being treated unjustly. This is where we need to be reminded of Buchanan's point in an important essay (1998). Buchanan, in effect, asks, "What precisely is the understanding of justice to which all these aggrieved individuals are appealing?" Have we had a social conversation in which we have come to a rich and nuanced and comprehensive social understanding of the conception of health care justice that we want to govern these very difficult situations where rationing and cost-control decisions must be made?

We object that decisions by insurance companies are often arbitrary, discriminatory, uncaring, and unfair. But this is disingenuous since we (citizens/future possible patients) have taken no responsibility for providing them with any guidance regarding how we believe these decisions ought to be made. We cannot provide that guidance if *we ourselves* have failed to engage in the deliberative conversations that would provide just and legitimate guidance to those insurance companies.

(8) A fair democratic deliberative process requires a commitment by all to reciprocity. Reciprocity is about cooperation among free and equal citizens, all of whom are equally worthy of respect. Rawls writes: "Cooperation involves the idea of fair terms of cooperation: these are terms that each participant may reasonably accept, provided that everyone else likewise accepts them. Fair terms of cooperation specify an idea of reciprocity: all who are engaged in cooperation and who do their part as the rules and procedure require, are to benefit in an appropriate way as assessed by a suitable benchmark of comparison" (1996, at 16). A commitment to reciprocity will mean that the same comprehensive package of health care benefits will be guaranteed to all in our society. In addition, the same set of rationing protocols will establish just limits with respect to that health care benefit package. Because we have to give one another reasons that are mutually acceptable for including or excluding any particular health service in particular clinical circumstances and because we ourselves

will have to live with the future consequences of our choices and because the deliberative process itself will educate us about the range and likelihood of various health vulnerabilities and because we all have bonds of affection and capacities for compassion that link us in complex ways to numerous others throughout society with a broad range of health problems and needs (thereby helping to correct excessive attention to our narrow health self-interests), a suitably managed deliberative process will likely yield "fair enough" terms of cooperation that are congruent with the requirements of one of the constitutional principles of health care justice, namely, the reciprocity principle. If the deliberative procedures and deliberative principles outlined here are scrupulously adhered to, it is very difficult to imagine how a rationing protocol that disadvantaged unjustly some identifiable group in our society would be legitimated as fair. The flip side of that concern is unfairly advantaging some distinct group, which, as we shall see, is a potential problem in the case of cancer patients and precision medicine.

How does it happen that some distinct group is advantaged or disadvantaged with regard to accessing costly innovative technologies? Recall a story from the 1990s regarding autologous bone marrow transplants in connection with breast cancer. At the time, this experimental intervention cost $150,000 per case. The belief was that this intervention might offer women a 10% chance of three-year survival. Insurance companies would deny these women coverage because the procedure was experimental. Women who were well educated and assertive threatened to bring in the media through their lawyers to embarrass these insurance companies. The tactic worked, at least for 41,000 women (Mello and Brennan, 2001). But the outcome was hundreds of millions of dollars in wasted resources and multiple injustices. Women who were more passive and less well educated simply accepted their fate. Should a just and caring society tolerate that outcome? Should the media be proud of itself for being the champion (only) of educated and assertive women?

One of the other consequences of the success of these women is that clinical trials aimed at definitively establishing the therapeutic value of these bone marrow transplants took extraordinarily long to complete. When the trials were completed and reported in 2001, this intervention proved to be no better than conventional, less costly therapies (Stadtmaurer et al., 2000). This lesson has gotten little attention outside academic circles, thereby undermining the need for a comprehensive deliberative conversation about health care justice, as opposed to isolated incidents that elicit media attention and (misguided) public sympathy.

We are faced with essentially the same problem with regard to these targeted cancer therapies. The clinical trials have been completed for many of these targeted cancer therapies, but the modest results are still hyped to the media, thereby generating exaggerated hope in the broad public (Horgan, 2020).[5] This "news" is followed by multiple television ads, as well as glossy ads in prominent medical journals, that drive home messages about the exaggerated effectiveness of these drugs.

(9) The results of the deliberative process must be *rationally justifiable* to all who would be affected by those results. Bohman (1996) offers a useful summative characterization of what he refers to as "public deliberation." It is "a dialogical process of exchanging reasons for the purpose of resolving problematic situations that cannot be settled without interpersonal coordination and cooperation" (at 27). This is a *dialogical* process. It is a process of democratic (public) inquiry focused on what is judged to be a public problem. Again, it is a public problem because a *public interest* is at stake. A public interest is something we all value that we cannot adequately advance or protect *unless we cooperate with one another to fashion a common resolution.*

The deliberative process should not be an adversarial process. Achieving the appropriate frame of mind in all participants requires presenting the rationing issue in a way that generates internal confusion within each participant, thereby motivating them to seek the help of others. Ultimately, a *practical* task must be accomplished, as opposed to a purely intellectual task. In the deliberative process we are not seeking truth; *we are seeking to construct a resolution to a public problem.* Often, there will be multiple possible resolutions for such problems, but each possible resolution represents a different mix of different values with a different set of consequences for different groups of individuals (though these are hypothetical patient groups in the

---

[5] Horgan concludes, "Physicians cannot bring about a shift toward conservative cancer medicine on their own. We consumers must help them." I take this as another endorsement for greater efforts to address these issues through rational democratic deliberation.

future to which current deliberators may or may not ever belong). Assessing these alternative options will typically become the substantive focus of this deliberative process. But, as noted, in a liberal society no single dominant value orders all other values, nor is there some dominant ordering of values that is *the* politically preferred ordering of values. However, when faced with a public problem that requires a cooperative resolution, individuals must find or create public values that *all can rationally endorse* as relevant for re-solving public problems, even if those values are not regarded as being espe-cially important in the private lives of some individuals.

The deliberative process advances *through giving one another reasons* for preferring one resolution over another to a specific public problem. This makes the process rational. Giving reasons to one another is essential to a deliberative process that is mutually respectful of our status as moral agents, as free and equal persons (Daniels and Sabin, 1997, 1998a, 1998b; Gutmann and Thompson, 2003, 2004; Fleck, 1992, 1994). This is the very opposite of a political process that is about using political power to impose one's will on another. Instead, this is about mutual education, mutual persuasion, and shared social problem-solving.

The reasons we give one another must be *public reasons* rooted in reason-able public values or public interests. The perspective we need to adopt is the perspective of citizens committed to preserving and enhancing a liberal plu-ralistic society in which we are all cooperative, mutually respectful members. Even if 90% of the country were Roman Catholic, if we still wanted to main-tain the liberal pluralistic political character of our society, we could not allow papal expectations to be among the reasons that could offer legitimate, reasonable support for or against any specific public policy.[6] Only public reasons can offer public justification for public policies aimed at resolving public problems.

What is characteristic of public reasons is that they can be endorsed as reasonable and legitimate from the perspective of multiple reasonable com-prehensive doctrines (religious and philosophic points of view). This phe-nomenon is what Rawls (1996) refers to as an "overlapping consensus." Such

---

[6] As Rawls would say, in a liberal pluralistic society, one of our two highest interests would be an interest in altering our most fundamental life commitments. That means a liberal pluralistic so-ciety would be committed to protecting the right of Roman Catholics to convert to being Baptists or Buddhists, the right of Republicans to become Social Democrats, and the right of meat lovers to be-come vegetarians.

a consensus is the essence of public reason; it is essential to the stability of a liberal pluralistic society. This is not something that is "given"; rather, it is something that needs to be constructed through sustained rational democratic deliberation (in a way that is analogous to the construction of science and scientific reason over the past 400 years as well as law and legal reason). What an overlapping consensus means is that adherents of diverse comprehensive doctrines can find reasons within their own comprehensive doctrines for supporting a broad range of public values that transcend all comprehensive doctrines (i.e., are neutral or agnostic with respect to the truth claims of those doctrines). This is what makes possible the creation of a political framework that is respectful of all reasonable comprehensive doctrines, where "reasonable" captures the idea that these comprehensive doctrines are respectful of other "reasonable" comprehensive doctrines, all of which endorse the social values and social practices that are integral to sustaining a liberal pluralistic democratic society.[7]

Justification of specific public policies occurs at two levels. The first is the level of the social values endorsed in that overlapping consensus. The second level is that of specific comprehensive doctrines. No doubt it will often enough be the case that specific public policies will not be endorsable from the perspective of a specific comprehensive doctrine; for example, orthodox Roman Catholics will not likely support public funding for pre-implantation genetic diagnosis aimed at identifying embryos harboring deleterious genetic mutations. Still, Roman Catholics could respect such a policy as reasonable and legitimate from the point of view of social values that were part of the overlapping consensus integral to the character of a liberal pluralistic society.[8]

Showing this sort of respect and acceptance would not be easy, especially for orthodox Catholics. Some reminders might elicit a tolerant response. Recall the Lakeberg conjoined twins case (Thomasma et al., 1996). These infants were born sharing a six-chamber heart. They were treated at Loyola

---

[7] This is what Joshua Cohen refers to as the "reasonable consensus test." For a fuller explanation and justification of the point I am making in this sentence, see Cohen's essay "Moral Pluralism and Political Consensus" (1993).

[8] A recent illustration of my point has to do with public funding for embryonic stem cell research that would use "excess embryos" from fertility clinics as sources of these embryonic stem cells. A number of prominent advocates for a strict right-to-life perspective have endorsed these policy proposals as being congruent with a "pro-life" position. Senator Orrin Hatch (R-Utah) would be one such example. The research offers the hope of cures for Alzheimer's disease and spinal cord injuries and other medically devastating disorders that severely diminish either length of life or quality of life.

University's Medical Center in Chicago. What was clear was that the twins could not survive beyond a year while sharing that malformed heart. The parents were uninsured and wanted everything done to save the lives of their twins. The only possible surgery required the surgical reconstruction of that malformed heart into a more normal heart that would go to one of the twins. That meant one twin had to be killed (a harsh term, admittedly) in order to have a 1% chance of saving the life of the other twin. This was going to involve radically innovative surgery. Loyola refused to do the surgery. The institution was ethically opposed to killing one twin to save the other. They also objected to the fact that their charity fund could be depleted by $1 million to cover the cost of surgery and recovery. They noted that they served the needs of an impoverished community on the west side of Chicago, that much more health good would be accomplished by addressing the certain needs of that community as opposed to spending it on a 1% chance of saving one twin. I bring up this example because, at one level, Loyola was appealing to recognized Catholic values but, at another level, the values could be endorsed by any reasonable liberal citizen. This is the sort of outcome that can be produced through a fair and well-constructed process of rational democratic deliberation.

What we need to articulate through the deliberative process are shared considered judgments of health care justice (reasons) that would justify various rationing protocols. Those reasons, however, will have legitimate persuasive power only if they are public reasons, only if they can be part of an overlapping consensus, only if they are sufficiently detached from any comprehensive doctrine. As citizen deliberators we are free and equal persons who must be mutually respectful in order to sustain in practice fair terms of cooperation. Mutual respect is about reciprocity; if a particular social rule that is constitutive of fair terms of cooperation binds you to behave in a certain way in certain circumstances, then I am equally bound by that rule in those circumstances.

Schauer (1995) gives a concise characterization of what the process of reason-giving is about in these deliberative contexts. He writes, "Just as making a promise induces reasonable reliance, giving a reason creates a prima facie commitment" (at 649). If I assert that it would be unjust and uncaring for you (my fellow citizens) to allow me to die from an inflamed appendix at risk of rupturing, then I am making the implicit claim that it would be unjust and uncaring for our society to allow *anyone* to die under those circumstances.

5.7. Just Caring: An Illustrative Example of Democratic Deliberation

How can our deliberative process yield outcomes (access and rationing protocols) that are just and legitimate? How expansive should a set of health benefits be that would be guaranteed to all in our society as a matter of justice? We started with treatment for appendicitis. No morally relevant plausible public reason could be given for denying anyone access to that needed treatment. We can justifiably generalize from this point: If anyone's life is threatened by a curable or ameliorable medical condition and we have available an effective and costworthy medical intervention that can save that person's life with an acceptable level of functioning, then justice requires that we assure access to such medical interventions for all in our society. This is what health policy analysts would refer to as "high-value" care (Moriates et al., 2015; Hausman, 2015).

Someone could argue for a more expansive generalization that would be some version of Daniels' (1985) fair equality of opportunity account of health care justice. In effect, the point would be that "bare life" (as in persistent vegetative state [PVS]) would not be judged by most of us as being worthy of special moral status. What counts, morally speaking, is protecting our capacity to function effectively. So the more general principle we ought to endorse would be: If practically significant functional abilities are threatened by a curable or ameliorable medical condition and we have available an effective and costworthy medical intervention that can save or restore those functional abilities, then justice requires that we assure access to such medical interventions for all in our society.

Both these generalizations will have fuzzy and controversial edges: What would be the minimal gain in life expectancy or functional capacity that would reasonably justify providing this life-saving or function-restoring technology, especially if it is very costly? Think of any of our wicked problems. Consider spending $475,000 at the front end for chimeric antigen receptor (CAR) T-cell therapy for some type of leukemia when we have a biomarker that predicts with 90% confidence that this patient will not survive a year. Or think of the $700,000 first-year rehabilitative costs associated with aiding someone who has become quadriplegic as a result of an accident. What would be the degree of effectiveness below 100% that would be the minimum necessary to reasonably justify our commitment to providing this technology? Think about the Lakeberg conjoined twin case where the cost was in excess of $1 million for a 1% chance of saving the life of one of the twins through surgical reconstruction of a six-chamber heart. Think about providing access to imiglucerase for Gaucher's disease at $300,000 per patient per year for an indefinite number of years. Or think about a number of drugs comparable to imiglucerase that are comparably costly and comparably effective for Pompe disease or Fabry or cystic fibrosis or hemophilia. This is precisely appropriate subject matter for the deliberative process. No experts can tell us the right thing to do with medical interventions in these fuzzy areas (though the deliberative process needs medical or scientific expertise). Empirical data will sometimes be helpful but not yield unique correct choices. Lots of possible choices within these fuzzy areas would become "just enough" if there is sufficient reasonable democratic agreement about those choices.

This last sentence might trigger the thought that the conception of justice for which we advocate is purely procedural. In other words, as long as the deliberative body is sufficiently inclusive or sufficiently representative, as long as no voices have been inappropriately squelched, as long as there has been no fraud or coercion or deception, then whatever result has been agreed upon will be "just enough" simply by virtue of the agreement being fairly achieved. However, I am not endorsing that conclusion. On the contrary, substantive justice-relevant considerations constrain the conversation in various ways.

Sometimes our reasons and reasoning have no implications beyond a very specific limited context; at other times our reasons and reasoning have spillover effects in a range of contexts. Let me illustrate each possibility. Consider the case of Alice and Betty, both in their early 40s; both need a liver transplant within the next two months, or they will die. We have only one liver to transplant. Alice has other medical problems and will survive only two years with the liver transplant; Betty may survive 20 years. Should we be maximizers or egalitarians in deciding who gets the liver? Should we flip a coin to determine who gets the liver, thereby demonstrating equal respect for the right to life of each? Or should we seek to maximize the medical good achieved for a social investment of $350,000, thereby giving the liver to Betty?

No overwhelmingly powerful arguments require us to go either way. There are good, justice-appropriate reasons for going either way. However, we cannot allow in practice a flip-flop back and forth between these rationales since that would permit all manner of morally irrelevant features of individuals to be determinative of an outcome, thereby masking injustices with a justice-relevant rationale. We need a social rule that says we will be either consistent maximizers or consistent egalitarians in such circumstances. The choice we make *in this very limited context* does not seem to have obvious implications for other medical contexts requiring distributional judgments with life-sustaining consequences.

Here is another transplant example that deserves more careful rational democratic deliberation. This pertains to heart transplants, which have a cost of about $500,000. Individuals move up the transplant list for both reasons of urgency and length of time on the list. We will imagine individuals on the list in their 50s and 60s. If one individual suddenly achieves urgent status, likely to die in the next two weeks if no transplant is provided, but a confident medical judgment concludes they are still salvageable, then they will be offered an LVAD at a cost of $250,000 to sustain them until a suitable heart becomes available. At that time, the LVAD is removed and the transplant goes forward. However, LVADs have improved over the past few years so that they can yield two to four extra years of life for these patients. That is less than what they would gain from a heart transplant, which generally offers a 75% chance of five-year survival and a 50% chance of ten-year survival. Still, there is a serious problem of health care justice here. Remember that heart transplants are an absolutely scarce good, roughly 2,700 per year in the United States. If patient A gets *both* the LVAD and the heart transplant, someone else will not get a heart transplant and will die prematurely. The LVAD option adds to the overall cost of transplantation and alters the order of survival on the transplant list. Would it be more just if patient A had to choose either to take the LVAD as "destination therapy" or to gamble that a last-minute matching heart will become available? This situation is another suitable candidate for a democratic deliberative process. What choice would emerge from the deliberative process as being "just enough" if deliberators imagined themselves, or those loved ones they cared about, in either situation? And, equally important, what would be the reasoning that was most supportive of that choice? Would it matter, for example, that not every patient on the transplant list would also be a candidate for an LVAD? In other words, if patient A gets the LVAD, then later a well-matched heart transplant, the person further down the list who would otherwise have gotten that transplant turns out not to be a candidate for the LVAD and dies. Should we collectively endorse that outcome as being "just enough"?

5.8. Rational Democratic Deliberation: The Justification Challenge

How do we know whether the outcomes of any particular deliberative process are well justified? How do we know that any particular proposal is "just enough"? Is it justified simply because it emerged from a fair and well-conducted deliberative process? Or are there substantive considerations that are a necessary feature of a well-justified outcome from the deliberative process? Daniels sees something of a conundrum here: If there are substantive criteria that are used to assess the justness or legitimacy of the deliberative process, then the deliberative process is otiose. On the other hand, if the relevant substantive criteria are unable to yield the "correct answer," then the outcome of the deliberative process ought to be the final word. To my mind this is a false dichotomy. The deliberative process itself must be constrained and shaped in various ways. Those constraints will not conclusively dictate the outcome of the deliberative process. If they were to do that, then Daniels would be correct. Instead, the broad constraints I have in mind are intended to identify ethically relevant or justice-relevant considerations that must be part of that specific deliberative conversation. More specifically, those constraints will include: (1) relevant scientific and social facts, (2) considered judgments of health care justice (and other relevant social values), (3) relevant past judgments that are precedent-like and presumptively require consistency, (4) constitutional principles of health care justice that establish the outer boundaries of any deliberative process, and (5) establishing a reasonable reflective equilibrium among competing justice-relevant considerations.

Recall that what initiates the need for such a deliberative effort is that we are ethically puzzled and confused as to what is the right policy choice to make, all things considered. For example, given the extraordinarily high front-end cost associated with CAR T-cell therapy ($475,000) for advanced blood cancers, would it be permissible as a matter of health care justice to deny individuals access to that therapy if we have a biomarker that would tell us with 90% confidence that this individual will not survive another year after receiving that therapy? We are ethically puzzled because one year is not a marginal benefit. Furthermore, how can a just and caring society allow someone to die for economic reasons when we have the technology that might give that individual an extra year of life? Isn't this the relevant moral logic that made it obligatory for us to create the end-stage renal disease program? Should not this same logic apply in the case of a patient needing CAR

T-cell therapy? Further, this patient has no alternative life-prolonging therapeutic options available. That adds to the moral urgency and necessity of our providing access to this technology. Moreover, assuming that our biomarker is reliable in its predictive use, there is a 10% chance this patient could survive more than a year. What if some patients in that 10% category were to gain two or three extra years of life? How can a society that cares about human life deny this patient that 10% chance? This is one side of the argument. Consider the other side as well.

CAR T-cell therapy is a very aggressive therapy. Depending upon the type of leukemia or lymphoma that we are talking about, anywhere from 30% to 50% of these patients will experience either cytokine release syndrome or severe neurologic effects that will require a substantial stay in the ICU at an additional cost of $200,000 or more. This is a medical and economic fact that cannot be ignored, especially if these patients are very unlikely to gain more than an extra year of life (Bach, 2018). Many health economists will say that we generally should not spend more than $100,000 per quality-adjusted life-year (QALY) gained. There might be ethically compelling grounds for ignoring that rule in specific circumstances. In this case we have a cost per QALY of $600,000 to $700,000. What would be the moral arguments that would justify our ignoring those numbers and providing the therapy anyway? To be clear, those arguments would have to be very specific to this situation and not generalized to other situations. This would be extremely difficult.

Recall the unintended consequences that emerged in connection with the dialysis program. It paid for dialysis *and* kidney transplants. That generated the obvious ethical question: If you are paying for kidney transplants, why not also heart or lung or liver transplants? After all, very well-insured individuals will have access to these transplants at private insurance expense, unlike individuals who are uninsured or underinsured. They will have no chance of gaining those extra life-years that others will gain from having private health insurance. Is that fair or just?

Going back to our CAR T-cell therapy example, how do we avoid opening the floodgates to our being ethically obligated to fund any technology that offers some significant gain in life expectancy no matter the cost? I will argue that we will make a serious mistake if we consider CAR T-cell therapy all by itself. We need to look at the broad spectrum of costly life-prolonging interventions to determine which ones we can afford and which ones need to be left to private resources and private decision-making. We need to do priority-setting, and some sense of justice must be included in a health care priority-setting process.

Someone might care to argue that it would be more just (from an egalitarian perspective) if we either gave everyone access to CAR T-cell therapy for whom it was "medically necessary" or else denied it to everyone, at least at social expense. Of course, the obvious follow-up question would be: What would justify excluding this intervention from a health care benefit package guaranteed to all in our society? Someone might offer a sufficientarian response: It is too far above a reasonable sufficiency threshold. Would compassion warrant social funding? However, that compassionate response would not be free. It would still require social resources. We would still have to inquire thoughtfully about all the other very expensive life-prolonging interventions that were above the sufficiency threshold. Were they all deserving social funding?[9] If not, what criteria were being invoked that justified choosing some and not others? In addition, what would justify making any such choices if there were patients with unmet health needs below the sufficiency threshold?

I now want to use CAR T-cell therapy to illustrate what I believe a process of wide reflective equilibrium must look like in order to justify specific decisions that might emerge from the deliberative process. The goal of the deliberative process is to get to a considered judgment of health care justice. Here are some possible considered judgments of health care justice pertinent to CAR T-cell therapy in the treatment of various blood-based cancers.

- The cost of CAR T-cell therapy should be part of a benefit package guaranteed to all who can derive any degree of therapeutic benefit.
- CAR T-cell therapy should be limited to individuals who will gain at least one extra year of life, that having been determined by a biomarker with 90% reliability.
- The cost of CAR T-cell therapy should be part of a benefit package guaranteed to all who can derive any degree of therapeutic benefit so long as they are less than 60 years of age.

---

[9] Recall the Cancer Fund created by the British government for those targeted cancer therapies that the National Institute for Clinical Excellence (NICE) had rejected. Why was there no such fund for expensive medications rejected by NICE for heart disease or rheumatoid arthritis or other costly medical conditions (Charlton and Rid, 2019; Rumbold et al., 2017; Claxton, 2015)? This illustrates how social beneficence can go astray, ethically speaking.

- CAR T-cell therapy should either go to everyone at social expense who can derive any degree of benefit from this therapy or to no one; we should not attempt to identify subpopulations for receipt of the therapy as such efforts are too likely to yield social discrimination, such as ageism.
- CAR T-cell therapy should only be a therapeutic option for those willing and able to pay for it, either through their own personal resources or through private health insurance, assuming such policies are available.

This list could get somewhat longer. What I would observe, however, is that none of these five options are ethically unreasonable, ethically unworthy of thoughtful democratic deliberation. Likewise, none of these five options are so ethically superior to all the other options that it would be pointless to expend effort on democratic deliberation, though the substantial majority of therapeutic interventions available today would quickly be endorsed as reasonable for inclusion in a benefit package guaranteed to all.[10]

How should judgments be justified within the deliberative process? Facts matter. Lots of facts (medical, economic, social, technical) can have a bearing on appropriate judgments of health care justice in specific circumstances. CAR T-cell therapy is extraordinarily expensive. Unlike the targeted cancer drugs that have monthly costs for as long as the drug is taken, the full cost of the intervention is up front. Heart transplants are like that as well, with a front-end cost of $500,000. However, we know statistically that 75% of those patients will survive five years with their transplant and 50% will survive 10 years or more. That brings the cost per QALY well below the $100,000 mark. Moreover, no transplant surgeon will offer a heart transplant to a patient whom they knew ahead of time would likely survive less than a year. We do not see such a judgment as inherently unjust; it seems to be widely accepted as reasonable.[11]

---

[10] Lots of medical interventions are very beneficial for the vast majority of patients who need those interventions. Consequently, they are included in a socially funded health care benefit package. However, that does not mean that each and every patient with the need for the intervention has a just claim to that intervention, especially if that intervention is very unlikely to yield any benefit for that patient in their very specific circumstances. These are judgments that must be made by physicians familiar with all the medical circumstances of that patient, though broad categories of limitations might be agreed to through the deliberative process.

[11] An individual might object, "That person could be me; I would want that extra year of life." This is where the deliberative process is helpful. Consider this response: "But it is just as likely that you would be the next eligible person on that transplant list, that you would now lose your chance of getting a heart transplant because that heart went to an individual who would only gain one extra year of life. In addition, you would have gotten five to 10 extra years of life. Do you still think that heart should go to someone who would only gain one extra year of life?"

This judgment regarding limited post-transplant survival is relevant to the question of whether CAR T-cell therapy ought to be provided to patients if we have a biomarker that can tell us with 90% confidence that this patient will not survive a year. Heart transplants represent an absolutely scarce resource, though CAR T-cell therapy is not. Both technologies are "last chance" therapies; no other interventions are available that would as effectively stave off death. Still, our egalitarian sensibilities are not offended when we deny a heart transplant to an end-stage cardiac patient who will live less than a year with a transplant. Still, some egalitarian sensibilities might be offended by having such a limitation with regard to CAR T-cell therapy for their blood cancer.

A majority of CAR T-cell patients will survive for two to four years, and there will again be some super-responders. What kind of ethical weight ought to be attached to these statistics? Why do 30% of these patients fail CAR T-cell therapy so quickly? Some scientific hypotheses might explain that outcome. Should we invest in medical research to fix this? This certainly looks like an ethically reasonable goal. One hypothesis is that the T cells that have been therapeutically turbocharged in the manufacturing process simply "poop out" after some limited period of time (Kasakovski et al., 2018). They are effective in controlling the cancer for that limited period of time, but they cannot defeat the cancer. Then we have the super-responders.

The reader will note that we have only talked about CAR T-cell therapy in connection with blood cancers (leukemias and lymphomas). However, research is seeking to apply this same technology to solid tumors. Again, biological barriers exist within solid tumors that impair the ability of these turbocharged T cells to get access to the cancer cells that comprise the solid tumor. However, research is occurring that is aimed at circumventing those barriers (Grens, 2019; Watanabe et al., 2018; Titov et al., 2020). We might see that as something hopeful. However, only 9.4% of all cancer deaths in the United States are related to leukemias, lymphomas, and myeloma. That means the aggregated cost of CAR T-cell therapy would increase by 900% if this therapy were equally effective in addressing various solid organ cancers.

Should these speculative outcomes of future research have any weight or relevance in a deliberative process aimed at determining what should count as just access to this therapy today? If, for example, we were to agree today that CAR T-cell therapy should be available at social expense to everyone who might derive any degree of benefit for their hematologic cancer, then how could we justifiably not committing to the same social coverage for CAR

T-cell therapy directed to solid organ cancers? That becomes a micro-wicked problem. We cannot simply cut off medical research aimed at finding ways for CAR T-cell therapies to attack solid tumors. The research is certainly not intrinsically ethically flawed. The research seems to be making steady progress. Public funding could be reduced, but if the research looked promising, private funds would take over for the public funds. If the research is successful, we would be faced with ever mounting health care expenditures that would make our overall problem of health care justice even more intractable.

We were talking about expanding CAR T-cell therapy to attacking cancers in solid organs. Barring outright failure of that research effort, I cannot imagine the ethical justification for failing to fund this technology if it had the success of CAR T-cell therapy for hematologic cancers. Furthermore, I am making the broad generalization that any life-prolonging therapy that is "effective enough" will command the social resources necessary for its therapeutic dissemination. We will most certainly face this challenge once a totally implantable artificial heart is available. The same will be true for the $2.1 million gene therapy for spinal muscular atrophy or for hemophilia, as well as the new $100,000 drugs for sickle cell anemia or the $300,000 drugs for various lysosomal storage diseases. What gets in the way of making those choices justly? They clearly offer some significant benefit for some patients, which is what creates a kind of ethical necessity, at least speaking from a descriptive ethics perspective (Kaufman, 2015). Sharon Kaufman is an anthropologist looking at the US health care system. Her point is that once these extraordinary treatments are regarded as part of "ordinary medicine," they acquire the status of being both medically and ethically "necessary," which is to say that it becomes virtually impossible to limit, much less dislodge them entirely, from the medical armamentarium. Still, we cannot afford that conclusion.

Given competing theories of justice, how are we supposed to get to social agreement that is "just enough" and "legitimate enough"? In the United States we simply deny the need for social agreement or for thinking about the rationing problem as a matter of justice. We reduce the problem to decisions made by employers regarding benefits. Benefits are freely given, and benefits can be freely reduced or taken away. Medicaid is largely left to the ideologic whims and political winds shaping the judgment of state legislators. Medicare pressures are largely in the direction of unregulated expansion. In the Medicare world, virtually no one is lobbying for restraint, which creates health care justice problems elsewhere in the health care system (i.e., cost-shifting to patients). The European Union has the same problem with trying to address rapidly expanding, costly medical technologies, as exemplified by the targeted cancer therapies, while trying to control overall health costs. In the case of the European Union this problem has posed a significant threat to its commitment to solidarity.

One option is to put in place governmentally sponsored organizations charged with addressing the "just caring" problem. The other option is to engage the broader public in addressing these issues through well-constructed processes of rational democratic deliberation.

We can start with the organizational approach. Those organizations can take either the form of temporally limited commissions, as in Norway, Sweden, and the Netherlands, or the form of permanent organizations, such as NICE in the United Kingdom or the Institute for Quality and Efficiency in Health Care (IQWiG) in Germany. Those referenced commissions have tended to produce reports advocating the use of very broad principles for rationing and cost control (Calltorp, 1999; Hofmann, 2013; Reckers-Droog, 2018; Berg et al., 2004; Norwegian Ministry of Health and Care Services, 2017). Those very broad principles are the practical equivalent of the theories of justice we have discussed. They are too broad and too abstract to effectively address our wicked rationing problems.

In contrast to those commissions, NICE and IQWiG do address very specific cost constraint challenges presented, for example, by the targeted cancer therapies. Those therapies are individually assessed from both a cost-effectiveness perspective and a straightforward effectiveness perspective. On this latter point, how much medical benefit is provided by this particular drug for the vast majority of patients with a specific medical condition? If the benefit is marginal, then even an inexpensive drug will be judged to be a low-value intervention. These are judgments that are made by a variety of experts (medical, basic sciences, epidemiology, economics) as opposed to elected politicians. That means their judgments are untainted by political pressures or partisanship. It means their judgments are as objective as possible. Their judgments will also reflect ethical commitments, most often utilitarian.

Recall that within the European Union a comprehensive package of health benefits is already provided to virtually all citizens. From a sufficientarian perspective, that represents a high threshold of sufficiency. In turn, that suggests that decisions regarding the targeted cancer therapies are matters of social beneficence "beyond the domain of justice." This would seem to imply that if every one of these targeted cancer therapies were rejected as unaffordable by NICE or IQWiG, no injustice would have occurred because their social funding would merely be a matter of social beneficence. If a primary concern in the European Union is preserving social solidarity, then denying social funding for all these drugs could be congruent with preserving social solidarity. However, the obvious consequence would be that either wealthy individuals would pay for these drugs or a private insurance market would emerge for the financially well off. The result would be the fracturing of solidarity.

In the United Kingdom, solidarity is not a social value that governs to any degree the decisions that emerge from NICE. The National Health Service (NHS) must operate with a fixed budget, along with the hospitals and commissioning groups whose funding comes from the NHS. Consequently, cost-effectiveness considerations play a dominant role in NICE's decisions, the general expectation being that these targeted cancer therapies must yield gains in QALYs for less than £30,000 per QALY, though in 2009 NICE increased its willingness to fund drugs used for terminally ill patients to £50,000 per QALY (Baker et al., 2018). This was followed in 2011 by the creation of the Cancer Drug Fund. The Cancer Drug Fund was actually purchasing QALYs that were costing £200,000 per QALY. Did this make sense? Was this either just or prudent? Did this reflect widely endorsed public values? Research carried out by Baker et al. (2018) gave a negative answer to this last question. In their survey research, only 4% of respondents endorsed NICE's decisions regarding enhanced funding for prolonging life with these targeted cancer therapies. This brings us back to the role of rational democratic deliberation in addressing the "just caring" problem and its wicked descendants.

5.9. Democratic Deliberation: Getting to Reflective Equilibrium

Why should we endorse relying upon rational democratic deliberation to address the "just caring" problem? Ultimately, democratic deliberation has utility and legitimacy if it can yield considered judgments of health care justice that are stable, well justified, and autonomously imposed. This last notion is what is most ethically critical and what is missing from NICE and the various EU commissions. Rationing decisions need to be collectively rationally self-imposed by those most likely to be affected by such decisions. Expertise of various kinds must be integral to the process. However, more important are the justice-relevant judgments that must be forged and justified through that deliberative process. This is a matter for public reason. Again, participants must assume the role of *citizens as such*. They must identify the relevant empirical information that is needed and the justice-relevant considerations pertinent to that problem, especially well-anchored considered judgments of health care justice. Then they need to propose possible considered judgments of health care justice that would address that specific rationing problem, which need to be integrated into a broader framework of health care justice aimed at achieving a wide reflective equilibrium. Every such judgment has wider ethically relevant implications that might have a destabilizing effect with regard to other rationing decisions. Finally, the whole deliberative process must occur within the boundaries established by what I refer to metaphorically as "constitutional principles of health care justice."

What prompts the need for sustained and comprehensive democratic deliberation is that we are unsure about how these considered judgments of health care justice apply in novel and complex situations. The dialysis example can easily generate and justify the idea that human life is priceless. However, that would yield outcomes that would be imprudent, unjust, and uncaring. Readers will recall the Baby K case, the anencephalic infant in Virginia sustained for 2.75 years at a cost of more than $1 million (Greenhouse, 1993). If every anencephalic infant were provided with this level of aggressive life-sustaining care, the annual costs would be more than $1 billion. Similar issues arise regarding the 25,000 PVS cases in the United States or the roughly one million late-stage Alzheimer patients.

We need resources for palliative care, for reducing or eliminating human suffering that is medically ameliorable but not life-threatening. Sacrificing palliative care for the sake of prolonging at great expense marginal lives would fail to generate a reflective equilibrium because it would require severely modifying or giving up other considered judgments of health care justice. The deliberative process must tease out the rationale behind these very firm considered judgments of health care justice to see what rational insight they can provide in addressing more complex and less clear rationing cases.

Let me offer a somewhat complex string of examples to illustrate what this process might look like. We (just and caring democratic citizens) are morally confident that no considerations of health care justice would require sustaining the life of an anencephalic infant at a cost of $1 million. I believe we are equally morally confident that if we were to list a large number of childhood life-threatening medical problems for which we have very costly but effective medical interventions, we would collectively agree that all these interventions ought to be high on our prioritization scheme. The dominant moral justification might be that of protecting fair equality of opportunity as well as equal concern and respect. Further, our judgment would be that justice would require *all children in the relevant medical circumstances* to have access to these costly but effective medical interventions. We would reject, as unjust, children in these circumstances having differential access because of the vagaries of the insurance market and the judgments of private employers, especially if those vagaries resulted in premature death or otherwise avoidable permanent disabilities for these children.

Consider funding for cystic fibrosis. It affects about 35,000 individuals in the United States. In 2019 the drug elexacaftor/tezacaftor/ivacaftor (Trikafta™) had been introduced at a cost of $310,000 per patient per year for the rest of an individual's life. For 30 years, the aggregated cost would be more than $9 million. Medical disagreement exists regarding the effectiveness of this drug. It does significantly improve lung function, which means reduced hospitalizations, which offsets some portion of the annual drug costs. Perhaps this results in increased life expectancy, though no empirical evidence supports that conclusion at present. There are mild to severe forms of the disease. The benefits might be marginal for individuals with milder forms of the disease. Should those individuals not be candidates for the drug? Would this be "just enough," a reasonable societal trade-off aimed at both reducing social costs and improving and prolonging the quality of lives. This is a matter for rational democratic deliberation. What would NOT be "just enough" is allowing each state through its Medicaid program to determine whether it would pay anything at all for this drug for children. That would fail the equal concern and respect test, as well as fair equality of opportunity.

I would expect that children with hemophilia would also have their medical costs covered, and this would be seen as a requirement for a just and caring society. As with cystic fibrosis, newer drugs for hemophilia A have been introduced with very high annual costs, for example, emicizumab-kxwh (Hemlibra™), which has an annual cost of $492,000. Roughly 20,000 individuals in the United States have hemophilia. This drug is a prophylactic intended to reduce substantially the average of 30 bleeds per year experienced by hemophiliacs (Miller, 2018). One research study demonstrated that this drug reduced bleeds by 96% and reduced *treated* bleeds by 68%, which means reduced costly hospitalizations (Mahlangu et al., 2018). These frequent bleeds are not just an annoyance. These bleeds do damage to joints and gradually reduce substantially quality of life and length of life for these patients. From the perspective of health care justice, this drug significantly protects fair equality of opportunity for these individuals. I think this drug would be approved through a fair democratic deliberative process.

Do we also believe that funding this drug would not disturb a certain reflective equilibrium with respect to health care justice? If the net cost of this drug for one patient each year were $400,000, the annual social cost for 16,000 patients would be $6.4 billion. We have to consider trade-offs. Each year in the United States, 847 infants are born with anencephaly. Should we have the rule that such infants would be provided with comfort care only and allowed to die? Given the nature of anencephaly, these infants have no life opportunities. This is tragic and regrettable, but those are the medical and social realities. Advocates for persons with disabilities might disagree with this proposal and this judgment. Would they argue that every one of these infants had a just claim to unlimited costly life-sustaining care? Would that same judgment apply to all individuals who have various disabilities, no matter how costly that intervention or how marginal that benefit? If they answered in the affirmative, they would be expecting unlimited access to health care resources for the population they represented at the expense of other patient populations. That is a perfect example of unreflective disequilibrium. No organized group of patients can demand unlimited access to health care resources for themselves at the expense of other patients. We are ethically obligated to spend $750,000 to rehabilitate an individual who has become a vent-dependent quadriplegic as a result of some terrible accident. We can restore this person to the normal opportunity range of our society. That is precisely what is not possible with an anencephalic infant or other infants born with devastating brain malformations or brain injuries.

Sickle cell disease (SCD) afflicts about 100,000 Americans, the vast majority of whom are African American. SCD is a horrible disease that reduces life expectancy by about 30 years and very adversely affects quality of life for the preceding 40 years. Twenty years have elapsed since a new drug was introduced to alleviate the symptoms of SCD. However, the drug, voxelotor, demonstrated significant disease-modifying potential (Thompson, 2019). More specifically, it reduced by almost 50% the frequency and intensity of the pain episodes, and it can prevent severe anemia that can lead to permanent brain damage. Clearly, this represents significant improvement in quality of life and length of life (i.e., life opportunities).

At almost the same time, the FDA approved another novel sickle cell drug, crizanlizumab-tmca (Pazdur, 2019). This drug is given as a monthly infusion. To be clear, neither of these drugs is curative. Both drugs must be taken for the rest of one's life. Both drugs have an annual cost of $100,000, with additional costs associated with infusion for the latter drug. I would again argue that a just and caring society ought to fund both of these drugs. The disease starts with very young children. Most of these patients are Black, a population in the United States that is often disadvantaged in multiple ways. These drugs are effective at significantly reducing disability and increasing life expectancy. Funding these drugs for this patient population demonstrates equal concern and respect where it has often been lacking in our society. Finally, if we have to rank various costly life-prolonging interventions, where would we rank these sickle cell drugs or cystic fibrosis drugs or hemophilia drugs relative to our targeted cancer therapies from the perspective of health care justice, whether egalitarian or utilitarian or prioritarian or sufficientarian? I think the obvious answer would be that the targeted cancer drugs would be somewhere below these other drugs, given the generally marginal benefits they yield.[12]

I can imagine that many of my fellow deliberators would be extremely sensitive to the health needs of children, especially those who were tragically doomed to survive for only a small number of years. If we were strongly opposed to taking dollars away from marginally treatable childhood health needs, then what adult medical needs would we give lower priority to in order to generate the dollars needed to fund these "costly" extraordinary childhood health needs? Implantable cardiac defibrillators (ICDs) at a cost of $40,000 each would be a case to consider. Research has shown that 81% of those devices never fire over a five-year period of time (when $20,000 batteries would need to be replaced). A T-wave alternans test could be used to determine who was least likely to have that device fire over the next two years. Such a test could save more than $2 billion per year by reducing by 60,000 the number of these devices implanted per year. But the moral cost of doing this is that about 800 individuals from among that 60,000 would die of an arrhythmic event who otherwise would have been saved. These, of course,

---

[12] Someone might call attention to the cost differences between these targeted cancer therapies and the hemophilia or cystic fibrosis drugs. However, that can be misleading. A recent three-drug combination for metastatic HER-2-positive breast cancer (trastuzumab, tucatinib, and capecitabine) has annual costs of $146,000, far below the $300,000 cost of the cystic fibrosis drugs. However, the incremental cost-effectiveness ratio of that three-drug combination is $699,000 because it yields only 0.21 additional QALYs relative to an alternate therapy (Wu et al., 2020).

are generally older individuals. The question for our deliberators is whether providing ICDs for these individuals who are *least likely* to benefit from them should be of lower priority than providing the medical resources needed by our more controversial childhood cases.

5.10. Priority-Setting, Wide Reflective Equilibrium, and Rational Democratic Deliberation: Addressing the Stability Problem

We want to elicit "considered judgments of health care justice" of suitable specificity that represent a sort of rule that would be used to fairly prioritize similar sorts of health care needs and treatment options. We also want to capture for future use the reasons and reasoning that were most successful in providing reasonable justification for awarding higher priority to one condition or treatment over another. This is what we need to maintain a reasonable reflective equilibrium over many years. What will happen in practice is that our earlier collective deliberative judgments will be further refined and specified by what we learn in later deliberative efforts. This is essentially how we contribute to the creation of substantive "public reason," as Rawls (1996) uses that term. That is, this is how we develop public reasons and public methods of reasoning that are suitable for citizens solving public problems in a liberal pluralistic society.

To return briefly to our last example, we might conclude that those very expensive hemophilia treatments deserve higher priority for funding than those marginally beneficial defibrillators. We might initially formulate our considered judgment of health care justice in this way: "Children faced with imminent death from some life-threatening disease process have a just claim to whatever medical interventions offer any chance of saving their lives even if the costs of that intervention are substantially higher than what we might spend for an adult in comparable medical circumstances." We might judge, as noted above, that the major justice-relevant reason for supporting this considered judgment is protecting fair equality of opportunity. These are not children who have virtually no effective opportunity to achieve or experience anything in life because of gross brain deformations; these are children who can in theory experience a considerable portion of the normal opportunity range in our society if we provide the medical resources they need in a timely way.

But then we call to mind the Child B (Jaymee Bowen) case in Great Britain (Butler, 1999, at 10; Ham, 1999). This was a young girl with a cancer that was not defeated by any of the usual cancer therapies. In addition, she had had a failed bone marrow transplant. She was now seeking a second bone marrow transplant at a cost of about $150,000 that would have virtually no chance of defeating her cancer or even giving her much additional disease-free life. The NHS denied her that funding. However, if these dismal prior probabilities of success are true for other children (marginal benefits, very high costs), then it would not be unjust to withhold funding for therapies for children threatened by imminent death when those therapies promised little medical gain. This is a concise example of how reflective equilibrium protects the fairness and the reasonableness of the deliberative process.

Some readers may see the reference to reflective equilibrium as something that sounds more like a philosophy seminar session than a deliberative process with which ordinary citizens can become fully engaged (Young, 2003). But the concept refers to a process of consistent reflective justification in the face of changing morally relevant considerations that are very much part of our lives as individual moral agents or as citizens struggling with complex policy issues as a community. To give a quick example, if someone contends that justice does not require funding protease inhibitors and fusion inhibitors for individuals whose immune systems have been seriously compromised by the AIDS virus (even though these drugs represent 10–30 extra years of life) but that justice requires funding these extraordinarily expensive cancer drugs at a cost of $150,000 for a course of therapy that might offer only extra months of life, then we would demand from that individual some coherent explanation of how those two moral judgments were compatible with one another. The AIDS drugs cost much less than the cancer drugs and are medically much more effective in prolonging life and protecting quality of life than any of these cancer drugs. What exactly would be the rationale that would justify the claim that both these moral judgments were right and just without at the same time disrupting massively what we might have regarded as fair and reasonable and settled judgments of health care justice related to numerous rationing situations? A legitimate concern would be that the judgment regarding the needs of AIDS patients reflected unjust discrimination.

There is nothing esoteric or academic about raising such a question. Our judgments of health care justice are related to one another in complex ways, which is best captured by speaking of a dynamic equilibrium among them. Any explanation offered to make morally compatible our two propositions above would necessarily be disruptive of a large number of other justice judgments, which would have to be revised or deleted until that equilibrium was re-established. We have already noted that a *dynamic* reflective equilibrium in matters of health care justice is inescapable because of the effects of emerging medical technologies, changing organizational structures and changing economic relationships. But we are generally capable of explaining to one another in ways regarded as fair and reasonable the refinements and rebalancings we collectively craft in our judgments of health care justice in response to these external pressures.

Our legal system (maybe an idealized version) provides a good analogy for understanding how wide reflective equilibrium in the context of rational democratic deliberation works. Our legal system is a social construction, but it is not an arbitrary construction either in its structure or in its workings. It is a system of checks and balances aimed at maintaining a kind of equilibrium among multiple reasonable social values that might be in conflict with one another in specific circumstances. The most "reflective" part of that system would be our courts. Courts have to resolve interpretive disagreements regarding how the laws apply to a particular social dispute. The laws themselves (somewhat ideally) represent shared social understandings about the scope and limits of social behavior in specific social and economic contexts. Our basic moral norms and judgments are also essentially shared social understandings about the scope and limits of the behavior of each of us in specific social contexts. Those shared ethical understandings may not be as formally formulated as are laws, but they are quite real features of our lives. But then new social facts, such as new medical technologies that are costly and marginally beneficial, may disrupt what had been easy and obvious applications of one of these widely shared ethical judgments. The same sort of thing happens in our legal system with emerging technologies, for example, the question of whether or not genes can be patented. A panel of judges in such matters would be the analogue of our deliberators: free and equal, mutually respectful.

Though conservative legal commentators will insist that judges may never "make laws," the social and political fact of the matter is that judges are often forced by the nature of a particular legal dispute and the "open" nature of the laws that apply to that dispute to render a decision that will create a novel precedent with the future force of law. Judges are expected to offer some legally reasonable resolution of every case brought before them because the problem must be resolved. Judges have "deliberative space" for creative work with the law to fashion novel resolutions when required. But that deliberative space is not "wide open." It is rationally constrained in multiple ways. A fair and reasonable and legitimate resolution will require that judges must be attentive to (1) the legally relevant case facts, (2) scientific information relevant to the case, (3) precedents that apply to the case (with reasons and reasonings that offer potential legal justification for resolving a case one way rather than another), (4) relevant laws whose ambiguity may have helped to precipitate the legal dispute in the first place, and (5) constitutional considerations that might require that one or another law pertinent to the case be invalidated but that always establish very firm boundaries for the deliberative space within which judges must work. These are the sorts of factors that require that a dynamic legal equilibrium be maintained.

Note that the equilibrium is not simply a matter of logical or interpretive coherence among legal concepts and other legal materials. That equilibrium is closely tied to our social/political/economic world in all its complexity. The pragmatic test of the justness and the reasonableness of any particular judicial resolution is that it does not trigger a number of other legal disputes. If it is a somewhat novel judgment that is rendered and it unsettles significant areas of what had been thought settled law without offering a legal explanation that can resettle those areas of law, then that judgment *might be* flawed. We are unlikely to be able to say with certainty that that judgment *is flawed* because it might take considerable additional deliberation to make that case.[13] The reader will recall civil rights legislation from the 1960s and the very widespread effects in terms of changed policy and practice it had, not to mention uncertainty and disputes about innumerable specific applications, such as all the issues around affirmative action. This same kind of equilibrium is what needs to be sustained in the deliberative conversations about issues of just health care rationing.

We saw how someone who proposed severe restrictions on funding protease inhibitors for HIV but expansive access to these extraordinarily expensive cancer drugs would cause an unreasonable and irresolvable sort of moral disequilibrium. This represents a legitimate constraint on the deliberative

---

[13] We see this same phenomenon in the practice of science. Scientists make some observations that are inconsistent with current scientific theory and that are resistant to being "explained away." Consequently, theories must be revised. In 1970 it was proposed that the continents actually move about the earth. This was greeted with great skepticism because it seems so "obvious" that the continents are immoveable. However, the theory of plate tectonics explained how that would happen, and that theory gradually became fully corroborated as scientists were now directed by that theory to make other observations that further confirmed that theory.

process to minimize the risk of moral error. I offered this as an easy and obvious illustration of my point. I could have used something less obvious, more controversial, more likely to require sustained subsequent deliberation (i.e., individuals whose health problems are a clear outcome of their behavioral choices).

If we considered a very wide range of cases that fit this generic rubric of personal responsibility for health, we might find the reflective equilibrium shifting a bit in response to this or that specific example. Some of that shift might be required by some of our more settled considered judgments of justice relevant to a specific case, but other portions of the shift would be precipitated by outcomes from the deliberative conversation. Some members of the deliberative group might make novel, morally convincing distinctions or offer insightful moral analogies that cause a shift in thinking. What this makes perfectly clear is that the outcome of the deliberative process is not predetermined (as a matter of excellent moral argument and analysis) to one legitimate outcome, relative to which all other proposals are erroneous. All the morally relevant considerations pertinent to some of the more complex rationing and justice issues we must address will still often be insufficient to yield a single *just and legitimate* considered moral judgment. The work of judges will often require legal creativity, and the work of our democratic deliberators will likewise often require (constrained) moral creativity.

5.11. Constitutional Principles of Health Care Justice: Delimiting Deliberation

We now turn to the final structural element in our understanding of the process of rational democratic deliberation and wide reflective equilibrium, what I have referred to as constitutional principles of health care justice. This is obviously a metaphorical use of the phrase. One of the key functions of these principles is to define the legitimate space of democratic deliberation. Some rationing proposals do not warrant deliberation because they violate in an obvious way one or another of these constitutional constraints. Some might see this as illiberal or elitist, but such concerns would be wide of the mark. Imagine someone proposing that we give serious thought to reinstituting slavery as a way of regaining our competitive edge in world labor markets. Such a proposal would be morally and constitutionally outrageous. There are no reasonable moral or legal justifications that can even be imagined by perverse philosophic minds to support such a proposal. Rejecting it out of hand is the only reasonable and liberally appropriate response. This is what Cohen (1993) and Rawls (1996) defend as a "reasonable pluralism." Likewise, if someone were to propose that AIDS patients should receive no health care at social expense that was related to any disease condition linked to their being HIV+, then this too would just as readily be justifiably rejected as an option for democratic deliberation.

These constitutional principles of health care justice are the most fundamental conditions that must be respected in order to have a well-ordered deliberative democracy capable of articulating and legitimating through the deliberative process a fully adequate pluralistic conception of health care justice congruent with public reason. I would identify the following constitutional principles of health care justice: a principle of equality, a principle of liberty, a principle of fair equality of opportunity, a publicity principle, a principle of respect for persons, a principle of liberal neutrality, and a principle of reciprocity. I make no claim that this list is complete, only that these principles seem necessary to sustain the effort to articulate a fully adequate pluralistic conception of health care justice. I will briefly explicate each of these principles. Philosophic readers will readily appreciate the fact that volumes have been written on each of these principles. I can only say enough about them to make clear their application in a deliberative process about health care justice and the problem of health care rationing.

Consider the publicity principle. This principle requires that our rationing policies and practices be the product of a public, visible decision-making process, including the reasons and reasoning behind a specific rationing or priority-setting decision. This is what builds trust and stability. This is what assures all that the process is fair and worthy of respect and acceptance, even when a particular decision is seen as adversely affecting the self-interests of an individual. This is what assures all that favoritism has not infected the process. This is what permits mutual education through the deliberative process and a broad sharing of critical perspectives, all of which is aimed at producing as fair and as informed an outcome as is reasonable.

Recall the advocates for the "virtues" of invisible rationing. These are virtues only Ayn Rand (fully insured) could love. Mechanic (1997) has argued for the view that physicians should not have to disclose to patients specific cost-control incentives that might shape their medical judgments, such as income-related penalties for doing "excessive" diagnostic testing. This has the "virtue" of avoiding difficult conversations with patients that might potentially undermine the patient's belief that the physician is loyal and trustworthy. Such denials of potentially beneficial care are easily accomplished because the mechanism of denial is silence. Consequently, a patient has nothing to assess or appeal as unfair. These are the sorts of practices that the publicity principle would identify as presumptively objectionable.

A research article on cancer and nursing home patients reported the following conclusion: "Very few cancer services are provided to Medicaid-insured nursing home patients, despite the fact that many of these patients likely experienced cancer-related symptoms and marked physical decline before diagnosis and death" (Bradley et al., 2008, at 21). There might be reasonable considerations of health care justice that would justify these practices and these outcomes. Most of these patients have significant co-morbidities that would cause many physicians to wonder whether it was either compassionate or just to institute treatment. What would be the strong considerations of health care justice that would *speak in favor* of saying such patients had a just claim to costly life-prolonging health care resources? My judgment is that it might be difficult to find such considerations.

Nevertheless, my other judgment is that these practices in any nursing home are presumptively unjust because they are clear violations of the publicity principle. I am certain that these nursing homes are not informing future possible patients or their family members that these are the practices of the nursing home and that these practices are primarily motivated by the desire to save money. The deliberative process itself is essential to justifying these nursing home rationing practices. This is what "full publicity" would require. The primary virtue of the deliberative process itself is that it permits all of us to articulate and legitimate rationing protocols for our future possible selves.

This brings us to the second of our constitutional principles, the autonomy principle. Individuals must have a reasonable and effective opportunity to decide for themselves as citizens which rationing/cost-control/priority-setting policies and practices are reasonable and just. Our health care system is a complex cooperative enterprise to which virtually all have contributed in multiple ways. It is a public interest and a shared social good. Our health care system is a *public interest* because it is essential to protecting the health of each and every one of us, and it is an interest we cannot adequately protect for ourselves simply *as individuals*. Consequently, complex cooperative behavior with all in our society is necessary to protect that interest. What this means in relation to our autonomy principle is that autonomy *cannot* mean that individuals have the right to take whatever they want from the health care system for any reason whatsoever. That yields the tragedy of the commons. Likewise, autonomy does *not* mean that individuals are free to not contribute to sustaining the health care system because they feel perfectly healthy. That generates the "free-riding" problem familiar to all political scientists. What we have in mind is the conception of autonomy that Rawls has articulated.

Rawls distinguishes "rational autonomy" from "full autonomy." Both are part of his overall conception of autonomy. Rational autonomy is about "having the moral power to form, to revise, and rationally to pursue a conception of the good" and "to deliberate in accordance with it" (1996, at 72). Full autonomy "is realized by citizens when they act from principles of justice that specify the fair terms of cooperation they would give themselves when fairly represented as free and equal citizens" (at 77). Rawls goes on to say that full autonomy is something realized by citizens in public life. Full autonomy is "realized by participating in society's public affairs and sharing in its collective self-determination over time" (at 78). This is the very opposite of the individualism that is potentially corrosive of the full autonomy Rawls regards as politically necessary to preserve just social institutions and policies. The fullest realization of autonomy requires the fullest realization of social justice. Full autonomy and social justice are synergistic, not antagonistic, values.

Rawls' "original position" description is intended to model what *rational* autonomy is and the conception of justice he argues would emerge from that position. The original position involves the use of a veil of ignorance. For Rawls that veil is very opaque in order to model the degree of impartiality required for a reasonable conception of justice to emerge from the deliberations. The vast majority of us are truly and naturally ignorant of our future health needs because so many potential health needs are a product of accident and the arbitrary collocation of circumstances (e.g., flying in a plane with a passenger with tuberculosis or COVID-19).

Imagine our individual above being diagnosed with cancer and having insurance only for heart disease. They realize how foolish they have been, so they now seek to purchase a more expansive health insurance plan but are turned down by all insurers. They claim that this represents an unjust restriction on their autonomy. However, what they are proposing would really be an unjust violation of the autonomy of everyone else who has invested in the insurance program for the past 40 years. If they were permitted to join now, they would be seeking to enjoy the benefits of this insurance plan without having borne their fair share of the costs. Further, if they were allowed to make such a choice (as a matter of respect for individual liberty), then all others would have the same right. And if all those others chose to exercise that right, there would be no insurance plan at all. All would have expressed their individual autonomy initially, only to find later that they had sacrificed both their individual autonomy as well as their chance for full autonomy.

What full autonomy requires is the sacrifice of purely self-interested individual autonomy that seeks to gain personal advantage at unjust cost to others. Consequently, in matters of health insurance and health care rationing, full autonomy requires that we come to agreement on a package of health care benefits that is just and prudent for all, where "all" includes all those future possible versions of myself that might come to be as a result of the health-related contingencies of the world. No socially affordable health insurance benefit package can maximize the likelihood that all citizens in our society will achieve a maximally medically possible life expectancy. But a reasonable and just health insurance benefit package that is a product of a fair deliberative process will maximize the opportunity for all citizens to achieve a reasonable life expectancy by having assured access to needed and effective and costworthy health care. That would represent full autonomy.

Our third constitutional principle would be a liberty principle. In brief, we want to maximize the right of individuals to make health care choices for themselves so long as those choices do not threaten the comparable rights of others or health care public interests. Thus, individuals do not have a liberty right in the midst of the current COVID-19 pandemic to refuse to wear masks or socially distance when in socially crowded spaces because they are creating a public health risk to both themselves and others. Likewise, government can justly and justifiably constrain the liberty rights of individuals to purchase "skinny" health plans as well as the rights of insurers to sell such plans. Inevitably, some of these individuals will find themselves unable to pay for necessary and effective life-saving care for themselves, which a compassionate society will feel obligated to provide anyway at unjust expense to others.[14] Individuals should be free to choose their health care providers so long as those choices do not threaten to undermine or

---

[14] We should note what otherwise ought to be obvious, namely, that the "need" for "skinny" plans does not exist in EU countries offering comprehensive health plans to all their citizens. It is because in the United States the cost of health insurance is widely individualized that less well-off individuals can only afford such "skinny" health insurance that such insurance is available. "Skinny" insurance offers only the illusion of coverage.

violate our shared understanding of health care justice. To illustrate this point and its limitations, if we had agreed for some range of mundane medical problems that primary care providers would be nurse practitioners and physician assistants (as a way of making more efficient use of the medical talents of physicians), then an individual who insisted on seeing a physician instead would have to pay the difference in cost for exercising this liberty right. This is not an unjust constraint on the liberty rights of anyone. Likewise, individuals would always have the liberty right to buy their way out of any rationing protocol *so long as their exercise of that right did not undermine or threaten the just claims of others to needed health care.* A rich person could not "outbid" a poorer individual for the last bed in the ICU or for a needed transplantable organ.

The liberty principle would also protect some specific range of liberty rights of health care providers, again, so long as the actual exercise of those rights did not threaten the justice commitments legitimated through the deliberative process. Thus, we would not be justified in outlawing all for-profit aspects of medicine as presumptively unjust. We must in each case consider the empirical evidence available to make a reasonable judgment. Should we permit physicians to own for-profit labs or imaging equipment or other such medically relevant services? It depends. Regulatory efforts might be effective in controlling overuse of such facilities and excess costs that might represent less than just claims on social resources.

Physician-owned for-profit specialty hospitals might be an easier call. These hospitals do generally represent a threat to the just distribution of health care resources. They generally take the best-insured and most profitable patients from community hospitals without accepting any responsibility for meeting comparable medical needs of patients with little or no ability to pay for needed care. Hence, the capacity of community hospitals to continue to provide high-quality care to all their patients is very much threatened by these for-profit physician-owned hospitals.

Insurers may demand the liberty right to turn away customers with potentially costly medical problems, but these are the sort of unjust practices that the liberty principle cannot possibly warrant. If such patients cannot (as a practical matter) be fairly spread across insurance plans, then for-profit insurance plans can be justly outlawed. What they would most clearly undermine is the protection of fair equality of opportunity for those who are medically least well off but clearly capable of benefiting from what medicine has to offer. Insurance companies may justifiably claim that they are

not charitable institutions. The justice-relevant implication of that asser-
tion is that a society does not need that type of business since it interferes
with our social capacity to be justly responsive to all our citizens' health
needs. To its credit, the Affordable Care Act did eliminate the practice of
insurance companies excluding individuals with potentially costly preexisting conditions who had to purchase insurance in the individual market
or small business market. The Kaiser Family Foundation (Claxton et al.,
2019) estimated that 54 million Americans under the age of 65 have preexisting conditions that would result in their being denied coverage if they
needed to use the individual insurance market prior to the passage of the
Affordable Care Act.

The equality principle is the fourth of our constitutional principles of
health care justice. This again will be a complex principle in practice. The
simple formal expression of the principle is that like cases should be treated
alike. Physicians will sometimes assert that no two patients are clinically alike.
The medical circumstances of every patient are unique. But if we take that as
an absolute medical truth, we risk never having any rules or guidelines that
would assure the fair and stable implementation of any rationing protocols.

There are lots and lots of *kinds of medical cases* sufficiently alike to warrant a similar medical response. Hence, what our equality principle will
mean in practice is that if we have a rationing protocol regarding access to
ICDs ($40,000 each) that limits them to those with specific results from a
T-wave alternans test, then exceptions will not be made (at social expense)
for individuals who are excessively anxious or especially demanding or affec-
tionately ingratiating. Any exceptions to any deliberatively legitimated just
rationing protocol must be made for explicit justice-warranted reasons available for review by some impartial party in a health plan.

Again, the primary reason from a structural perspective why the deliberative process can yield just rationing protocols is that deliberators are making
these decisions for their own future possible selves. All are subject to the
same rationing protocols in the same (roughly) clinical circumstances. This
is how we respect one another as moral equals. There cannot be blue-collar
and white-collar and gold-collar rationing protocols that correlate with socioeconomic status. Medicine is complex, and medical problems are complex. There will be legitimate exceptions to many rationing protocols, but
those exceptions themselves must be clearly warranted by the relevant medical or scientific evidence and clear considered judgments of health care justice. Being a powerful politician or prominent CEO or lovable sports star or

quirky philosopher are all irrelevant characteristics that would not warrant any exception to any rationing protocol.

The objection will be raised that rich individuals can buy their way out of any particular rationing protocol. That seems to threaten the fairness and stability of any system of health care rationing. However, if we have created a fair and reasonable set of rationing protocols congruent with a reasonable level of social resources we are willing to dedicate to the meeting of health care needs in our society, then no one among our democratic deliberators is made worse off by allowing the wealthy to buy these exemptions for themselves. Recall that the vast majority of rationing protocols constructed through the deliberative process would be aimed at denying our future possible selves what we rationally judged to be very marginally beneficial excessively costly health care. That is, we have in effect said to ourselves that we would not use our own money to buy such health care for ourselves. Further, from a justice perspective, if I regard such marginal care as a bad buy with my money, then I have no moral or political right to commandeer the money of others to buy such care for myself. If other individuals choose to make that purchase for themselves, then I am not morally harmed by that choice. We are a free society. Wealthy people choose to spend their money on many ridiculous things. If they wish to spend that same money on cancer drugs that cost $100,000 for several extra months of life, then that should not be objectionable as long as it is a wholly private expenditure (no tax breaks) and no one is made worse off by permitting that purchase.

I can imagine some potential complications that might have to be resolved through the deliberative process. If someone has purchased one of those expensive cancer drugs and then suffers complications associated with that therapy which we would ordinarily regard as covered health care services in the national benefit package, does justice then require that we cover those expenses from social resources, or would justice require that individuals be responsible for those additional costs as well (the argument being that, but for their purchase of that marginal therapy, it was unlikely that either they or us would have been faced with these additional costly medical consequences)? Perhaps this is one way in which we might think about this challenge. What if that individual recovers from a supposed terminal cancer? Years later they have a serious cardiac problem. Would we, citizens of a just and caring society, be ethically justified in refusing that individual all medical care at social expense along with the explanation, "You were supposed to be dead. We no longer have any obligation to meet your health care needs. They are now entirely your personal financial responsibility." At the very least, this would be harsh. This person would still be owed equal concern and respect, especially because they had not done anything that was itself unjust. Our social policies permitted them to make that choice.

Our fifth constitutional principle would be that of protecting fair and effective equality of opportunity. Our core moral intuition is that we ought to be responsive to health care needs. But the language of needs in social practice is open to wide and morally unmanageable interpretation. The health needs that matter (as far as justice is concerned) are those that are linked to protecting fair and effective equality of opportunity. Daniels (1985) uses the notion of equality of opportunity broadly. Among the major moral advantages of this broad conception of opportunity is that older retired individuals or persons with a wide range of disabilities are not at risk of having their health needs ignored because they may not be economically productive members of society.

What I have just explicated is the "fair" part of equality of opportunity. But we need to take equally seriously (as a matter of justice) the "effective" part. Effectiveness can fail at either end of the medical encounter. Effectiveness may fail because the technology itself may yield little objective clinical benefit. If an antidepressant lifts the experience of depression by only 20% in only 10% of patients who are given the drug, that drug is not very effective at increasing or protecting the experiential opportunities of depressed patients who take it.

Effectiveness can also fail at the patient end of the clinical encounter. That is, a particular medical intervention may very often have dramatic life-prolonging or quality of life–ameliorating effects. But in particular types of patients who are in particular types of clinical circumstances, its effectiveness may be barely detectable in terms of protecting or enhancing the experiential opportunities of those patients.

Another type of patient-centered failure might be related to the genotype of a patient. Some patients may have genotypes that are either especially responsive or especially non-responsive to certain drugs. If we focus our attention on patients who are poorly responsive to a certain drug because of their genotype, then this may be *unfortunate*, but it is not obviously unjust if we have a rationing protocol that would deny them access to that drug at social expense. This challenge might be most socially distressing when the drugs we are talking about are regarded as "last chance" therapies that are extraordinarily costly. But that social distress is not equivalent to justified moral distress.

As we saw above in our cardiac/cancer genotype example, it would be especially distressing when such drugs work very well for some segment of this patient population but barely work at all in some larger portion of that patient population. It feels psychologically uncomfortable that we would provide social resources to a portion of this patient group and deny them to another portion of the group where the likelihood of a positive response was very low. This will prove to be especially true with regard to many of our targeted cancer therapies, particularly as we discover more reliable predictive biomarkers associated with the use of these drugs. Despite these psychological feelings, it would not be unjust if such a rationing/distributional protocol that relied upon some of these predictive biomarkers were adopted and legitimated through the democratic deliberative process. We can say that the "same patients with the same medical condition" were not treated equally. But there were these morally relevant differences between the groups, and our principle of protecting fair and effective equality of opportunity would provide a presumptive moral warrant for such a choice. Again, we remind the reader that the deliberative process is taking place (generally) when the vast majority of deliberators are ignorant of their future possible medical circumstances. Thus, in this case deliberators could be in either the genetically favored group or the genetically disfavored group. Consequently, whatever their judgment might be, it will not be flawed so far as impartiality is concerned. The protocol would be fair and legitimate. It would not violate any of our constitutional principles of health care justice, nor would it be especially disruptive so far as reflective equilibrium was concerned.

Our sixth constitutional principle of health care justice is a principle of respect for persons. There are two major aspects to this principle: (1) respect for cultural and religious differences among patients related to health care needs and (2) respect for patients as ends in themselves who should not be used by others for their ends. With regard to our first point, our general social rule (as a liberal pluralistic society) ought to be to accommodate special health care needs related to the cultural or religious commitments of patients *so long as the accommodation of those needs does not threaten the just claims of other patients to have their health needs met.* Thus, we respect the rights of Jehovah's Witness patients to refuse blood transfusions for surgery, and we will often modify surgical procedures in ways designed to minimize blood loss in order to maximally protect their lives while respecting their religious commitments.

By way of contrast, one of our newer drugs is a genetically engineered version of factor VII, which is very effective at achieving rapid blood clotting. This is an extraordinarily expensive drug that can cost $100,000 for an episode of bleeding. Some hemophiliacs will have a clear (no alternative) need for this drug to save their lives, and they will have a presumptive just claim to that resource at social expense. If a Jehovah's Witness patient is aware of this drug, is undergoing major surgery with a substantial risk of bleeding out, but does not want to die and does not want a blood transfusion either, then (I argue) they would have no just claim to factor VII at social expense. Our unwillingness to provide this drug to them does not represent any disrespect for their religious beliefs; it represents instead the flip side of our liberal commitments to respect diverse religious views by insisting that we will not provide public subsidies for the support of an individual's religious beliefs (especially if those subsidies were provided at the expense of other just health care claims).

The other aspect of our principle of respect for persons is that patients should not be used as means to satisfy the objectives of others. We cannot permit any coerced health care bargains. We cannot permit any cost-control protocols or practices that would threaten the integrity of the commitment of physicians to the just medical interests of their patients. We cannot permit cost-control mechanisms aimed at patients that motivate patients to deny themselves needed beneficial health care, especially if such cost-control mechanisms would have their most effective impact on patients who were among the financially least well off. One of the major lessons from the Rand experiments was that cost controls aimed at patients work, but they work in a very non-discriminating way. That is, patients deny themselves what from a medical point of view are both beneficial and non-beneficial health care services (and these are decisions they typically make for themselves without the benefit of medical judgment because the decision very often is whether or not to show up in a doctor's office). These sorts of self-denials of care will often be a mix of just and unjust self-denials.

Deliberative democratic conversations about health care rationing are also forms of self-denial, but this is collectively informed self-denial shaped by the specific moral norms of justice endorsed in that process (and relevant medical information). To the extent that rationing protocols that are a product of the deliberative conversation are congruent with our constitutional principles of health care justice, they will reflect mutual respect among free and equal deliberators. That is, no one is being denied needed health care to achieve social objectives unrelated to health care justice. From the perspective of the moral integrity of physicians, their compliance with these protocols does not represent any morally objectionable compromise of their commitments to their patients.[15] But cost-control mechanisms that somewhat indiscriminately incentivize physicians to save money by providing less care (without the specific guidance of democratically legitimated just rationing protocols) risk random injustices due to the essentially private way in which physicians would make these judgments.[16]

Our seventh constitutional principle of health care justice is a principle of liberal neutrality. Just rationing protocols must be rationally justified through public reason. Just rationing protocols must not reflect as their justification deep religious or comprehensive views. Thus, a rationing protocol that would deny public funding for contraceptives or for various forms of assisted reproduction or for pre-implantation genetic diagnosis (when there was a known prior risk of having a child with a serious genetic disorder) because such procedures would be offensive to Roman Catholics or those committed to a right-to-life perspective would be presumptively violative of our liberal neutrality principle. These are not public reasons. Having said that, the reader should understand that such health care services must not necessarily be part of a just comprehensive package of health benefits guaranteed to all in our society. An argument based in public reason must be made for the inclusion of any of these services in a national health benefit package. Further, if that argument is made successfully, then the additional argument must be made regarding their priority status. Relative to protease inhibitors for HIV+ patients or relative to these very expensive cancer drugs in patients with metastatic disease or relative to those drugs that might stave off macular degeneration in the elderly or relative to patients in end-stage heart failure who need an artificial heart, is it more important or less important (as a matter of health care justice) that we fund access to pre-implantation genetic diagnosis for a couple at risk of having a child with a serious genetic disorder

---

[15] Here I reject the views of Tilburt and Cassell (2013), who want to make a sharp distinction between parsimonious care and health care rationing, which allows them to claim that physicians must never make rationing decisions at the bedside. However, health care rationing decisions that are justly democratically endorsed must ultimately be carried out by physicians at the bedside (Fleck, 2016a).

[16] Very worrisome is a recent trend for "investment groups" to buy up medical practices that are seen as being especially profitable. This has gotten the attention of the American College of Physicians, which has issued a policy paper soundly criticizing a range of business practices seen as a threat to the moral integrity of physicians and their responsibility for a more just health care system (DeCamp and Sulmasy, 2021).

at a cost of $40,000 per successful pregnancy? For now, we only raise these questions as a way of illustrating the applicability of this principle.

Our eighth constitutional principle of health care justice is a principle of reciprocity. Reciprocity is about cooperation among free and equal citizens. Rawls writes:

> Cooperation involves the idea of fair terms of cooperation: these are terms that each participant may reasonably accept, provided that everyone else likewise accepts them. Fair terms of cooperation specify an idea of reciprocity: all who are engaged in cooperation and who do their part as the rules and procedure require, are to benefit in an appropriate way as assessed by a suitable benchmark of comparison. (1996, at 16)

What a commitment to reciprocity will mean in practice is that the same comprehensive package of health care benefits will be guaranteed to all in our society and that the same set of rationing protocols and the same priority scheme will establish just limits with respect to that health care benefit package. Because we have to give one another reasons that are mutually acceptable for including or excluding any particular health service in particular clinical circumstances and because we ourselves will have to live with the future consequences of our choices and because the deliberative process itself will educate us about the range and likelihood of various health vulnerabilities and because we all have bonds of affection and capacities for compassion that link us in complex ways to numerous others throughout society with a broad range of health problems and needs (thereby helping to correct excessive attention to our narrow health self-interests), a suitably managed deliberative process will likely yield "fair enough" terms of cooperation that are congruent with the requirements of the reciprocity principle. If the deliberative procedures and deliberative principles outlined here are scrupulously adhered to, no rationing protocol would be legitimated as fair that disadvantaged some identifiable group in our society.

This completes an overview of my understanding of the role of rational democratic deliberation in addressing complex problems of health care rationing in a liberal pluralistic society. The challenge now is to apply this model to the wicked rationing problems I have identified in connection with precision medicine. That will be the task of our next chapter.

6

Rational Democratic Deliberation

Disciplining Wicked Challenges Justly

6.1. Organizing Precisely a Flexible Deliberative Process

In this chapter I hope to accomplish two goals. First, I want to describe what I actually do by way of preparing an audience for deliberating about some of the problems of health care justice related to precision medicine. Keep in mind that my goal is to have the same audience for as many as 10 to 12 two-hour sessions. Second, I want to provide a somewhat compressed surrogate deliberative process regarding all of the wicked problems I described in earlier chapters. I refer to it as a "surrogate" deliberative process because all the deliberation is occurring in my head by a mind that has absorbed an enormous number of articles and perspectives regarding problems of health care justice, now focused on the specific challenges posed by precision medicine. What I want to illustrate is a reasonable reflective equilibrium regarding each problem I discuss. There will be no *ideal* reflective equilibrium with respect to any of these problems. What Rawls (1996) refers to as the "burdens of judgment," the "strains of commitment," and respect for a "reasonable value pluralism" all conspire to yield most often several potential reflective equilibria points with respect to a particular rationing problem that would be "roughly just" or "just enough." Any of those points could be legitimated through a fair deliberative process. Of course, other deliberative proposals might not even be "roughly just."

I usually seek to recruit 25–35 individuals for a deliberative project. I typically seek a diversity of perspectives: politically liberal or conservative perspectives, health professionals versus non-health professionals, racial/ethnic diversity, professional versus non-professional backgrounds, some age distribution, a random distribution of personal health problems for self or others. I am not seeking to "represent" the community as a whole, which

Precision Medicine and Distributive Justice. Leonard M. Fleck, Oxford University Press. © Oxford University Press 2022.
DOI: 10.1093/oso/9780197647721.003.0006

is meaningless. I typically recruit participants by speaking to various social groups at their regularly scheduled meetings where I would talk about the "just caring" problem. I paint a statistical picture of that problem. I emphasize the role of emerging medical technologies in generating and exacerbating that problem. I identify the values that incline us to want to address all the health problems that afflict individuals, and I call attention to their desire to control their insurance and tax dollars going to health care. I deliberately seek to dissuade them from dismissing the problem by blaming any number of greedy villains, whether pharmaceutical companies or physicians or hospitals or insurers.

This effort at dissuasion may strike some of my academic readers as being problematic. It looks like I am biasing the conversation; I contend that I am keeping the conversation honest. I am seeking to prevent collective self-deception. To illustrate, since pharmaceutical companies tend to be regarded as the greediest of the villains, I will note that in 2020 total health spending in the United States on pharmaceuticals was about $430 billion with a net profit of 18%. If I were elected president, I would force all these companies to become non-profits. That would save consumers $77 billion. However, this is a one-time savings. Given current trends, overall health care costs from 2020 to 2021 would still increase by about $220 billion, roughly an increase of 6%. Those increases would have been largely driven by ongoing developments in medical technology in every area of medicine. That tells me (and I tell the audience) that the problem we are addressing through the deliberative process is inside us, as David Eddy (1996) and many others have argued. Recognizing this is what motivates the need for the democratic deliberative process. We have to agree on limits, we need to define reasonable trade-offs, and we have to do this fairly and compassionately.

This is how I recruit participants. I use a more detailed version on the first night that includes some of the ethical issues generated by precision medicine. We generally provide participants with readings for each session, nothing too philosophically complicated, including case accounts from national papers, such as the *New York Times* or the *Washington Post*. We also provide handouts with a focal problem for discussion for the next week and questions intended to provoke critical thinking. We encourage them to share these focal problems with friends and family and co-workers to see what sorts of preliminary reactions they might elicit. For example, we would ask them whether they would endorse a chimeric antigen receptor (CAR) T-cell immunotherapy rationing protocol, as discussed in Chapter 5.

Those handouts provide ethical language that they could readily understand but that might not occur spontaneously to them during a discussion. We preface a series of value statements with these two questions: (1) What should be the fundamental social/political/ethical values that shape health care policy in the United States, most especially the problems of health care cost containment and access? (2) How should these values be balanced in relation to one another? For example, when should we sacrifice some liberty (the individual mandate) for the sake of improving equality of access for all to needed health care, especially individuals with preexisting conditions? Below is the actual list of values and value statements that are provided to participants.

- **Treat everyone justly or fairly.** What do you think it ought to mean to treat everyone justly or fairly when it comes to health care needs, especially very expensive health care needs?
- **Treat everyone with equal concern and respect.** No one should be the victim of discrimination when it comes to health needs. Everyone with appendicitis should have assured access to the surgery necessary to treat that medical condition. If two individuals of roughly the same age need cardiac bypass surgery at a cost of $70,000 to Medicare but one of them has an indefinite life expectancy while the other has a pancreatic cancer likely to be terminal in less than six months, should "equal concern and respect" require both to receive bypass surgery? Why or why not?
- **Treat everyone with compassion (as you would wish to be treated if you were in their shoes).** Does this mean that patients have the right to receive any sort of health care that they want, no matter how much the cost, no matter how small the likely benefit?
- **Provide health care cost-effectively.** What should count as a standard for reasonable health care costs for an intervention? Must this same standard apply to all health care interventions? Some health policy experts say we (society) should pay no more than $50,000 to buy a high-quality extra year of life. Others would up that figure to $100,000. Here is what that means. If a cancer drug costs $100,000 and on average provides someone with metastatic cancer an extra three months of life, then the cost-effectiveness of that drug is $400,000. Some individuals with the very same metastatic cancer (but with different genetic features) might survive two or more years if given that same drug for $100,000. That means the cost-effectiveness of that drug for them

is $50,000. Question: Are you ethically comfortable with an insurance company that would deny this drug to the first patient but provide it to the second patient?

- **Respect freedom of choice for all**. Some insurance companies bargain with physicians for 20%–30% discounts from their normal fees. They then can offer less expensive insurance to individuals or employers. This is what is referred to as a "narrow" network of health care providers. Patients with that insurance plan cannot choose any physician or surgeon they might want for their care at the expense of that plan. Question: Is that an unjust or wrongful constraint on free choice by patients? If an insurance plan says it will only pay for a generic drug that is almost as good as a brand name drug (in order to save money for everyone in that plan), is that a wrongful or unjust constraint on free choice by patients?

- **Assure access to needed care, most especially for those who are medically least well off**. This norm is about both justice and compassion. We ought to be especially sensitive to the needs of those with very serious health care needs that threaten either a premature death or greatly diminished quality of life. But if we need to be mindful of controlling health care costs and if we think we should collectively pay for only effective health care that can save a life or restore quality of life, then maybe we should distinguish between patients who are medically least well off who can be restored to health (even at very great expense) and those whose illness is virtually certain to kill them (end-stage cancers or end-stage heart disease or end-stage emphysema, etc.) but who might gain extra days or weeks of life at enormous expense. Question: Would you endorse this distinction as ethically acceptable? That is, would you endorse having your health plan pay for the care that patients need in the first category but only pay for "comfort care" or "hospice care" for those in the second category?

- **Assure access for all to a "basic" or "adequate" level of care** (as opposed to the best care medically possible). Many health policy experts will argue that no society can afford to pay for the very best health care technologically possible for everyone in that society. Still, they will add that it is unjust to have 30 million individuals without health insurance, that is, without *assured* access to needed health care. They will conclude that a just and caring society ought to guarantee everyone a comprehensive package of "basic" or "adequate" health care interventions.

Question: What do you believe must be included in that "basic" or "adequate" benefit package guaranteed to everyone? Would you, for example, exclude from that package the $250,000 left ventricular assist device for patients with late-stage heart failure? Would you exclude $100,000 cancer drugs for patients with metastatic cancer if those drugs yielded only extra months of life? Would you exclude a $300,000 drug, imiglucerase, for a child with a disease called Gaucher's (it replaces a critical missing enzyme) that would be needed every year for the rest of that child's life? In other words, 15 years of that drug would cost $4.5 million. Would you exclude a $100,000 anti-hemophilic factor (factor VIII) for children with hemophilia that would cost $2 million to buy 20 years for that child?

- **Take seriously social solidarity.** "Social solidarity" is a European notion. It basically means "we are all in this together; we are all vulnerable to life-threatening diseases or quality of life–sapping disabilities; we all need to share the risks and costs with one another." This attitude is what underlies a commitment to universal health care in most European countries. Question: Do you want to see this same value reflected in health policy choices in the United States? If so, what should social solidarity look like when we need to control health care costs?

- **Respect human life as priceless.** Many will argue that we should never put a price on human life, that if we have the technological ability to save or prolong human life, then we are ethically obligated to use that technology for that desperate patient, no matter what the cost. The practical implication of commitment to this value is that it would not be morally or politically acceptable to control health care costs by denying anyone any health care that yielded any small gain in life expectancy. Question: What would be other acceptable ways to control health care costs? Would you deny patients very expensive pain medications in order to transfer those dollars to health care interventions aimed at prolonging life, such as expensive cancer drugs or left ventricular assist devices?

- **Respect cultural and religious differences.** This is a very fundamental American value. It is also a cheap value but not always. Question: If someone is a Jehovah's Witness (they will refuse blood transfusions because of what they see as a prohibition in the Bible) and if they need a surgery where there is a risk that they might bleed out and die without a transfusion, should they have a moral or legal right to demand instead a $100,000 blood-clotting protein, proconvertin or factor VII, that would be provided at expense by your insurance company or Medicare or Medicaid? Likewise, if someone is deeply committed to a right-to-life perspective, should they have a moral and legal right to demand a $150,000 drug for their metastatic cancer paid for by your health plan that everyone else in your plan would be denied if they had the same metastatic cancer and needed the same drug? How does this norm fit with our "equal treatment" or "fair treatment" norm?

- **Minimize administrative costs in the system.** In Europe and Canada, administrative expenses for the health care system are 6%–10% of all health care dollars. Medicare in the United States has about 6% administrative costs. The private health insurance sector in the United States has average administrative costs of 16%–22% of every health care dollar (though some put that figure at 31% [Himmelstein et al., 2020]). Administrative costs do not pay for any health care. We have very high administrative costs because we have more than 1,000 health insurance companies with dozens of plans with numerous co-payments, deductibles, coverage rules, profit for stockholders, etc., that add to that administrative expense. A single-payer system (same health plan, same rules for everyone) would save enormous sums, but that does represent a sacrifice of some individual liberty (there would be no other health plan you could choose), though you could use any doctor or hospital that had room for you that you wanted (no narrow networks). Question: What other ways of controlling administrative costs would you endorse that would not be so politically dramatic (but that would save $100 billion per year)?

- **Expect individuals to take more responsibility for their health.** Many costly health problems are related to bad health choices individuals have made (i.e., lung cancer and smoking, diabetes and heart problems related to bad dietary choices, orthopedic problems [hips and knees] related to extensive running and excessive exercise). Is it fair that you, who have been fairly thoughtful about your health-related behaviors, should have to pay the excessive health care costs of those who have been thoughtless regarding their health-related behaviors? Question: What is it ethically and politically reasonable to do by way of encouraging or requiring better health choices by individuals? Should they be expected to pay a much higher premium for health insurance or pay individually for more of the cost of the care that they need? Would this be an unjust intrusion on individual liberty? How would we non-arbitrarily distinguish costly health problems that are a product of both behavior and complex genetic vulnerability from health problems that are a product of pure irresponsible patient choice? What would be the additional administrative costs necessary to monitor all that individual behavior and assess the costs fairly?

- **Avoid funding very costly, very marginally beneficial health care tests or treatments**. If we have only limited resources (money) and virtually unlimited health care needs, then it seems reasonable to fund the most health benefits at the lowest cost. What would be the consequences of using this principle to govern where we spend our health care dollars? Some health care interventions are very costly ($200,000+), but they effectively save lives from premature death. Other health care interventions are very costly (late stages of a terminal illness), but those interventions only postpone death briefly. Is that a wise use of social resources? However, these are the patients who are among the "medically least well off," who generally command compassion. Also, physicians will tell you that it is difficult to predict with certainty that THIS patient will not survive this hospitalization. Question: What is the right policy choice to make, all things considered, when we need to control health care costs?

  The above example is dramatic. There are thousands of more mundane examples. Almost everyone has suffered at one time or other a really awful headache. It might be a brain tumor. You might want your doctor to do a magnetic resonance imaging (MRI) scan to rule out a brain tumor at a cost of $1,400 to Medicare or your insurance plan. Given the number of really bad headaches in the United States each year, that would quickly add up to billions of dollars of costs that yielded little actual medical benefit. Question: Would you be willing to accept your physician's judgment that it was extremely unlikely that your headache was the result of a brain tumor, and therefore, they will not order the MRI you wanted because that would be a waste of money?

- **Maximize health benefits gained for every dollar spent**. As taxpayers and insurance premium payers you do not want unlimited sums of your money spent on health care. There must be limits. Recall that in any given year 5% of patients will use 50% of the health care dollars spent in that year. Some will have their lives saved from those very large expenditures; others will die despite those very large expenditures. If we can predict with 90% confidence who will belong in this latter group, then what choices would you regard as being ethically acceptable with regard to limiting their access to very expensive care? A lot of very expensive health care treatments are associated with chronic degenerative conditions (heart disease, cancer, chronic obstructive pulmonary disease [COPD], liver disease), especially near the end of life. Would you endorse taking money from very expensive life-prolonging care for these conditions and reallocate it to more aggressive health care prevention aimed at reducing the incidence and severity of these conditions?

This is the material distributed to deliberative participants to give them ethically relevant considerations for addressing a range of health care rationing issues. I do mention to them the various theories of justice, but I avoid any lecturing regarding these theories. The material captures the distinctive features of each of the theories of justice commonly discussed. This is introductory material. Hence, I put off health care justice issues related to the needs of persons with various disabilities as well as issues related to health care disparities or the social determinants of health. They get attention at later stages of the dialogue process.

6.2. Just Deliberations: Tafamidis

Our goal in the remainder of this chapter is to conduct in an experimental mode examples of democratic deliberation regarding all of our wicked rationing problems. What justice-relevant considerations should determine which particular interventions ought to be included in a comprehensive health care benefit package assured to all in our society? Recall that inclusion will be only in a qualified mode. No one has a just claim to a therapy that will yield little benefit in specific medical circumstances, even though others might garner substantial benefit. Our primary focal points are the therapies and interventions associated with precision medicine. However, we will also need to discuss various interventions outside the domain of precision medicine primarily for a comparative perspective. Our bottom line in each case is determining whether the inclusion or qualified inclusion of some intervention preserves a reasonable, stable enough, just enough, reflective equilibrium, as opposed to generating a somewhat chaotic disequilibrium in our understanding of health care justice and health care social beneficence.

We start with a drug called tafamadis. It is used to treat a very specific form of heart failure called transthyretin amyloid cardiomyopathy (ATTR-CM). Approximately 100,000–150,000 patients in the United States have this version of heart failure, out of roughly 6.5 million current heart failure patients, with annual increases of 600,000. The cost of this drug is $225,000 per patient per year (O'Riordan, 2020). This is a drug, like the multiple sclerosis drugs, that could be taken (in theory) for several years. Note that only 4% of patients with this condition are correctly identified as having this condition. Instead, they are simply identified as heart failure patients, and they are treated with relatively inexpensive drugs. It is estimated that 13% of heart failure patients have ATTR-CM. This raises a provocative question so far as basic clinical ethics is concerned. Should all patients now identified generically as heart failure patients undergo more sophisticated diagnostic testing to identify correctly those with this very specific version of heart failure, potentially adding $32 billion per year to the cost of treating these patients (Kazi et al., 2020), the assumption being that all the patients identified as having ATTR-CM would have access to tafamidis? Powerful economic considerations would likely speak against such an effort. Would considerations of health care justice make such an effort ethically obligatory?

Recall that a small percentage of these patients would already be correctly diagnosed by a few astute clinicians. Would health care justice, all things considered, be best preserved if this drug were not offered to any of these patients? This sounds like a plausible option. However, in the arena of targeted cancer therapies and immunotherapies, all manner of genetic testing is being done to identify patients whose tumors have specific genetic mutations likely to elicit a beneficial response with some novel drug. This information is not being hidden from these patients. Why should such information be withheld from cardiac patients who would stand to benefit from tafamidis? One response would be that the cost-effectiveness analysis by Kazi et al. (2020) found that the use of this drug with these patients would have an incremental cost of about $1,135,000 and an incremental cost-effectiveness ratio (ICER) of $880,000 with a range of $697,000–$1,564,000. This is in comparison to the current standard of care provided to these patients at a cost of $16,000.

The average age of patients with this form of heart failure is 74 years. The median gain in life expectancy with this drug is about 1.5 years.

The question for democratic deliberation would be this: Would it be unjust if we excluded tafamidis from our benefit package? Tafamidis does yield some clinical benefit. How should we assess that? The median gain in life expectancy is 1.5 years. However, to achieve that gain, annual costs to a health care budget would be $32 billion. Is this an unreasonable distortion in health care spending priorities for that marginal gain in life expectancy? However, this is a median number. Projections put the gain in life expectancy for 20% of these patients at four years, clearly a more significant benefit. But it would still cost $32 billion per year to save those lives since, at present, we have no way to distinguish short-term survivors from long-term survivors.

Consider a thought experiment. Considerable research is looking for predictive biomarkers to better determine the most appropriate therapy for a patient. But biomarkers can also be used to achieve better (more just) uses of limited health care resources. More specifically, assume we have a biomarker that can predict with 90% reliability which of these patients will fall below that median mark. Should our deliberators endorse the use of that biomarker to reduce by 50% the social cost of tafamidis? That still leaves $16 billion for those patients who would only gain two to three years of life expectancy. If one of our ethical reference points is seeking to preserve equal concern and respect for all, then would we more clearly satisfy that egalitarian concern by denying social funding for this drug for everyone? Insurance companies, if so motivated, could offer a rider that some number of financially well-off individuals could purchase. I would not see this as violating our egalitarian sense of health care justice since no one who is unable to afford such an insurance product would be worse off as a result of this product.[1]

The annual cost of the drug itself is very high, not to mention the cost-effectiveness numbers. If approved, this could open the floodgates to every costly, marginally beneficial drug on the market. That would result in some state of justice-relevant chaotic disequilibrium. Sometimes we ought to

---

[1] No insurance company would be likely to offer such a "stand-alone" product. An insurance company would offer an insurance product that covered multiple medical interventions such as this (i.e., very high cost interventions excluded from social insurance that typically yielded only marginal benefits). These companies would insist on the right to exclude individuals with preexisting conditions. Should our deliberators endorse permitting such policies as not unjust?

ignore those cost and cost-effectiveness numbers. We saw in Chapters 3 and 4 that the enzyme replacement drugs for Pompe disease, Fabry disease, Gaucher's, and several others have costs of $200,000–$300,000 per patient per year. These are drugs that would be required for a lifetime. They seem to be very effective in that they restore enough of the missing enzyme that the deleterious effects of these diseases are minimized, and individuals may achieve something closer to a normal life expectancy. However, this is precisely what cannot be said with regard to tafamidis.

Tafamidis is used to treat a terminal condition. It will prolong life to a moderate degree, roughly 1.5–4 years for most patients. Should it be justice-relevant that the average age of these patients is 74? If we look at this from the perspective of Daniels' fair equality of opportunity account, then these patients would already have achieved a normal life expectancy. In his 1988 volume *Am I My Parents' Keeper* he suggested a thought experiment intended to justify age-based health care rationing under some circumstances. He imagined younger individuals concerned about the uncertainties associated with having health insurance over a lifetime and the risks of a life-threatening illness. Such individuals would want to maximize the likelihood of their achieving a normal life expectancy. This would require a willingness to give up some number of very expensive, life-prolonging therapies beyond, say, age 75 so that those resources could be transferred to their younger self in order to maximize their life expectancy. This looks like an option that would be both just and prudent. Given this perspective, tafamidis looks like something that would be given up *autonomously*. Those same resources could also be used to cover the costs of the enzyme replacement drugs needed for children with the relevant disorders.[2]

This is a wicked problem. While ATTR-CM will largely affect much older individuals, we must note that in most cases it has a genetic cause, a mutation in the TTR gene. The inheritance is dominant, but the gene can be mutated in a number of different ways. In some cases, the mutation will not result in this disorder. In other cases, the onset of the disease may be at a younger age, perhaps an individual's 40s or 50s. That raises this justice-relevant question: Should such an outcome be regarded as merely unfortunate, not justice-relevant. That would mean that tafamidis would not be

---

[2] Daniels himself is mindful that this is an interesting thought experiment that does yield moral insight. However, it is not readily achievable in the US health care system with its highly fragmented system of health care financing.

provided to these patients at social expense. Alternatively, if we agree with the above argument built on Daniels' work, should we make an exception to this rationing protocol and provide social funding for this drug to these younger individuals? Should this seem just and compassionate to our democratic deliberators?

There would remain a possible ragged edge problem. Where is the age-based line beyond which tafamidis would not be provided at social expense? This can be an impossibly arbitrary problem. In this case, our deliberators could choose 65 as a reasonable limit since access to the drug at that point would likely get an individual close to 70, which would be "just enough." We have already noted that ATTR-CM is a terminal condition. Tafamidis is the only therapeutic option that can lengthen the terminal phase of this condition. Consequently, it can be regarded as a "last chance" therapy. The question for our deliberators, however, is whether that characterization of the drug should have justice-relevant consequences.

Are we obligated to ignore the cost of providing this therapy because it is the only chance these patients have for some additional gain in life? Some deliberator might invoke the rule of rescue to justify providing tafamidis. However, we have already seen that the logic of this argument does not apply to terminally ill patients. We could prolong the lives of those ATTR-CM patients for $32 billion per year. However, what would we owe all the other terminally ill patients (heart patients, cancer patients, COPD patients, liver patients, dialysis patients, end-stage diabetic patients, and so on) for whom we also have very expensive, marginally beneficial, last chance therapies that could extend their lives somewhat longer? No reasonable person could endorse the conclusion that these patients have unlimited just claims on health care resources.

The direct opposite conclusion would not be rationally or justly endorsable either (i.e., no terminally ill person ever had a just claim to any expensive life-prolonging therapies). Distinctions need to be made. Children with various advanced leukemias would be correctly described as having a terminal illness. Thirty years ago, most of them would have died. Today, 70%–80% of them are actually cured of their leukemia, though it is at very substantial expense, sometimes exceeding $1 million. I have to believe that our democratic deliberators would judge that these children had a just claim to these social resources, certainly a much stronger just claim than our ATTR-CM patients. The dominant reason for this conclusion would be that most of these children have the opportunity to achieve a normal life expectancy. This is a conclusion I would see endorsed by utilitarian, egalitarian, prioritarian, and sufficientarian considerations of health care justice, the sort of overlapping consensus that would have strong justificatory power.

A critic might point out that a significant number of these children will acquire another cancer in early adulthood, perhaps related to the aggressiveness of the therapy that saved their lives as children (Constine et al., 2020). Some of these adults will die from that later cancer; others may again be cured, perhaps at substantial expense. In either case, these individuals would have just claims to the resources needed to save or prolong their lives in these latter circumstances. One further clarification: Some children will regrettably be faced with a cancer (or comparable medical problem) that has clearly become incurable, and death is imminent (within months or less). If some very expensive quasi-experimental medical intervention is available that has a small chance of offering extra weeks of life, I would argue, as a deliberator, that child would have no just claim to that intervention. If that intervention cost $250,000, those saved resources could be redirected to actually saving the lives of salvageable children. Again, this conclusion could be endorsed from the perspectives of utilitarians, egalitarians, prioritarians, and sufficientarians.

As a democratic deliberator, my conclusion would be that appealing to either the "last chance" rationale or the "rule of rescue" rationale would be insufficient to justify funding from social resources tafamidis for these ATTR-CM patients. Additional considerations that would speak against social funding for tafamidis would be the cost of the drug itself, the aggregate cost of providing this drug to all ATTR-CM patients, and cost-effectiveness considerations. Calling attention to the $300,000 per year we spend to address some childhood life-threatening conditions in an effort to make the cost of tafamidis seem more reasonable will have no moral weight. As noted already, the situations of those children and ATTR-CM patients are too radically different to permit any justice-relevant comparisons.

6.3. Some Wicked Prefatory Comments

Let's consider more directly the wicked problems related to precision medicine. First, the literature on precision medicine is enormous. There are now more than 150 of these targeted therapies or immunotherapies that have Food and Drug Administration (FDA) approval and some degree of effectiveness in addressing specific cancers with very specific genetic mutations. I will address representative drugs and their genetic cancer drivers for major cancers, such as lung cancer, melanoma, breast cancer, and colorectal cancers. Later in this chapter, I will discuss the various immunotherapies that are designed to address hematologic cancers (i.e., leukemias, lymphomas, and so on).

Second, I want to remind the reader that our primary focus is on the problem of justice with regard to health care rationing and precision medicine. I will also want to address these issues from the perspective of obligatory social beneficence, which I do in the following chapter. Numerous bioethicists and physician researchers in oncology see this as a problem that needs to be addressed. Many politicians, bureaucrats, and health care administrators might not see this as a problem *to be publicly addressed*. This goes back to the problem of invisible rationing.

Consider that there might be 45,000 metastatic lung cancer patients with an EGFR mutation driving their cancer who could benefit with a median gain of nine extra months of life from one of these $150,000 targeted cancer therapies. That would add $6.8 billion annually to the cost of health care. Does that represent a just claim on social resources? My critic will contend that the cost figure is a gross exaggeration because no more than 20%–30% of those patients would have the insurance to cover the cost of those targeted therapies. However, this bypasses entirely the problem of health care justice; this is essentially a libertarian response. Justice-relevant considerations of reciprocity as well as equal concern and respect would require that these patients all have access to this targeted therapy if any of them have access at social expense, the assumption being that all would have an equal opportunity for benefit. Certainly, egalitarian and prioritarian conceptions of health care justice would require that.

Third, the discussion that is integral to democratic deliberation occurs at the population level, at the level of policy. But the care provided by physicians is patient-centered. Goldstein and Den (2019) call attention to the definition of patient-centered care endorsed by the Institute of Medicine, namely, "providing care that is respectful of, and responsive to, individual patient preferences, needs, and values and ensuring that patient values guide all clinical decisions" (at 288). How is that supposed to square with justice-relevant limitations on access to some of these targeted therapies? They call attention to some research regarding nivolumab, a checkpoint inhibitor, and PD-1/PD-L1 expression in metastatic lung cancer. What the research showed was that PD-L1 positivity greater than 5% in the cancer cells resulted in 26% of those patients having a response. (I remind the reader that "having a response" is a very weak therapeutic effect.) Nivolumab did not seem to have any effect with regard to either progression-free survival or overall survival. Approval was denied because chemotherapy could achieve this same result at a fraction of the cost. Researchers did some data mining and found that patients whose tumor cells were 50% positive for PD-L1 did achieve some degree of progression-free survival (which implied nothing regarding overall survival). It appears that these patients would not receive this modest benefit because approval was denied overall. Goldstein and Den (2019) conclude, "Providing that side effects were minimal, most individual patients with a fatal disease would likely wish to receive a therapy that has biological plausibility, even if it lacked robust clinical evidence" (at 289). Respecting such patient preferences, however, would undermine just efforts to control overall health care costs. To elaborate on what Goldstein and Den conclude, imagine an oncologist caring for a patient and saying, "I can either treat you with chemotherapy or this targeted cancer therapy. You will get the same result so far as survival is concerned but you would be spared the awful side effects of chemotherapy with the targeted therapy. You have great insurance that will pay for either choice." Obviously, patients without great insurance would not have that choice. What policy should be chosen in this regard through our deliberative process with which physicians could be ethically comfortable?

Fourth, virtually all of these targeted cancer therapies are now described as "orphan drugs." In the United States, this designation means that fewer than 200,000 patients in a year would have need of the drug, that they have a serious illness, and that no other effective therapy is available. Drug companies were free to set whatever price they judged reasonable to cover their research and development costs. Diseases such as Pompe disease or Gaucher disease occur in about 400 births per year. These are enzyme replacement disorders for which we now have drugs that cost $300,000 per year. No one imagined in 1985 what precision medicine was going to yield. Researchers know today that cancer is not a single disease. Instead, it is really 200 or more diseases, with each type defined by a specific genetic mutation that is the primary driver of a cancer. To illustrate, these are the known driver mutations for lung adenocarcinoma: KRAS, 25%; EGFR, 15%; ALK, 8%; BRAF, 5%; PIK3CA, 3%; MET, 3%; ERBB2, 3%; MEK 1, 1%; NRAS, 1%; ROS, 1%; RET, 1%; other 33% (Garraway, 2013). There are targeted therapies for many, but not all, of these driver mutations. Each one of them is regarded as an orphan drug because each of these genetic driver mutations is taken to define a different disease entity. The obvious consequence of this is the very high price for these drugs, as well as very high profit margin, something legislators in 1985 never imagined.

Should our democratic deliberators endorse all of these targeted therapies for inclusion in a comprehensive benefit package guaranteed to all Americans simply because these are "effective enough" orphan drugs and might be regarded as a "last chance" therapy? However, that is not an accurate characterization of the overall situation of these patients. Recall my discussion of cancer drug resistance in Chapter 2.

Imagine a non-small cell lung cancer that is EGFR-positive. It will first be treated with gefitinib. But the cancer will mutate after months, and that drug will become ineffective. Even though this was allegedly the "only" drug that could treat that cancer, the now mutated and progressing cancer will be treated with afatinib or dacotinib, which are other tyrosine kinase inhibitors (TKIs). These too will encounter resistance after months, primarily because of the emergence of the T790M mutation. Osimertinib would then be used as another orphan drug because it is especially effective against that T790M mutation (Remon et al., 2018; Wang et al., 2016; Yu et al., 2015). However, it too will ultimately fail. These patients will have been given multiple "last chance" interventions. What should our democratic deliberators conclude? At the very least, they should conclude that the language of "last chance therapies," certainly in this context, should carry no determinative moral weight in judging the just claims of these patients.

Fifth, considerable political pressure has been applied to the FDA to "fast-track" approval of many of these targeted cancer therapies. What "fast-tracking" means is that a lower level of evidence is judged acceptable for approval. The "real" effectiveness of these drugs should be measured by overall survival. However, it would take years to acquire this information. Consequently, surrogate end points are employed, namely, progression-free survival. This is a reasonable surrogate standard that sometimes correlates with overall survival and at other times does not. This cannot be known at the time of FDA approval. To adjust for that, the FDA will require post-marketing research for seven years or more to gain a better picture of a drug's overall effectiveness. As you might surmise, pharmaceutical companies do not have a lot of motivation for doing this research: Nothing can be gained, and much can be lost if effectiveness in the real world is much less than in the experimental setting or if nasty side effects are identified. Roughly 40% of pharmaceutical companies fail to comply with this FDA requirement (Salcher-Konrad et al., 2020).

We go back to the initial reasons for creating a fast-track option. These are patients with a terminal illness. If we have to wait extra years for a stronger form of evidence-based approval, those patients will have died. However, there is a justice-relevant problem here. If use of the drug in a real-world setting with less than the "ideal" patients needed in an experimental setting results in only very marginally beneficial therapeutic gains and if it would be five or more years later before any post-marketing studies are available, the drug is entrenched in clinical practice. This might be a poor use of limited health care resources, but nevertheless it would be virtually impossible to remove the drug from the market. That would require some truly devastating side effects. If dozens of such very costly drugs remain on the market, each generating billions of dollars in annual sales for a pharmaceutical company, that is a problem of health care justice. This is what is emerging as a substantial problem with FDA approval of aducanumab for early-stage, mild Alzheimer's (Fleck, 2021).[3] Pharmaceutical companies will claim to be advocates for these patients, emphasizing the benefits of these drugs being sacrificed for the sake of some abstract moral or economic ideal related to imagined future possible patients.

---

[3] Biogen has set the cost of aducanumab at $56,000 per year. At present (2021), 3.1 million mild Alzheimer patients would be eligible for the drug at an aggregated cost of $173 billion per year, plus another $15,000 per patient for the monthly infusion costs, plus another $15,000 per patient for positron emission tomographic scans to identify brain swelling or brain bleeds that are side effects for 40% of patients. That yields potential first-year aggregated costs of $258 billion. Aducanumab does reduce β-amyloid in the brain, but functional benefit (cognitive or behavioral) is extremely marginal. The FDA would allow Biogen nine years to complete post-approval clinical trials.

6.4. Wicked Problems, Wicked Analyses, Wicked Deliberation

6.4.1. Combinations of Targeted Therapies: More Benefit? More Cost?

Recall our earlier discussion in Chapter 2 regarding cancer drug resistance. One way of responding to that problem is the so-called AIDS strategy, using two or three drugs in combination or sequentially to better manage the cancer and increase survival. One example of that is using either a doublet for BRAF-mutant colon cancer (encorafenib and cetuximab) or a triplet that added the MEK inhibitor binimetinib. Both these combinations yielded a median survival gain for patients who responded of 9.3 months. In the control arm the median gain in survival was 5.9 months. This represents a net gain of 3.4 months (Kopetz et al., 2019). The cost per month for the doublet is $23,000, and that for the triplet is $32,000. The annual cost for the doublet would be $280,000. The annual cost in the control arm would be $52,000. Response rates with the doublet were 20%, and those with the triplet were 27%. What this means is that we need to multiply by five the annual cost of the doublet for each 3.4 months of net gain we would hope to achieve, or $1.4 million. The ICER cost per quality-adjusted life-year (QALY) would be $4.65 million.

My recommendation to our democratic deliberators would be funding only the control arm. The cost of either targeted treatment is excessive in both absolute and relative terms for the very marginal gains in life expectancy. This is mostly an older patient population, which is not an endorsement of ageism. Our deliberators could do a Daniels experiment and ask whether they would accept a risk of an earlier death at a younger age from some disease for which they could not afford the therapy in order to preserve their access to this doublet combination were they to have a BRAF-mutated colon cancer. I think the answer to that question is obvious. Someone can ask rhetorically, "Who would not want the last three months of their life?" However, this is misleading. It makes it sound as if it is the day before you die, you are told about this drug, which you are denied, and then you die. The medical reality is that you would be aware of your impending death roughly nine months earlier. This doublet would give you a 20% chance of three extra months of life beyond that.

If you argued that a just and caring society was ethically obligated to cover the cost of this treatment for a future possible you, then you would be logically and ethically committed to paying for such end-of-life therapies for an enormous number of extremely costly future possible versions of you, not to mention an enormous number of future actual others who would have these costly needs. This is what reciprocity would require in a just and caring society.

Finally, the triplet combination resulted in 27% of those patients gaining those 3.4 extra months of life, though the cost per month would be $32,000 rather than $23,000. Our erstwhile objector would have to endorse choosing the triplet combination and these additional costs, even though it yielded exactly the same amount of therapeutic benefit for that greater cost. However, 7% more individuals would be the beneficiaries of that extra cost, which is what would seem to make it ethically obligatory, given the position of our objector. Still, extra costs without corresponding benefits are hardly reasonable. Further, as the researchers note, the addition of that third drug increased the frequency and severity of adverse events, which would have their own costs.

6.4.2. Just Trade-offs: Optional or Obligatory

Our next item for discussion is the OncoType DX 21-gene expression assay. For women with early-stage breast cancer, HER2-negative and node-negative, this assay can determine whether chemotherapy post-surgery will be necessary (Sparano et al., 2015). Roughly 100,000 women each year would be in this category, and 70% of them would be told, as a result of the assay, that they could safely skip chemotherapy. What "safely" means is that those women would have a 10% chance of recurrence, though that recurrence would be treatable. The cost of the assay is $5,000. Hence, the annual social cost of the assay would be $500 million. However, the average total cost of chemotherapy is $50,000. The assay could generate a savings of $3.5 billion each year. Our justice-relevant question is this: Should our democratic deliberators approve a protocol that would deny chemotherapy at social expense to the 70% of these women who were informed by the assay that they did not need chemotherapy?

If some of these women were very anxious about the risk of recurrence, they would still be able to receive chemotherapy at their own expense.

This would be an impossible financial burden. Does that represent an injustice? Recent research suggests that $700 billion in health care spending in the United States is wasteful (Shrank et al., 2019; Figueroa et al., 2020). Would this proposed protocol represent an annual reduction in such wasteful spending of $3.5 billion? No one can have a just claim to wasteful health care.

What makes something *wasteful* health care? One response would be that it was not *medically necessary*. Is the chemotherapy medically necessary for women in the 70% cohort? It will yield no medical benefit at all for the vast majority of them, but it would involve some significant suffering. However, as noted, 10% of them will have a recurrence of their cancer. Keep in mind that some portion of the women in the 30% cohort who have chemotherapy will still have a recurrence of their cancer. Chemotherapy is no guarantee of a cure.

Let us consider the 10% who have a recurrence in the 70% group. What if a fraction of 1% of those women end up with a cancer that becomes metastatic and terminal? We would know this statistically, though we could not identify those women before the fact. Should that alter the judgment of our deliberators regarding this proposed protocol? Would it no longer be appropriate to judge the chemotherapy *wasteful* for those women in the 70% group who wanted it? Would they have a just claim to the therapy then? How should our deliberators respond?

To eliminate any male bias, I will restrict our deliberators to be exclusively female. The fundamental question they would have to ask themselves is whether higher-priority health care needs represented a more just and more efficient use of the $3.5 billion in savings from this protocol. An affirmative answer would be endorsed by both utilitarians and prioritarians. The women in this 70% cohort are not among those who are least well off. They are actually quite fortunate because the surgery would likely have cured their cancer, and the assay would spare them chemotherapy. From an egalitarian perspective, the anxious women in the 70% cohort are not being denied equal concern and respect. We have to remember that at an earlier point in time, when they were behind a future health status veil of ignorance and forced to address the "just caring" problem, they would likely regard chemotherapy in these circumstances as a low-value option. They would have been members of our all-female deliberative group. The women in the 70% cohort would cover the entire racial/ethnic and socioeconomic spectrum. Hence, there would be no reason to suspect discrimination.

Perhaps the number of women who would still want chemotherapy would be relatively small. The costs would be bearable. Perhaps some appeal to respect for patient autonomy is implicit in this argument. However, this would set a terrible precedent that would very much disrupt anything we regarded as a just reflective equilibrium. To explain, what would justify our restricting the making of this exception to this situation alone? Why would we not have to make a comparable exception for every just rationing protocol that might emerge from the deliberative process? If we think of this as a matter of either compassion or respect for patient autonomy, we will in effect be subverting our commitment to health care justice in making these collective choices. To be sure, at times exceptions to a rationing protocol will be warranted, but those exceptions will have to be very well justified and shown to be congruent with our overall sense of health care justice.

6.4.3. The Super-Responder Challenge: Must We Maximize?

I next consider the challenges posed by super-responders. This is one of our more complex wicked challenges. Recall our faculty member with a gastric cancer, diagnosed at Stage IV and given six months to a year to live. However, his cancer was found to be HER2-positive and responsive to trastuzumab. He is alive 11 years later. It has cost $170,000 per year for an infusion every three weeks. The aggregate cost of his care thus far has been $1.7 million. He was part of a cohort of patients with the same condition. All the other members of that cohort died after two years of treatment. No one knows why he has survived this long. He was 70 years old in 2020. Question: Does he have a just claim to all these health care resources?

I cannot imagine our democratic deliberators answering this last question negatively. This has been a very effective therapy. He has been very fortunate. Still, a very strict (hard-hearted) cost-effectiveness analyst might raise an objection. That $170,000 figure is far above that $100,000 limit. How can that be justified? The cost-effectiveness analyst will ask whether we are setting a precedent. Would every metastatic cancer patient have a just claim for multiple years to $170,000 worth of cancer therapy? More broadly, would every patient faced with a terminal diagnosis be entitled to life-prolonging care that cost as much as $170,000 per year?

Roughly, 600,000 cancer patients die each year in the United States. If there were seven cohorts of such patients, with each patient in each cohort receiving $170,000 worth of care, the annual aggregated cost would be $714 billion. This would be absurdly unaffordable. Recall the drugs that cost $200,000–$300,000 per year for children with these very rare diseases. Having made that exception to our cost-effectiveness criteria, why would that not justify $170,000 per year for our gastric cancer super-responder? One obvious response would be that they are children, these drugs seem to be very effective, and they may be able to achieve something close to a normal life expectancy. Cancer patients, in contrast, tend to be much older. Hence, we need a stronger rationale than that.

Here is another scenario to consider. It is a philosopher's scenario, but it might have analytic value. We have 1,000 patients with this HER2-positive gastric cancer. After the fact, so to speak, we know 950 of them will die with a net gain in life expectancy of six months after being on trastuzumab for a year, another 40 will achieve a net gain of one year in life expectancy, and the remaining 10 will be super-responders who each gain at least seven extra years of life. The real cost of purchasing that six months for the 950 patients will be $340,000 each when annualized, which would be very objectionable from a cost-effectiveness perspective. However, we have no way of knowing before the fact who those 950 individuals will be. Would it be acceptable, as a matter of health care justice, to deny all 1,000 of those patients access to trastuzumab at social expense? That would save $170 million. However, we would be sacrificing the extended lives that would otherwise have been available to our 10 super-responders. This is something that we would know statistically to be true. We would have no way of knowing who those 10 individuals might have been. Would such a social choice be tragic and unfortunate, but not unjust, if this were a rationing protocol endorsed through a process of rational democratic deliberation? I remind the reader that such a protocol would have been endorsed from behind a health status veil of ignorance. All the deliberators would know that in the future they (or a loved one) could be that patient with the HER2-positive gastric cancer, perhaps the one who might have gained at least seven extra years of life, though that would be an extremely remote chance. However, the deliberators would know that the dollars saved could be redirected to other higher-priority therapies that would yield more life-years sustained at lower cost, and there was a greater chance that they or their loved ones could benefit as a result of that choice.

If we switch to a more realistic scenario, acceptably just options are somewhat murkier. In the real world, we would find a survival continuum stretching from four months of life expectancy gained to more than seven years. The distribution would be heavily weighted toward the lower end. The vast majority of these patients would gain no more than two extra years of life. Perhaps 1% of them would gain those seven extra years of life. As things are now, we have no idea who would be in the super-responder cluster. However, research is seeking biomarkers that would identify those patients before the fact. The scenario we next need to consider is one in which we have done just that. Would only those individuals have a presumptive just claim to that $170,000 worth of treatment for as many years as they were able to benefit? This is a much more challenging problem of health care justice.

Just to provide some arbitrary contextual numbers, assume that 80% of the patients in our cohort of 1,000 will gain six months to a year of additional life; the next 19% would gain up to two years, perhaps slightly more; and then we have our super-responders whom we have identified with some biomarker with 90% confidence the identification is correct. What makes this so ethically challenging? We know who the super-responders will be. If we agreed earlier that these super-responders had a just claim to the resources necessary to sustain their lives for all those years, then it is clear we would be obligated to sustain their lives in this scenario as well. It would appear to be unthinkable to simply allow these patients to die when we have available a drug that can sustain their lives for many years. These are identifiable individuals. I assume it would be equally unthinkable to choose not to identify these individuals by not testing for the relevant biomarker. Trastuzumab is very expensive, but it is not something absolutely scarce. The moral logic here is what required us to create the amendments to the Medicare program for end-stage renal disease patients at a cost today of $90,000 per patient per year. For these very same reasons it would be unjust to say to the super-responders that it was up to them to pay for this drug.

Having agreed to save the super-responders, what position should a just and caring society, our democratic deliberators, take with regard to all the other members of this cohort? The two years that could be gained by the other 19% of this cohort is a significant gain in life expectancy. It would seem harsh and uncaring if we required those individuals to find the resources needed to purchase those two years themselves. Perhaps we would find it ethically painful but ethically acceptable to say that to the 80% of the cohort that would gain only six months to an extra year of life. However, by hypothesis, we have no way of identifying who might be in the two-year cohort and who might be in the six-month cohort. All of these individuals are faced with a terminal prognosis. They can justifiably be included among the medically least well off from a prioritarian perspective. From a utilitarian perspective this might not look like a wise use of limited resources, given the opportunity to save $170 million for higher-priority health care needs where we could save more life-years at a lower cost.

Egalitarians might find themselves internally conflicted. They could be ethically comfortable with providing trastuzumab for either everyone in this cohort or no one. However, for the reasons stated above, it would be ethically problematic to include in the "no one" category our super-responders. Our deliberators could choose to fund care for the super-responders but deny funding for everyone else in that cohort. Utilitarian considerations might motivate such a choice. However, such a choice would not necessarily be anti-egalitarian. Reasons of justice and compassion would seem to necessitate saving the super-responders. Being a super-responder would seem to be an entirely random event. The rich and the poor, the young and the old, the socially prominent and the socially invisible would all have an equal likelihood of being a super-responder. To that extent, egalitarian sensibilities would be respected.

We need to note, however, that there are super-responders across the entire spectrum of cancer. We can find biomarkers for super-responders among numerous other types of cancer. If we agreed as democratic deliberators that it was not unjust to sacrifice those gastric cancer patients who might gain two extra years of life for the sake of saving $170 million, then would consistency require the same judgment regarding all these other cancer types that were comparable enough to the gastric cancer case? It is noteworthy that most of the new targeted cancer therapies are now being priced in the $150,000–$180,000 range as an annual cost or for a course of treatment.

While we ponder that last point, we need to consider another wicked aspect of this problem in the real world, as opposed to my neat hypothetical world. These targeted cancer therapies are regarded as orphan drugs. They are typically put on a fast track for approval, though the degree of benefit may be uncertain, hence the need for post-marketing research. Do we then imagine discovering what we hypothesized in our gastric cancer example? That creates an ethically awkward situation. The drug is already "out there" and being taken by patients who are getting some degree of life prolongation. There is a steady stream of patients in each of these cancer pipelines. Suddenly, we would have to stop social funding for this drug as a result of our deliberative process. We would not literally rip this out of the medicine cabinets (or out of the arms) of patients who were already on the drug. But we would deny the drug to any newly diagnosed patients with a specific cancer, though those patients would be aware of their friends who were benefiting from the drug, perhaps with a gain of almost two extra years of life. This transition would be ethically easier if we had discovered some horrible side effects that required pulling the drug from the market or that the drug yielded very little benefit for the vast majority of patients. However, this is exactly what is not true. Nothing new at all has been discovered with regard to the drug itself. Instead, what was discovered was that the drug was not such a wise use of social resources. This is not a rationale that new patients in these circumstances will find terribly convincing, congruent with what they would regard as a just and caring society.[4]

We can expand on our scenario in yet another way. We noted in Chapter 2 that a major goal of cancer research with respect to metastatic patients was to give them several extra years of life with a reasonable quality. We want to create many more super-responders. Instead of individuals being *natural* super-responders for entirely unknown reasons, these super-responders would be a product of scientific ingenuity. Not every patient with metastatic breast cancer or metastatic melanoma or metastatic lung cancer or metastatic colon cancer will benefit from this strategy, at least in the foreseeable future. Still, significant numbers will benefit. We can consider several possible scenarios. To put things in context, there were 143,000 lung cancer deaths in the United States in 2019, 7,000 deaths from melanoma, 43,000 deaths from breast cancer, and 53,000 deaths from colorectal cancer. Another relevant statistic would be five-year relative survival rates with metastatic colorectal cancer (14.3%), metastatic breast cancer (28.1%), metastatic melanoma (4%), and metastatic lung cancer (5.8%).[5] These are the cancer patients with

---

[4] One way of avoiding this scenario is to have an entity such as the National Institute for Clinical Excellence (NICE) make all of these decisions regarding these cancer drugs in as objective a way as possible *before* the drug is clinically available. One of the virtues of NICE is that it is wholly independent of government as well as lobbying efforts by interested parties. Moreover, its decisions are final. That is essential to its independence. The government cannot override its decisions (Charlton, 2020). However, the government did create the Cancer Drug Fund as a way of skirting NICE's negative decisions with respect to specific drugs (Epanomeritakis, 2019). It is unclear what just and reasonable criteria the keepers of this fund used to disperse the available funds, thereby creating something akin to a lottery.

[5] All of these statistics come from the National Cancer Institute: Surveillance, Epidemiology and End Results Program. See https://seer.cancer.gov/statfacts/ (accessed Nov. 3, 2020).

each of these cancers who survive with metastatic disease for five years given available therapies for the period 2014–2018.

In our hypothetical scenarios I want to imagine that our goal is to bring up to 50% the number of metastatic cancer patients who survive for five years. Note that as things are now, most of these metastatic cancer patients will only survive a year or two. Hence, we will need to increase their life expectancy by 3–4 years, with the likely consequences that other metastatic cancer patients who already survive five years might see their life expectancy increase to 7–8 years or more. To appreciate the ethical challenges, recall that we agreed we were ethically obligated to provide the resources necessary to sustain the lives of our super-responders, most certainly when we knew who they were before the fact. To be clear, what we are in effect doing is creating a very large cohort of super-responders, which would be an extremely costly enterprise if we were successful.

We can imagine three main scenarios. First, let us start with what I will call our *black* scenario. From the whole cohort of metastatic lung cancer patients, we have no idea which patients might prove to be among the relative super-responders who gain three or more extra years of life from our use of multiple targeted therapies. What we do know is that each life-year gained will cost $175,000. Consequently, if we wish to maximize the number of individuals who are able to achieve five-year life expectancies with metastatic disease, we will be required to provide our enhanced targeted therapies to *all the patients* with a specific cancer. This would be a very costly strategy, given that 143,000 patients die each year of lung cancer in the United States.

Second, for our *black and white* scenario, assume that we can identify one or more biomarkers that predict correctly 80%–90% of the time those individuals who are most likely to gain the most life-years from our advanced targeted therapy strategy. Consequently, half the patients in any of these disease categories would be denied access to these enhanced targeted therapies at social expense. Since our biomarker predictors are only 80%–90% accurate, this will mean that some number of individuals denied access to this therapy at social expense would have become super–responders. This strategy would presumably reduce by 50% the social cost of caring for these patients, though that will require sacrificing the lives (life-years) of some potential super-responders. We have no way of knowing who they would have been. In this respect identifiable lives are not sacrificed, but we would need to consider whether describing them as "merely" statistical lives dissolves any health care justice issue.

In our third scenario, our *black and white and gray* scenario, we have biomarkers that tell us which patients are least likely to be strong responders to our enhanced targeted therapies. That would be 35% of the cohort. A different set of biomarkers identify with a high degree of confidence the individuals who will most likely be super-responders to our enhanced targeted therapies. That is another 35% of the cohort. The middle 30% yields mixed results from our biomarkers. Some are a bit more likely to be strong responders; others are a bit less likely. There is considerable interpretive uncertainty. The differences are such that it would be ethically perilous to allow these small predicted differences to determine who would receive or be denied the enhanced targeted therapies.[6] What is the just choice to make, all things considered? If we treat everyone, then we are certain to save all the super-responders. But we will waste considerable social resources on the poor responders, though they might gain an extra year or two they would not otherwise have gained. Alternatively, we can choose to treat no one in the gray group, thereby saving considerable sums of resources, though sacrificing the potential super-responders in that group. Again, they are not *identified* or visible lost lives and life-years, but they will nevertheless be real life-years. Would we be able to achieve "rough justice" with a compromise of sorts, namely, through the use of a lottery: Half the gray area's patients receive the enhanced targeted therapy; the other half are denied it?

For the sake of simplicity, we will again assume our cohort is comprised of 1,000 metastatic cancer patients. Our enhanced targeted therapy strategy will cost about $175,000 per life-year gained. Recall that more than 600,000 individuals die of cancer each year in the United States. Hence, the overall goal we have in mind for these hypothetical scenarios is giving 300,000 of these individuals five extra life-years. In our first scenario, the *black* scenario, all 1,000 patients would receive the enhanced targeted therapy for an aggregated cost of $175 million in Year 1. In Year 2 we would only have 750 patients, with an aggregated cost of $132 million. In Years 3, 4, and 5 we would have 500 patients, with an aggregated cost of $88 million each year. In Year 5 and every year thereafter the aggregated cost of each survival cohort would be $670 million. If we extrapolate that to the cohort of 300,000 metastatic cancer patients we would hope to help, the cost in Year

---

[6] See Frances Kamm (1993, at 101–05) and what she refers to as the principle of irrelevant utilities. In brief, some differences are so small or uncertain when assessing the justness of allocating some scarce life-saving resources that it would be unjust to use such small differences to make such allocations with such major consequences for individuals on the basis of those differences.

5 and every year thereafter would be $201 billion for this first scenario. In our second scenario, the *black and white* scenario, only half the patients will receive the enhanced targeted therapy over the five years. For the group of 1,000 patients, the annual cost would be $88 million, the five-year aggregated cost would be $440 million, and the five-year cost for the cohort of 300,000 would be $132 billion that year and every year thereafter. In our third scenario, the *black and white and gray* scenario, the top 35% would cost $310 million in Year 5 and $93 billion for the cohort of 300,000 in Year 5 and every year thereafter. These numbers also represent the savings from not covering at all the bottom 35%. If we choose not to cover the middle 30%, that almost doubles the savings; if we cover the middle 30%, that almost doubles the cost. These are the cost figures and options that our democratic deliberators would need to consider. Finally, the actual cost of cancer care in the United States was $173 billion for 2021. What this figure says is that most of these scenarios would more than double the cost of cancer care in the United States. This is not intrinsically ethically objectionable. But it would require raising taxes and/or insurance premiums unless savings could be extracted from other areas of medical need.

How should our deliberators assess these three scenarios? Egalitarians would be most satisfied with the first scenario because everyone would be given an opportunity to benefit from these enhanced targeted therapies. However, we would need to recognize that this would be a very narrow egalitarian perspective. The broader egalitarian perspective would require looking over every area of medicine, especially those areas where numerous patients would be faced with terminal conditions that could be treated with extraordinarily expensive life-prolonging care. I cannot imagine any justice-based argument that would give special ethical standing for health care resources such that we would be ethically obligated to meet all cancer needs before we addressed the needs of cardiac patients or patients with late-stage lung disease or Parkinson's or rheumatoid arthritis or amyotrophic lateral sclerosis, and so on. Again, this entire hypothetical strategy aimed at increasing substantially the life expectancy of cancer patients would be the result of very large research investments, some public, some private. In either case, a justice-based justification would be required for these research investments, especially if nothing comparable were made available in other areas of medicine.

Utilitarians would likely not be ethically comfortable with this first scenario. Too much money would be spent for only very marginal benefits. They might be more ethically comfortable with our second scenario, though the entire scenario exceeds the $100,000 cost-effectiveness criteria per life-year gained. The libertarian perspective has some relevance across all three scenarios. The question our deliberators need to ask themselves is: When is it permissible from the perspective of health care justice to say that social resources should not be used to pay for this specific care, that private resources and private insurance should be an option for patients who wish to choose that option and can afford to choose that option? An affirmative answer is easy when the anticipated benefits are very marginal and extraordinarily costly. Requiring $100,000 for a chance at three extra months of life would be a clear example. But in our second scenario, the half of that patient cohort judged ineligible for our enhanced targeted therapies would be a complex mixture of patients whose potential gain in life expectancy would be anywhere from three months to two years. My suspicion is that as we get beyond the one-year mark for survival gain, most of our deliberators would be uncomfortable with sacrificing all those potentially salvageable life-years. However, by hypothesis, we had no test or biomarker that could reliably identify the survival potential for individuals in the lower half of the spectrum. All our biomarker could tell us was that this other cluster of patients was very likely to be something close to super-responders.

Again, patients in this bottom half of Scenario 2 are not turned out to the hospital parking lot to die. They would still have the option of chemotherapy, though the side effects at this stage would be substantial and debilitating. Should that elicit moral discomfort in our deliberators? Most problematic would be the "gray group" in our third scenario. This is a complex mix of patients. Some might be somewhat marginal responders. Most of them would gain two or three extra years of life. Some of them might be true super-responders that our biomarkers failed to identify. The argument they could make to our deliberators (some of whom could be in that gray group at some point in the future) is that each life-year saved in this group costs the same $175,000 that will be spent on the super-responders. Their life-years do not represent an exaggerated cost relative to the costs of all the other life-years saved. Further, the super-responders are very fortunate to gain all those additional life-years at social expense; it would be unjust and uncaring, a failure to demonstrate equal concern and respect, for the gray group individuals to be denied the same degree of social support. This strikes me as a compelling argument, at least as long as the deliberators accept the $175,000 per life-year saved in this context as reasonable and just.

6.4.4. Ragged Edges and Rough Justice

We return to the actual world of oncology, which is more complex and fuzzier than the hypothetical scenarios I sketched above. Here our deliberators must address the ragged edge or "line-drawing" problem. In different clinical contexts tumor mutational burden, high microsatellite instability (MSI), and PD-1/PD-L1 expression greater than 50% are all regarded as predictive of longer progression-free survival and overall survival. In all of these cases, however, standard clinical practice demonstrates that patients fall in various degrees below the standard but still have a somewhat significant response to the targeted therapy. Let me provide a couple of examples.

In the KEYNOTE-042 trial patients were treated with either pembrolizumab, a checkpoint inhibitor, or chemotherapy. These were patients with advanced or metastatic non-small cell lung cancer. Patients were divided into three groups: those with a tumor proportion score (TPS) greater than 50%, a score of 20%–49%, and a score greater than 1% but less than 20%. A course of treatment with pembrolizumab would cost $156,000. Median overall survival in the pembrolizumab group with a TPS greater than 50% was 20.2 months compared to chemotherapy at 12.2 months. That represents a median gain in life expectancy of 8 months. In the group with a TPS of 20%–49% median survival was 17.7 months in the pembrolizumab group versus 13.0 months in the chemotherapy group, a median gain of 4.7 months. In the final group, median overall survival with pembrolizumab was 16.7 months versus 12.1 months for chemotherapy, a net gain of 4.6 months (Mok et al., 2019).

These numbers can be a little misleading, as two cautious critics noted in a commentary that accompanied this article (Smit and deLangen, 2019). They called attention to the survival curves included in the article itself (see below). There is an unequivocal survival benefit for patients in the pembrolizumab group with a TPS greater than 50%. But in the other two groups, the survival curves actually cross at one point, which is to say that the chemotherapy patients for some portion of the survival curve actually did better than the pembrolizumab patients. Further, for most of the survival curve the differences between the two groups are not very large. How should our democratic deliberators respond to this situation?

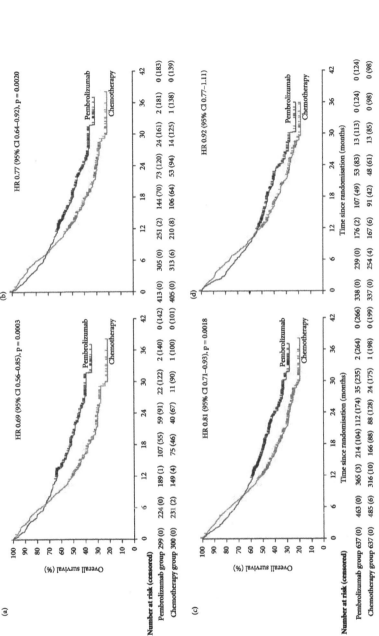

"Kaplan–Meier survival curves for non-small-cell lung cancer patients treated with either pembrolizumab or chemotherapy"

Note: We need to make sure that these graphs include text below the graphs in the article that explain what "A", "B", "C" and "D" are about.

CI, confidence interval; HR, hazard ratio

[Reprinted with permission from the Lancet]

Smit and deLangen (2019) suggest that individual patients should be allowed to make their own choice as to which therapeutic route they might prefer. This has obvious ethical appeal in terms of respect for patient autonomy. What precisely is the choice they are faced with? For some portion of the survival curves patients who choose chemotherapy might actually have a reduced chance of dying prematurely, though this would require accepting the significantly diminished quality of life associated with chemotherapy. Pembrolizumab will have fewer problematic side effects and, for most patients, will yield a small gain in life expectancy. Why not let patients choose? The cost of pembrolizumab would be about four times the cost of chemotherapy for roughly something close to the same outcome. That is a problem of health care justice. Are those quality-of-life gains sufficient to justify the excess costs associated with pembrolizumab? Or does this really represent a waste of health care resources (i.e., spending a lot more money for something very close in terms of survival gains)?

Our deliberators in a utilitarian frame of mind could not endorse what they would regard as a waste of resources. In an egalitarian frame of mind, perplexity would be the order of the day. On the one hand, patients with a TPS score greater than 50% did have a greater gain in overall survival with pembrolizumab than any patient with a lower TPS score. This was not a huge difference, but perhaps it was enough to justify the additional costs associated with pembrolizumab. On the other hand, it might not feel fair, say, in the cases of patients with a TPS score in the 40%–49% range that they would be denied the opportunity for some additional survival gain and quality-of-life gain because they missed that 50% mark. This is our ragged edge/line-drawing problem. Deliberators thinking like egalitarians might see abolishing that line as the easiest way out of this problem. They could either deny everyone pembrolizumab in this scenario (a hard bullet to bite), or they could give everyone access to pembrolizumab at social expense (which might represent unjust and unjustified waste). However, we again must remember that this discussion has implications far beyond this single scenario. This is where reflective equilibrium comes in.

Dozens and dozens of other scenarios can be readily identified in which PD1/PD-L1 expression or tumor mutational burden or high MSI might serve as a biomarker for providing or withholding one or more of these targeted cancer therapies. Consequently, we can hardly imagine abolishing the dividing line in the case of pembrolizumab and non-small cell lung cancer *only in that case and no others* where a comparable dividing line would be suggested. This would require a powerful justification. Without such a justification and with no line drawing in all these other cases, the likelihood would be an enormous waste of health care resources for very marginal and uncertain benefits. At this point our deliberators could assume a libertarian frame of mind and suggest that the waste of social resources could be eliminated by simply saying that anyone who wanted one of these targeted therapies instead of chemotherapy for their metastatic cancer could pay for it themselves (or could have purchased some special form of insurance that would pay these costs). This could be regarded as a legitimate example of "rough justice." The financially well off would be purchasing this marginal gain in life expectancy, but it would not be at the expense of those less financially well off, especially if it were the case that our democratic deliberators had collectively decided that the funds thereby saved could be better allocated to meeting other life-prolonging or quality of life–enhancing health care needs for all. This outcome would actually be congruent with the justice-based intuitions of our deliberators, whether those intuitions were of an egalitarian, utilitarian, or prioritarian sort. Again, this represents what Rawls would refer to as an "overlapping consensus," which represents the sort of justification that needs to be achieved in a liberal, pluralistic society with competing conceptions of health care justice.

We could also describe this as a pluralistic outcome of a *political* conception of health care justice. In other words, even though I describe our deliberators as adopting a utilitarian or egalitarian or prioritarian perspective in assessing a specific rationing issue, they are not really assessing these specific challenges from the perspective of the comprehensive doctrine that is identified as utilitarianism or egalitarianism. Instead, they are appealing to the core values integral to those perspectives but separable from those perspectives, such as maximizing efficiency for the sake of all or giving due consideration to those who are least well off health-wise or assuring that all patients are entitled to equal concern and respect. These are reasonable values that any reasonable person can endorse apart from any comprehensive doctrine to which they might be committed.

I want to continue our discussion of ragged edges and line drawing in connection with three other biomarkers related to cancer prognosis. These are the notions of tumor mutational burden (TMB), high MSI, and mismatch repair (MMR) deficiency. The context for this discussion will again be the checkpoint inhibitors and other forms of immunotherapy. TMB is almost self-explanatory. It refers to the fact that in metastatic cancer the cellular machinery is so disrupted that as these cancer cells multiply, they develop an increasing number of mutations. What will strike many non-cancer researchers as odd is that cancer cells with a very high mutational burden are more vulnerable to attack by various immunotherapies than cancer cells with a low mutational burden. The apparent reason is that having more targets in these cells makes them more vulnerable to attack by the immune system (though this still does not result in cure). The "microsatellite" in MSI refers to a number of repeated DNA bases that are different from what the microsatellite was when it was inherited. Again, a hallmark of cancer is the presence of these mutations and aberrations in the cellular machinery that result in unchecked growth of these cells. MSI is indicative of MMR deficiency. There are specific genes whose job it is to repair the internal cellular machinery when something goes amiss. When these genes are damaged and cannot do their job, mutations in daughter cells go uncorrected.

These three biomarkers are seen as having predictive value for determining whether or not checkpoint inhibitors might be beneficial for patients with several different types of metastatic cancer. Their value is easy to grasp if they indicate either that a patient is very unlikely to benefit from these drugs or that a strong likelihood exists of their benefiting significantly. Money is saved, which has justice-relevant consequences, and unnecessary suffering is avoided. Unfortunately, these biomarkers also create some significant gray areas. "Tumor mutational burden (TMB) appears to be an important independent biomarker to identify patients with hypermutated colorectal cancer tumors with microsatellite instability (MSI) who are likely to respond to immune checkpoint inhibitors" (Fuerst, 2019). To be precise, a TMB of 41 mutations per megabase or greater yielded progression-free survival with a median of 18 months when treated with a PD-1 inhibitor. If TMB was below 37 mutations per megabase, the median gain in progression-free survival was just two months. The researchers concluded, "The implication, he said, is that patients with MSI and high TMB should consider receiving immunotherapy as their first treatment. Those with MSI and low TMB (less than 37 mutations/Mb) should be considered for chemotherapy rather than immunotherapy as their first treatment option" (Fuerst, 2019). However, there is that gray area between 37 and 41 mutations per megabase.

To add to the ethical challenges, one of the researchers suggested that some patients close to that 37 number might have a better median response than someone closer to 29 or 31 mutations per megabase. That researcher added that not all MSI-high colorectal cancers are created equal; lots of other factors might determine response and resistance, and we seem to have little understanding of those other factors. How then should our deliberators respond to this scenario? Again, the researchers emphasize that chemotherapy is available as a treatment option that will likely prove more beneficial than treatment with any checkpoint inhibitor. They suggest that patients in or close to that gray area might be offered a choice. However, this raises the same problem that we discussed above.

Treatment with the checkpoint inhibitors will cost at least four times more than treatment with chemotherapy, and we have no way of knowing before the fact that those additional costs would be just or justified. This situation is somewhat more challenging than the situation with pembrolizumab and non-small cell lung cancer. In that earlier situation the median survival differences were not that great. In this case, the median survival differences are great, 18 months versus two months. Our deliberators might like to believe that median survival in that gray area group of patients ought to be closer to 18 months than two months of survival. That is not an irrational belief. Our deliberators might judge that a strict utilitarian commitment would not warrant accepting that belief, but compassion might be the ethically safer course of action. This would be another example of rough justice. In effect, our deliberators in this case would reject the libertarian option of requiring patients in the gray area to pay for their care with their own funds (or private insurance funds). One of the virtues of the libertarian option in these sorts of situations where a line must be drawn is that it is "thick space" that separates socially funded health care from health care that is not socially funded (and that even private insurance would be unwilling to fund). However, when a very thin, sharp line separates those two domains, individuals very close to that line (but on the non–socially funded side) will demand that they too deserve compassionate treatment because they are so close to that line and might benefit significantly if provided those social resources.

6.4.5. Lazarus Patients: Can We Afford Them?

One of the more wicked problems our deliberators need to address is one that includes the "Lazarus effect." Several variations are possible. Prior to the precision medicine era, oncologists would often offer chemotherapy to their patients who were very near death. This practice has been subjected to harsh ethical criticism, either for reasons of harm to patients or for reasons of health care justice. These are patients who are denied timely access to hospice care, who are often perceived to end up dying a less than dignified death as a result of all the side effects associated with the chemotherapy. However, on rare occasions, one of these patients springs back to life as a result of that last dose of chemotherapy. They are not cured, but they are given an extra year or two of life that no one ever expected. They are like Lazarus in the Gospel stories. The difference, of course, is that no one else died a horrible death in order for Lazarus to be brought back to life. In these end-of-life cancer situations we can readily imagine that several hundred such patients would have to undergo very late aggressive cancer treatment in order to get one Lazarus survivor.[7] Is that an ethically acceptable trade-off? Who should be responsible for making these decisions? Should this be a pure medical decision? Is this a matter of shared decision-making? Should desperate patients be offered the opportunity to make such choices? We will have to put all those traditional clinical ethics questions aside. I want to examine some Lazarus issues in the context of precision medicine.

Recent medical reports address the issue of potential Lazarus patients with certain biomarkers, such as high MSI (Pietrantonio et al., 2020). These are actually patients with what is termed "poor performance status." They are somewhat near death; they seem to have little in the way of physiological reserve. These are patients who would never be included in a clinical trial. Consequently, no one really knows how these patients might respond to a checkpoint inhibitor if their disease exhibits biomarker traits that would otherwise be predictive of a positive response to one of these drugs. In this reported research, which was retrospective, 27 patients were identified with diverse tumor types. These were all patients with poor performance status, but they all had MSI-high cancers, which were treated with a PD-1 or PD-L1 inhibitor as salvage immunotherapy. Nine of those patients (33%) responded to the treatment, and three of those responses were complete responses (meaning no detectable cancer, which is not the same as a cure). In brief, three of these patients were beneficiaries of the Lazarus effect with a median gain in survival of 18 months. How should our deliberators interpret these results?

This was a retrospective study, which suggests that these results would not be duplicated with this level of success if this were done prospectively. For

---

[7] I have not been able to find any actual statistics, though everything I have read suggests these are very rare events.

discussion purposes, let me create this scenario. The authors of this study suggest that patients with very high TMB, MSI, or MMR and poor performance status should be given the option of salvage immunotherapy as opposed to hospice and comfort care. One advantage of these checkpoint inhibitors is that they are less toxic than chemotherapy. Still, in my hypothetical scenario we will imagine that 5% of a patient cohort experiences the Lazarus effect and has a median gain in life expectancy of 18 months. Is this outcome such that the whole practice ought to be socially funded?

In the research cited, median progression-free survival was just 3.5 months. In my hypothetical scenario it would take the cost of treating 19 patients to achieve one Lazarus effect patient. The current cost of these checkpoint inhibitors is $156,000 per year or $13,000 per month. If the average use of this drug were for six months, then the cost of one Lazarus survivor would be $1.52 million. These would be mostly older patients. This would almost certainly have to be a matter of low priority relative to the health care needs of other cancer patients who could achieve much more health benefit at a much lower cost. Consequently, it is difficult to imagine utilitarians, egalitarians, or prioritarians endorsing the use of social funds for the benefit of these potential Lazarus patients. Instead, this is another situation in which the libertarian option would be acceptable as a matter of "rough justice." That is, individuals with the financial resources could either pay for this gamble with their own funds or else have had enough foresight and enough anxiety about this cancer scenario that they would have purchased some form of private supplementary insurance far in advance of such a situation. This strikes me as a reasonable conclusion our democratic deliberators could endorse for their future possible selves as well as their loved ones.

6.4.6. Rare Cancer Drivers: Can We Afford the Cost of Searching?

I next address a different version of the Lazarus effect, patients who have very rare drivers of their cancer. The problem is that clinicians do not know that the primary driver of these cancers is some very rare mutation. Consequently, these patients are treated with some targeted therapy that will prove to be less effective. From the perspective of these authors (Steenhuysen and Burger, 2019), the deaths of these patients would be premature. They could be rescued for some additional life if only the right drug were provided to them. In order for that to happen, however, insurers would have to be willing to fund next-generation sequencing (NGS) of these tumors in order to find these very rare mutations. The cost of NGS will be about $5000. This is not an outrageous sum of money for some very sophisticated testing.

The authors specifically call attention to a type of mutation, NTRK fusion, that is very rare but that can be treated with a novel targeted therapy, larotrectinib. One of the distinctive features of these NTRK fusion mutations is that they are tumor-agnostic. They will be found in more than 20 different types of cancer. However, their rarity is a problem: 0.23% in a cohort of patients with non-small cell lung cancer, 0.35% in a cohort of patients with colorectal carcinomas, and 0.27% in a cohort of patients with various solid tumors (Solomon and Hechtman, 2019). What these numbers mean is that in order to find one patient with an NTRK fusion driver mutation of their cancer you would need to test 400 patients at a cost of $5,000 each. That is $2 million worth of testing. To be clear, the NGS platforms used for this purpose would all be multi-gene panels, perhaps looking for 70 different mutations that might be targetable. If larotrectinib is given to these patients, one study (Drilon et al., 2018) showed that 55% of these patients would have progression-free survival at one year (though, as with most metastatic disease, resistance eventually occurred). The cost of larotrectinib is $32,800 per month, which would be almost $400,000 for each of those patients who survived one year with their cancer. How should our deliberators assess this overall situation, that is, the rarity of the mutation, the aggregated cost of doing multi-gene NGS, the cost of the drug, and the limitations of the test?

Consider this hypothetical scenario. What will strike many as problematic from a health care justice perspective is the very high cost of saving one life-year. However, what if larotrectinib were extremely effective? What if 80% of the patients who needed this drug gained 10 extra years of life, all else remaining the same? Our deliberators might see social funding of these costs as a matter of health care justice. They would also attach urgency to the need to do NGS to identify all the patients with NTRK fusions who might potentially benefit from this drug. I remind the reader that there are no clinical signs of this mutation and that this mutation occurs across numerous types of tumors. In other words, active investigation will be necessary to identify these patients.

In my hypothetical scenario, 80% of these patients were going to gain 10 extra years of life. What about the other 20%? We will say that they will only gain one extra year of life, and we can identify before the fact who those unfortunate patients would be. Would we be justified in denying these patients access to this drug at social expense? I think the obvious answer would be in the negative. If we endorsed as a matter of health care justice social funding for each of the 10 extra years of life at a cost of $400,000 for the 10-year survivors, then nothing would justify our not providing that same funding for those who would gain only one extra year of life. This is straightforward ethical consistency. Part of what is driving our overall reasoning is that we regard it as unthinkable to sacrifice those 10 extra years of life for each of those patients when we have this drug with that very high degree of effectiveness.

Consider another scenario aimed at refining our intuitions further. What if only 10% of a cohort of identified NTRK patients were predicted to gain five extra years of life? All the other patients would gain six to 18 months of life. This may be thought of as a variant of our super-responder problem. Consider two versions of this scenario. In Version 1 we have no way of identifying who the five-year survivors would be. In Version 2 we have a biomarker that can predict with 90% accuracy who the five-year survivors will be. What options would our deliberators regard as requiring funding as a matter of health care justice?

In Version 1 we would have two choices: We could provide the drug to everyone for as long as it proved medically beneficial, or we could deny the drug to everyone. What would justify denying the drug to everyone? The overall gains in life expectancy are marginal, especially relative to the costs. We would be sacrificing the potential five-year survivors as a rationing decision. That does represent a significant loss of life. Egalitarians could again reason, given limited resources and unlimited health care needs, that many more life-years could be saved at a lower cost with the resources saved by denying this drug to these patients. Assuming that rationale is reasonable, deliberators could choose the libertarian option as a matter of rough justice. That is, they would understand that a future possible version of themselves (or a loved one) could have a cancer harboring an NTRK fusion mutation, and they would be denied social funding for larotrectinib. If they were especially anxious about that risk, they would have to purchase private health insurance to cover that risk. However, if they judged that the cost of such insurance would be substantial, keeping in mind that any such insurance product would have to cover numerous such rare but very costly health problems, then they would simply be making a reasonable self-imposed rationing decision. Nothing about such a choice would be unjust.

The other choice in this context would be to fund the drug for everyone. This could be seen as a compassionate response, something morally permissible. However, a justice issue would still need to be addressed. If our deliberators made that choice, would they also be committed to providing comparable resources for every other rare tumor mutation for which an expensive targeted therapy was available? If they balked at this consequence, they would have to be able to articulate some justice-relevant compelling reason why the NTRK fusion mutation was ethically special and warranted making it a funding exception. No such rationale is obvious, at least for now.

In Version 2 we have a biomarker that allows us to identify the five-year survivors with 90% confidence. They represent only 10% of the cohort. Still, sacrificing five years of life for each of these individuals as a result of a deliberate social decision seems unconscionable. This is one situation in which the "rule of rescue" imperative could be justifiably invoked. These are identified individuals at risk of premature death who can be easily rescued with a drug that is readily available. A critic (with a heart of stone) might focus on the fact that we are talking about "identified" individuals. We could, such a critic argues, just not bother looking for the biomarker that would identify these individuals, just pretend that we were completely unaware of the biomarker and its utility. This would be disingenuous and would represent a failure to accord these patients equal concern and respect. We may conclude at this point that justice and compassion required providing social funding for larotrectinib for these five-year survivors.

If we fund the five-year survivors, could we then deny social funding to everyone else whose survival would be in the six- to 18-month range? This would strike many of our deliberators as intuitively unfair. Each life-year saved cost the same $400,000, whether in a one-year survivor or a five-year survivor. Each five-year survivor was going to cost $2 million. It just seems wrong, stingy I suppose, to deny social funding for those one-year survivors. Could our deliberators choose the libertarian option for the whole cohort, as discussed above? In theory, our deliberators could agree to that option. However, this situation is arguably different from the earlier situation in Version 1. In Version 1 we have no way of identifying before the fact who those five-year survivors might be. We would only discover it after the fact. In Version 2 we know who the five-year survivors will be; they are identified individuals. That seems to justifiably invoke the rule of rescue. However, this might not be as compelling an argument as it first appears. The relevant fact (by hypothesis) is that we know 10% of the individuals in this cohort will be five-year survivors if they have social funding for the drug. As some have argued (Brock, 2015; Daniels, 2015), there is not an intrinsic ethical difference between saving identified lives and saving statistical lives when it comes to making resource allocation decisions.[8]

The example to which Daniels calls our attention is that of the 33 Chilean miners who were trapped underground for almost three months and required an enormous, technologically sophisticated rescue effort. If someone were to say in that situation, "This is really tragic; we must not allow this to happen again. Therefore, instead of spending money to save these 33 men, let us use the same amount of money to improve mine safety dramatically and save the lives of more miners in the future," they would likely be judged to be ethically incompetent and completely lacking in basic human decency. Of course, we ought to be spending money on costworthy mine safety measures. However, no matter what we spent on mine safety, we would still be ethically obligated to make a sustained effort to save the lives of miners trapped in similar circumstances. How does this comparison relate to our larotrectinib scenario?

The larotrectinib patients who will only survive six to 18 months are in many respects like the trapped miners. They are faced with a death that can at least be delayed if they are "rescued." Imagine, for example, that we are halfway through our rescue effort for the miners. We learn that some weird virus in the mine has infected all those miners and will cause their death in six to 18 months. I think our shared considered moral judgment would be that we were still obligated to finish the rescue effort, as opposed to calling off the effort, saying a few prayers, and letting that mine be their grave. In the case of the larotrectinib patients who would be five-year survivors, it seems ethically problematic and presumptively unjust to "rescue" the five-year survivors and allow the others to die prematurely. Again, to return to the mine analogy, we could not imagine saving those miners we were sure were not infected by that weird virus and allowing the rest to die inside the mine, though they could each gain six to 18 extra months of life. Relatively speaking, only a small amount of extra effort would be required to save all the miners. It would seem that the same is true with regard to the larotrectinib

---

[8] The context for this conclusion is most often the "treatment versus prevention" distinction. Some will argue that treatment must always have ethical priority because identified lives are at stake, whereas prevention involves "merely" statistical lives. Defending that distinction typically results in underfunding preventive health care efforts, which is a problem of health care justice. Menzel (2012) is for this reason a strong critic of assigning an intrinsic ethical distinction between identified and statistical lives for purposes of health care resource allocations.

scenario. There is no shortage of the drug. Egalitarian considerations would require providing the drug to all these patients, especially if we intend to provide it to the five-year survivors. That would put the libertarian option off the table, though this requires a bit more in the way of critical argument.

Recall my suggestion that our deliberators might consider and endorse the libertarian option in one version of our scenario. I suggested that as a justice-mandated necessity if social funding for shorter-term survivors was going to be approved. I also suggested that such social support in this case would require opening the floodgates to funding all these other targeted therapies for very rare mutations. That would result in a misallocation of limited health care resources that was neither just nor prudent. However, the alternative argument is that our scenario in Version 2 has some justice-relevant distinctive features, specifically, knowing that there were these identifiable before the fact five-year survivors who represented 10% of that cohort. I remind the reader that that was a hypothetical scenario. If it were a real-world scenario, then I would say our deliberators would be obligated as a matter of justice to provide larotrectinib to all the patients with that NTRK mutation. However, the precise scenario I have described might be very rare in the real world. If that were the case, our deliberators would not have to be concerned about having to make extraordinary financial commitments for purposes of prolonging the lives of patients with very rare cancer mutations.

We need to push our analysis a couple of steps further. In earlier chapters we called attention to the existence of super-responders. As things are now, we do not have biomarkers that will identify these super-responders before the fact. Also, relative to any specifiable cohort of metastatic cancer patients, they will represent a tiny percentage of that cohort. This is justice-relevant. It might well be the case that in any cohort of specifiable metastatic cancer patients, we would find a tiny number of super-responders. Would we be ethically obligated to fund very expensive targeted therapies for everyone in that cohort who would only gain extra months of life in order to save the super-responders? The answer I believe our deliberators ought to give would be negative. This is a conclusion I believe could be endorsed by our deliberators who might adopt for analytic purposes a utilitarian, moderate egalitarian, or prioritarian perspective. This is where very often a libertarian option would be ethically reasonable, roughly just.

Note that what I am emphasizing is that the vast majority of patients in any of these cohorts would gain only extra months of life at enormous social expense, say, $150,000 for those extra months. Assuming that what I hypothesized in that last sentence is true, then if we were able to identify before the fact who the tiny number of super-responders might be, we could provide those individuals with the expensive targeted therapies they needed for extra years of life without having any obligation to provide that drug at social expense to all of the other members of that cancer cohort. This would be because the targeted therapy would do too little good at too high a price for everyone else in that cohort. Again, in my hypothetical scenario, all the other members of that cohort were going to gain six to 18 extra months of life. We would have to leave to our deliberators a judgment about how much gain in life expectancy of good quality was necessary in order to make a just claim on social resources. My own inclination would be to say that it ought to be a confident year, nothing less than that.

Let me illustrate this last point with a recent article reporting on the KEYNOTE-355 trial. This trial was looking at the combination of pembrolizumab and chemotherapy against chemotherapy plus placebo in a cohort of women with metastatic triple-negative breast cancer that also showed PD-L1 expression. Median progression-free survival was 9.7 months in the experimental arm and 5.6 months in the placebo group (Cortes et al., 2020). This is a difference of only four months for a drug that costs $156,000 per year. I will add that this was given accelerated approval by the FDA. I will also note that there are very few treatment options available for women with metastatic triple-negative breast cancer. That makes this a last chance therapy in a strict sense. Is that sufficient to justify social funding for this drug combination?

I would argue that our deliberators ought to give a negative answer to that question. The problem is that for every metastatic cancer diagnosis there will be a last chance therapy. Some of those therapies may yield significant gains in life expectancy, even at great cost. Those would make a reasonable just claim on social resources. Others, however, could make no such claim. Imagine that we have good reason to believe that within this metastatic triple-negative breast cancer cohort a very small number of individuals could be super-responders. If we cannot identify them before the fact, then they would not have access to this drug combination at social expense. If those individuals could be identified before the fact, perhaps as individuals who would gain five extra years of life, they would make a presumptive just claim to social resources. However, that would not generate any just claims for social resources by anyone else in the cohort.

We should note that this last conclusion might give rise to the belief that identified lives do in fact make stronger claims on life-sustaining resources than statistical lives. That would be a mistaken conclusion. What is morally determinative in this last situation is that the identified individuals will gain multiple years of additional life. We can illustrate this point more dramatically with the example of PCSK9 inhibitors, introduced in Chapter 4 in this volume. Recall that those drugs dramatically reduce low-density lipoprotein (LDL), bad cholesterol, with the ultimate goal of reducing fatal and non-fatal heart attacks and strokes. The drug costs about $6,000 per year, and patients would be taking it for the rest of their lives. There are 19 million Americans who have LDL levels above 130 mg/dl, which is when a statin is needed to reduce the risk of a heart attack or stroke. However, the patients who can benefit the most from this drug are those with LDL above 220 mg/dl, which will most often be patients with very high cholesterol for genetic reasons or patients with serious advanced heart disease (Board et al., 2020). In many respects these patients can be described as super-responders in the domain of heart disease. They are at risk for the highest number of strokes and heart attacks and the greatest number of potential life-years lost. Consequently, they would have presumptive just claims to these drugs at social expense.

Patients below 220 mg/dl would also benefit from having access to these drugs with fewer strokes and heart attacks and lost life-years. But those numbers would decline substantially as we moved from the 220 mark to the 130 mark, and the cost per heart attack or stroke avoided would rise dramatically. These are all statistical lives. Some of these individuals might even be super-responders who are at risk of losing many life-years or preserving those life-years. However, we could achieve those results only if as a society we were willing to fund these drugs for all 19 million individuals with significantly elevated LDL. At $6,000 per patient, the aggregate annual cost would be $114 billion. This would be neither a reasonable nor a just social expense, given numerous other health care needs where much more benefit could be accomplished for certain at much lower cost for each life-year saved (Hlatky, Kazi, 2017).

We are giving up statistical lives, and we are saving some identified lives with the highest risk levels for stroke or heart attacks. But we are not concluding that the identified lives as identified lives are ethically more important than the statistical lives we are sacrificing. Instead, we are concluding that considerations of justice and effectiveness are what justify saving those identified lives and refusing to spend $114 billion on those additional life-years that could be saved by funding PCSK9s for all 19 million individuals. What needs to be kept in mind is that the risk of heart attacks and strokes (some fatal) for those with LDL above 130 mg/dl but below 220 mg/dl is relatively small. In 2020, for example, 805,000 Americans had a heart attack. However, the vast majority of those heart attacks would have nothing to do with LDL levels.[9] That is, they would not have been prevented by any of these patients being on PCSK9s. For strokes, the comparable annual figure is 795,000. Again, multiple causes account for these strokes, only some of which could be prevented by reducing LDL (Giugliano et al., 2020). Still, we have to concede that several thousand deaths could be prevented each year if we were more generous in permitting social funding for PCSK9s above the 130 mg/dl level. This is a ragged edge problem. A line needs to be drawn somewhere. We should readily admit that PCSK9s could also save lives (prevent heart attacks and strokes with LDL below 130 mg/dl). However, the outcomes in these circumstances would be very marginal and extremely costly (in the millions) per heart attack or stroke prevented) (Schmidt et al., 2020). Here too we (citizens in a just and caring society) could be accused of "sacrificing" lives for the sake of money. It matters, however, if these are choices that we collectively make through democratic deliberation, given limited resources and unlimited health care needs. In that deliberative process each of us would recognize that we are accepting that risk for our own future possible selves. We are not imposing that risk on others and sparing ourselves. That is, we are not violating our commitment to equal concern and respect for all.

Finally, recall the justifying role of wide reflective equilibrium. We have already made considered moral judgments in this regard when, for example, we chose not to provide funding that would separate all grade-level railroad crossings. Twelve hundred lives are lost each year at those crossings, often because drivers either try to beat the train to the crossing or go around crossing gates. We could deny drivers such tempting options by separating

---

[9] Additional factors contributing to heart attacks and strokes would be high blood pressure, diabetes, stress, a very bad diet, lack of exercise, smoking, and so on (Reiter-Brennan et al., 2020). If nothing is done with regard to these other factors that increase risk for heart attacks or strokes, then the PCSK9s would only alter these outcomes very marginally.

with overpasses or underpasses such crossings, though that would be at extraordinary (and unwarranted) expense. Decisions that we make regarding societally funded access to these PCSK9s are exactly like judgments we make regarding these railroad crossings. The same will be true when we make comparable decisions regarding very expensive targeted therapies that we can confidently predict will yield only marginal benefit.

6.5. Super-Responders: Can Aspirational Precision Medicine Generate Actual Ethical Commitments?

Our next wicked problem concerns the use of multiple targeted therapies with the intent of gaining greater life expectancy by more effectively countering cancer drug resistance. The goal is to create as many metastatic cancer "super-responders" as possible. Curing metastatic cancer is not something foreseeable on the medical horizon. Providing many of these patients with four to six extra years of life may be medically achievable. Here would be the first of our wicked problems. We have already provided strong arguments in favor of saying that we would be ethically obligated to provide the social resources necessary to support this achievement. This was ethically and economically non-problematic because super-responders are rare. Hence, even very high lifetime costs for these patients are affordable in the aggregate because these patients are small in number. However, cohorts of metastatic cancer patients in the millions could be created through success with combining these targeted immunotherapies, and the cost per life-year gained could easily be in the $150,000 to $300,000 range.

6.5.1. Precision Medicine and Non-Small Cell Lung Cancer

A good example of the issue of expanding costly cohorts would be the combination of ipilimumab and nivolumab in the Checkmate 227 trial (Courtney et al., 2020) used to treat non-small cell lung cancer. That two-drug combination has a monthly cost of $26,500, which is an annual cost of $318,000. This combination yielded improved effectiveness of 0.55 QALY compared to chemotherapy, which yields an ICER of $413,400/QALY (Courtney et al., 2020). The authors also noted that if we stayed with nivolumab as monotherapy for these patients, compared to chemotherapy, then the QALY gain would be so small that the ICER would be $1,885,400/QALY. However, the annual hard dollar cost for nivolumab would be $156,000. What this means is that the combination yields substantial improvement in effectiveness along with a doubling of cost to achieve that additional effectiveness.[10]

In another analysis of this same trial (Hellman et al., 2019), the median duration of survival for patients with PD-L1 expression greater than 1% was 17.1 months for patients given nivolumab plus ipilimumab and 14.9 months for patients given chemotherapy. This is a difference in median survival of slightly more than two months. Overall survival rates for the experimental group were 62.6% at one year and 40.0% at two years, while for the chemotherapy group those rates were at 56.2% one year and 32.8% at two years. These are not large survival differences. The annual cost of chemotherapy for these patients would be about $30,000 or $60,000 for the two-year survivors. The annual cost of the nivolumab and ipilimumab combination is $318,000, or $636,000 for the two-year survivors. The question for our deliberators is whether the overall survival gain is sufficiently large to justify a 10-fold increase in the cost of achieving that gain. We will put that question on hold while we consider some other metastatic cancers, similar statistics, and costs.

Again, to put this into an economic perspective, 155,000 individuals die of lung cancer each year in the United States. Roughly 30% of those patients have a targetable mutation that defines their cancer, EGFR (15%) and ALK (8%), just to name two. Those tumors are treated with TKIs. Another 50% of these patients can be treated with checkpoint inhibitors, such as pembrolizumab, nivolumab, or ipilimumab. The remaining patients may not have a cancer with a targetable mutation, or other factors might disqualify them from the checkpoint inhibitors. Roughly 78,000 of these lung cancer patients would be eligible for the checkpoint inhibitors, of whom 31,200 would derive somewhat marginal benefit; that is, they would gain a little more than or a little less than one extra year of life. This is the group that we would ask our deliberators to deny nivolumab/ipilimumab combination therapy at social expense. Such a denial would generate annual savings of $9.2 billion.

---

[10] This drug combination, Opdivo® and Yervoy®, is the subject of a 90-second commercial that has aired Sunday mornings on *Meet the Press*. The themes of the commercial are "A Chance to Live Longer," "A Chance for More Big Hugs," and "A Chance for More Together Time." Though the side effects are listed very rapidly and are serious, neither cost nor projected gain in survival is addressed.
https://www.youtube.com/watch?v=DU_pGlNfPGE (accessed 4/29/2022).

In what context should we locate this question for purposes of fair argument and analysis. We would be denying 31,200 individuals, some of whom would be our future possible selves, an additional year of life. We do have some reference points for making this decision. Patients with end-stage organ disease needing a major organ transplant will be denied access to the transplant list if we are medically confident they will not survive another year with that transplanted organ. This might also be true if predicted survival is less than two years, the key argument being that 75% of these patients ought to survive five years and 50% ought to survive 10 years. I take it that our deliberators endorse this practice as fair and reasonable, given that they could imagine themselves as potential 10-year survivors denied those 10 years in favor of someone who would only survive one year.

However, this organ transplantation comparison is with a resource that is absolutely scarce; the nivolumab/ipilimumab combination is not absolutely scarce. Moreover, we think of patients with end-stage heart disease or liver disease or HIV, and we imagine physicians would often know when these patients are facing their last year of life. Still, we provide them with life-sustaining care that might cost $40,000 for that last year of life, as opposed to saying to them that they can only have comfort care. Why not the same commitment to our lung cancer patients? Of course, there is one major difference: That last year of life will cost $318,000 per patient and more than $9 billion per year.

Another way to look at the question is to ask whether we would endorse as reasonable and just a demand by a patient for some therapy that would give them an extra year of life for $1 million. This would be at social expense. One ethically reasonable response would be: What makes you so ethically special that we (citizens of a just and caring society) are obligated as a matter of either justice or social beneficence to provide you with those resources? It is difficult to imagine any ethically compelling response to that question. The same point can be made with regard to the $318,000 cost.

I have been a critic of a sufficientarian conception of health care justice (Fleck, 2016b). Still, we must have an ethically defensible basis for saying what is "enough" when seeking to make just allocations of limited health care resources. It is not just the $318,000 number that is determinative of what is beyond sufficiency; it is the whole context around that number. We saw earlier that some hemophilia patients might require $300,000 worth of care for each of many years. However, these are individuals with an indefinite life expectancy of many years of reasonable quality. Effectiveness matters, morally speaking. This is precisely what is lacking for our lung cancer patients; they are in their last year of life.

Another example to reinforce our main point would be the future of patients with end-stage heart failure. They will have the option of getting an artificial heart implanted at a cost of $500,000. The expectation is that such patients would gain five extra years of life of reasonable quality. However, some of these heart patients will have an advanced cancer that might kill them in two years or some other comparable medical problem. They would justly be denied access to an artificial heart at social expense because of its limited effectiveness in their situation. We can readily imagine our democratic deliberators endorsing such a rationing protocol with respect to access to the artificial heart. They could imagine their future possible selves being in either of those two situations, though their present self (whatever its future health status might be) would have to begin to pay for that future possibility for themselves right now because there would be present "others" who would have that need right now. This is the same point that can be made with regard to our lung cancer patients who could possibly benefit from the checkpoint inhibitors combination therapy. Our deliberators are making rationing decisions in these cases; they are making trade-offs. What makes such decisions just and reasonable is that they are autonomously self-imposed rationing decisions. To return for a moment to our potential $9 billion in annual savings, our deliberators could also be thinking that they would want those resources redirected toward some of those very expensive cancer interventions that yield many extra years of reasonable life for these cancer patients, among whom might be their future possible selves.

One of the problems that has to be addressed with regard to using multiple drugs in combination to treat metastatic cancer is that each life-year saved is much more costly than previous life-years saved. In addition, more life-years are saved. This brings about one of those situations where some health policy analysts would say we are "doing better and feeling worse." That is, we are saving more life-years but at a cost to society that is increasing injustices and inequities in accessing needed health care, as well as other social problems. Consider the drug osimertinib. It is a TKI used in connection with metastatic non-small cell lung cancer with EGFR mutations. It started out as a third-generation TKI. It was used after two prior generations of TKIs had failed because of cancer drug resistance. Gefitinib and erlotinib were first-generation

TKIs for non-small cell lung cancer that were typically defeated by the emergence of the T790M mutation in EGFR roughly 50% of the time. Osimertinib was effective at controlling that mutation. More recently, the argument has been made on the basis of clinical research that osimertinib ought to be the first-line treatment for lung cancer with EGFR mutations (Remon and Lopes, 2020).

In the FLAURA trial the osimertinib cohort achieved median overall survival as first-line therapy of 38.6 months, while the comparator arm with either erlotinib or gefitinib achieved median overall survival of 31.8 months (Ramalingam et al., 2020). What creates one of our wicked problems is that the annual cost of either erlotinib or gefitinib is roughly $95,000, while the annual cost of osimertinib is $177,000, twice as much per life-year saved. In addition, osimertinib will have more serious side effects, manageable but themselves costly. The medical reason for this change in recommendation might be that osimertinib prevents the emergence of the T790M mutation from the beginning of treatment, and this seems to result in longer overall survival for more patients. From the perspective of a political conception of health care justice, I would expect our deliberators would endorse this outcome, whether from utilitarian, prioritarian, or egalitarian perspectives. The background understanding is that this judgment only reflects this self-contained situation. However, the larger problem of health care justice is not self-contained. This same pattern is emerging in many major areas of therapy for metastatic cancer.

In an essay I wrote several years ago (Fleck, 2013) I considered this semi-hypothetical scenario. At that time there were already recommendations in the cancer literature that attacking metastatic cancer would require using multiple cancer therapies either in combination or sequentially. The recognition was that a genuine cure was unlikely but that providing these patients with many extra years of life of reasonable quality was achievable. What I hypothesized as the goal was five extra years of life for each of the 600,000 cancer patients who die each year in the United States at a cost of $100,000 per life-year saved. Assuming that five-year success rate, the cohort of cancer patients being treated increases each year until we have a cohort of three million metastatic cancer patients being treated. The aggregated cost of this scenario would be $300 billion per year. However, as my osimertinib example illustrates, I underestimated substantially the cost of saving all those extra life-years. It looks like the cost will be much closer to $200,000 per life-year saved, or $600 billion per year!

6.5.2. Precision Medicine and Melanoma

Before trying to sort out some of the complexities of health care justice associated with this emerging trend, let me offer some documentation of the trend itself. In one report (Topalian et al., 2019) the PD-L1 inhibitor nivolumab was used to treat patients with advanced melanoma, renal cell carcinoma, and non-small cell lung cancer. Five-year survival rates were estimated to be 34.2% for the melanoma patients, 27.7% for the renal cell carcinoma patients, and 15.6% for the non-small cell lung cancer patients (though I need to add that this last figure has dramatically improved to at least 25% with the combination of nivolumab and ipilimumab in situations where there is high PD-L1 expression [Garon et al., 2019]).

Pembrolizumab is another drug used to treat melanoma that expresses PD-L1. For treatment-naïve patients with metastatic disease and PD-L1 expression greater than 50%, three-year survival was 51% and four-year survival was 48% (Robert et al., 2017). Predicted five-year survival would be above 40% (Hamid et al., 2019). These are patients who have experienced what is described as a "durable complete response" to treatment. This is not a cure, though many of these patients will survive beyond five years. The cost of pembrolizumab is $156,000 per year. Median time receiving the drug was two years, though some patients received the drug for as long as four years. At least 60% of these patients were able to stop the drug after two years and maintain that complete response. However, the other 40% had progression of their cancer one or two years after stopping pembrolizumab. They could go back to pembrolizumab, but the best they could then achieve was a partial response to their cancer. What is unknown is whether they would have maintained that complete response had they remained on pembrolizumab beyond that two-year mark.

Could we (citizens in a just and caring society) justly say to these patients, "A majority of you with metastatic melanoma will achieve a complete response with two years of treatment and remain that way into the indefinite future, perhaps five years or longer. However, 40% of you will have disease progression after an additional year or two. We have no way of knowing who belongs in either group. Some of you could still have disease progression even if you remained on pembrolizumab for another year or two. If we wanted to maximize the likelihood of prolonged survival for the entire cohort, we could keep everyone on pembrolizumab for four years, which would double the cost of pembrolizumab treatment in each cohort. Roughly 12,000 patients will die of melanoma each year in the United States. The four-year cost of this treatment per patient would be $624,000. We will pay the entire cost for those first two years. If you wish to continue treatment beyond that, you will need to somehow pay privately." Should our democratic deliberators accept this conclusion?

There is nothing invidiously discriminatory about this proposal. All would be equally at risk of progression or non-progression. Further, for those who did progress, we would pay the additional costs of whatever therapy was available that was reasonably effective. Hence, those who were financially less well off would not be disadvantaged; they would receive at social expense whatever the best available treatment was. What they are being denied are those two additional years of pembrolizumab at social expense. Consider that if we did fund four years of pembrolizumab for all these melanoma patients, 60% of them would derive no known benefit from that substantial additional expense. The vast majority of them would achieve five-year survival and maintain that complete response. This is another example of rough justice, which I believe our deliberators ought to endorse. Some relatively wealthy individuals will purchase pembrolizumab for those extra two years with their own resources. That does not violate the just claims of those who could not afford such a purchase. Those patients are no worse off as a result of that purchase.

6.5.3. Precision Medicine, Breast Cancer, and Therapeutic Proliferation

We turn next to the treatment of women with breast cancer whose cancer is HER2$^+$, roughly 20% of all women who are diagnosed with breast cancer. They too had a poor prognosis with metastatic disease, at least prior to trastuzumab. In 2019, 272,000 women were diagnosed with breast cancer in the United States, and 43,000 died of their breast cancer. Roughly 8,100 of those women would have been diagnosed with HER2$^+$ breast cancer. As expected, trastuzumab had limited efficacy. At that point women were treated with a combination of pertuzumab, trastuzumab, and a taxane. Median survival with this combination was 56.9 months compared to the control group, which was 39.4 months (Durkee et al., 2015). That represented a gain in the combination group of 1.8 life-years at a cost of $472,668 per life-year gained. The actual annual cost of this drug combination is about $160,000, still a very high price for each life-year gained. It might be societally affordable when the aggregate number of patients is relatively small; it is severely problematic for both ethical and economic reasons when we are talking about millions of patients in the aggregate. Bach (2015) offers the following comment regarding this issue:

> One approach to thinking about this problem is hinted at in the [American Society of Clinical Oncology] value framework, and it is essentially the notion that we should be willing to pay at higher levels for each unit of health benefit when the condition is rapidly fatal otherwise. Put another way, we should value treatments more when they forestall death more directly and immediately, meaning that a month of life gained for someone with a life expectancy of a few months has higher value than a month gained for someone with a life expectancy of several years (at 889).

This comment has some ethical attractiveness from the perspective of compassion, but it needs critical assessment from the perspective of health care justice.

Recall that Bach's comment was in 2015 when pertuzumab represented a last chance therapy. That has since been followed by a second-line therapy, trastuzumab emtansine (T-DM1), and then a third-line therapy that added tucatinib to trastuzumab and capecitabine. That second-line therapy was reported in the EMILIA trial, which resulted in a median gain in overall survival (relative to lapatinib) of 5.8 months (Le et al., 2016). What was reported as the lifetime total cost of that therapy was $276,447. The comparable cost for the lapatinib arm was $214,541. The ICER from the EMILIA trial was $220,835/QALY gained. What makes drawing out the justice-relevant implications of these numbers important is that invasive disease occurred in 12.2% of the patients who received T-DM1 and 22.2% of the patients in the lapatinib arm. That meant that at three years 88.3% of the T-DM1 patients were free of invasive disease, while in the lapatinib arm the comparable figure was 77.0% (Minckwitz et al., 2019). The authors concluded that this meant a 50% reduction in the risk of death or invasive disease for patients in the T-DM1 group. I take that to mean that at the five-year mark somewhere in the vicinity of 85% of the T-DM1 patients were still alive and stable relative to their cancer. The remainder of the patients in both those groups would go on to that third-line option for metastatic HER2$^+$ breast cancer.

In the tucatinib group median progression-free survival was 7.6 months, and in the control group (lapatinib) it was 5.4 months (Wu et al., 2020). Median overall survival was 21.9 months in the tucatintib group and 17.7 months in the control group. At one-year progression-free survival was 33% in the tucatinib group and 12.3% in the control group (Murthy et al., 2020). The cost of tucatinib is $18,000 per month, or $210,000 for one year, plus the costs of administration and side effects. The relatively small median gains in overall survival generated an ICER of $699,976 (Wu et al., 2020). Again, those are not dollars actually spent by anyone. That number allows us to make comparisons of the cost-effectiveness of various drugs relative to one another.

Women may also have triple-negative breast cancer, breast cancer related to the BRCA1 or BRCA2 gene mutations, HER2-negative breast cancer, or hormone-positive or hormone-negative breast cancers, all of which can be treated with various targeted therapies or immunotherapies with various degrees of effectiveness. In general, if a woman has metastatic breast cancer of whatever type, she will have a 27% chance of surviving five years. Given the pace of scientific advances, this figure will rise quickly, perhaps to 50% or higher by 2025. Achieving that result will not be inexpensive.

A recently approved drug for triple-negative breast cancer is sacituzumab, which has a cost of $273,700 per year. In a recent trial, median progression-free survival was 5.5 months and median overall survival was 13.0 months (Bardia et al., 2019). The median age of patients in this trial was 55. All of the patients were heavily pretreated, including treatment with checkpoint inhibitors. I mention this last point because the authors suggest that a check-point inhibitor offered in combination with sacituzumab might extend survival further, though at substantial cost. That could push the cost of that combination for a year to over $400,000.[11]

Consider this hypothetical. Suppose that these combinations were successful and yielded a median gain in overall survival of two years, roughly at a cost of $200,000 per year. Should our democratic deliberators approve this therapy for social funding as a matter of health care justice? The average age of women with this diagnosis is 55, well short of a normal life expectancy.

---

[11] Readers might wonder what is so important about being a first-line therapy, as opposed to a third-line therapy. The short answer is that more women would be candidates for the drug, likely for more years, which adds to the profitability of the drug. From a societal perspective and a health care justice perspective, each of those earlier gained life-years will cost $400,000 rather than $150,000 or $273,000.

These combinations will not yield a cure. These women will still be faced with a premature death. This might be a sufficiently compelling rationale for justifying placing these women in a special category for purposes of the just allocation of health care resources. Some deliberators might point to our apparent willingness to pay $300,000 per patient per year to prolong the lives of cystic fibrosis patients or hemophilia patients. These would be costs for many years in these latter cases, whereas these women with triple-negative breast cancer (for now) could not realistically hope for more than three or four years of additional life. Other deliberators might call attention to the fact that cystic fibrosis and hemophilia patients are much younger than these women, suggesting that the "have not lived a full life" rationale is not as ethically compelling as we might think. In addition, age 55 is a median number.

Some women (maybe not that many) will be over age 70 at the time of diagnosis. Should our deliberators endorse the idea that these women would not have access to this therapy at social expense because they had already achieved a full life? Of course, proposing that limitation would have implications for other women with other forms of breast cancer who were already over the age of 70 at the time of diagnosis with metastatic disease. Moral consistency would seem to require our denying those women access to the very expensive targeted therapies and immunotherapies available to treat their cancer, at least at social expense. The implications would necessarily extend beyond breast cancer; otherwise, it would seem that women alone were being subjected to this age-based limitation so far as cancer treatment was concerned. However, a relatively hard age limit for accessing these therapies would likely lack a compelling enough justification for our deliberators. Sometimes age limits are justifiable. In general, patients over the age of 70, for example, are not candidates for organ transplantation, primarily because those organs are a very scarce resource and many younger patients will have that need, without which they will die very prematurely. By way of contrast, older patients will have access to the COVID vaccine *before* younger patients who are otherwise healthy. They are at much greater risk of death from a COVID infection. In this situation, trying to argue that we should passively accept the deaths of patients in their 80s or 90s from COVID because they have lived a full life seems morally obtuse. The COVID vaccine will be scarce, but this will be a temporary scarcity measurable in months during which younger individuals will be better able to bear that risk, assuming they adhere to the normal public health self-protection measures.

6.6. Precision Medicine: When Is Enough, Enough?

Consider next a wicked problem I would describe as a "drip, drip" justice problem. No single drip is problematic so far as health care justice is concerned. However, the accumulation of drips will create a mess unless the drips are managed at their source. Patients with metastatic cancer are faced with a terminal outcome. It would be tragic if we had nothing to offer. However, with all these targeted therapies and immunotherapies that have various degrees of effectiveness, we are confronted with a prima facie ethical obligation for which thoughts and prayers would be an unacceptably meager substitute.

Imatinib and trastuzumab were among the earliest targeted therapies that proved to be reasonably effective. They helped relatively small, defined populations of patients. They were very costly, but the aggregated cost to society was not unreasonable or unbearable. Then came additional targeted therapies that targeted other drivers of various cancers, still small in number. They were not equally effective in all patients whose cancer bore an EGFR mutation or an ALK translocation or a HER2$^+$ mutation, but we had no ability to identify beneficiaries among these patients. With passing years, many more of these drugs were available for treating more cancers with many different mutations driving that cancer. Each combination of a targeted therapy and a driver mutation (or some form of immunotherapy) applied to a relatively small group of patients, though at substantial cost for each patient treated. If we had already agreed that social resources were justly allocated to the cluster of patients needing imatinib or trastuzumab, then we could hardly deny those same resources to other clusters of patients with other mutations who could benefit to any degree from vemurafenib or ponatinib or pembrolizumab or ipilimumab or atezolizumab or everolimus or cetuximab or bevacizumab or ramucirumab or nivolumab or tucatinib or erdafitinib or pertuzumab or idelalisib or bortezomib or osimertinib or ceritinib, and so on.[12]

There are now over 150 of these FDA-approved targeted therapies or immunotherapies. Each represents a costly "drip." If these drugs yielded gains in life expectancy measurable in weeks or months at very substantial

---

[12] The interested reader can go to the following website for a very long list of all these drugs and the cancers they are used to treat: https://www.cancer.gov/about-cancer/treatment/types/targeted-therapies/targeted-therapies-fact-sheet

cost, it would be easy for our deliberators to conclude that this use of social resources was neither just nor prudent. However, what we have witnessed most recently is the use of these drugs sequentially or in combinations that have yielded an extra two years of life, and often five extra years of life, for at least a significant fraction of any patient cohort. The costs are substantial at the level of the individual patient and very substantial at the level of an aggregated cohort of patients. Still, each cohort taken individually does not yield an unbearable financial or ethical burden for society. However, as the number of these cohorts increases with additional targeted therapies and therapeutic targets, the financial burden becomes both ethically and economically challenging. As noted above, if all 600,000 metastatic cancer patients were given $200,000 drugs for five years, the aggregated annual cost would be $600 billion. If all this transpired in the space of a year, we would have a substantial economic and ethical health care crisis. Instead, we are moving in the direction of that result with relatively small steps. What prevents us from not taking one of those steps?[13]

Consider another example. As reported in the *New England Journal of Medicine* (Drilon et al., 2020), selpercatanib has been very effective in treating RET fusion-positive non-small cell lung cancer. The drug elicited a therapeutic response in 64% of these patients, and the median duration of that response was 17.5 months. Estimated progression-free survival for 25% of these patients was put at 27 months, which, of course, means they would continue to survive with a progressing cancer for some time after that. The cost of this drug is $20,600 per month, or about $247,000 per year, or more than $560,000 for the 25% of these patients who made it out to 27 months. Only 1%–2% of non-small cell lung cancer patients would have this RET fusion. Should our deliberators deny this cluster of patients social funding to cover these costs? Should this be another therapeutic option that would be relegated to the purchase of private health insurance for those willing and able to purchase such insurance (again, very far in advance of any diagnosis of this cancer)?

---

[13] Few health policy analysts are concerned about the economic demands of cancer patients wanting these hyper-expensive therapies. This is because a substantial majority of these patients are uninsured or underinsured. If the likely benefits of all these interventions were very marginal, no concerns of justice would be raised. As we have documented, however, the benefits of many of these interventions are increasing steadily. Consequently, there are problems of health care justice which ought not to be hidden or ignored by the complexities and limitations of our fragmented health insurance non-system.

The problem, so far as health care justice is concerned, is that our deliberators might have already approved 50 other targeted therapies or combinations thereof. What would justify denying social funding for this one? These patients have no other therapeutic alternative. The cost per life-year gained is very high. However, our deliberators may already have approved drug combinations for other cancer patients with even higher costs, often because these combinations yielded gains in life expectancy of five years or more for a substantial portion of that cohort of patients. Very few of these RET patients would be likely to gain five extra years of life, but a significant number would gain at least three extra years of life. That is not a gain that can be readily overlooked as not being ethically weighty. As noted earlier, as a society we are ethically and economically comfortable with paying $88,000 per year for patients on renal dialysis with a resulting gain in life expectancy of 7 to 10 years at a potential aggregated cost of $880,000. Patients who are HIV-positive may be on drugs for 30 years at a cost of $35,000 per year, which can yield an aggregated cost of $1 million or more per patient. The "remaining lifetime" costs for these RET patients will be far below either of those numbers.

The Affordable Care Act eliminated lifetime limits in insurance contracts. This was a welcome reform. In general, health care needs are distributed randomly and with considerable heterogeneity. Some individuals will have enormous needs that are very costly to address effectively. It would be neither just nor caring if we were to suddenly stop meeting those needs because the cost of meeting those needs exceeded some arbitrary limit. This would be the practical equivalent of putting such patients out in the hospital parking lot to die. However, this is the moral logic that prevents us from putting in place hard limits on access to these targeted cancer therapies and immuno-therapies so long as they yield some significant degree of benefit for patients (or a significant number of patients within a cluster of patients). When we look at the way in which care is provided to multiple sclerosis patients or patients in heart failure or patients with diabetes or patients with any number of other chronic degenerative conditions, treatment continues so long as there is evidence of benefit to the patient. However, very often the benefit that is achieved, especially in the late stages of a chronic degenerative condition, is very far from being cost-effective from a societal perspective, which makes it all the more difficult to apply strict cost-effectiveness criteria in the case of cancer patients. This is really the heart of the wicked problems we face in connection with precision medicine.

6.7. CAR T-Cell Therapies: Medical Miracle, Ethical Abyss?

Numerous variants of CAR T-cell therapy are emerging. These variants are seen as necessary to address the limitations of the first two commercially manufactured CAR T cells, tisagenlecleucel (Kymriah°) and axicabtagene ciloleucel (Yescarta°). Both of these interventions have had notable success with blood-borne cancers, leukemias, and lymphomas. But they have not been curative. Two major problems with these therapies have been potency and persistence (Majzner and Mackall, 2019). Potency is about these manufactured T cells not being numerous enough and powerful enough to overcome all the barriers to attacking a cancer completely. The T cells need to multiply rapidly inside the body to maximize their effectiveness. Persistence is about T cells not enduring long enough to kill all the cancer cells that need to be killed. This is referred to as the problem of "T-cell exhaustion." In short, the T cells need to work long enough and hard enough to kill all the cancer cells that are circulating in the body.

In addition, both these drugs have significant and costly side effects at the time of administration, either various neurotoxicities or cytokine release syndrome. The latter has been reported in 20%–50% of all patients in various trials. We have also noted the front-end cost of these drugs: $475,000 in the case of Kymriah and $375,000 in the case of Yescarta. These numbers reflect only the cost of these drugs (removing them from a patient, reengineering them to attack specific features of these cancer cells, and producing them in sufficient quantity before being reinfused into a patient).[14] Everything associated with the reinfusion process adds another $40,000–$60,000 to the overall cost of the procedure. If a patient is faced with a more serious version of cytokine release syndrome, that will add several hundreds of thousands of dollars in cost for the intensive care unit care needed to save the life of that patient. This raises a distinct problem of health care justice relative to other targeted therapies and immunotherapies. Those latter therapies all have monthly costs. Once it is clear the drug is no longer effective, that therapy ceases along with its costs. However, with CAR T-cell therapies, all the cost is up front. If the vast majority of these patients gained at least five additional life-years, that would justify these front-end costs. However, roughly 30% of

[14] CAR T cells are designed to attack B-cell lymphomas, more specifically CD-19, which is found on these cells but not on healthy cells (Holstein and Lunning, 2020). However, if some of these B cells fail to exhibit CD-19, they survive the T-cell attack, which allows the cancer to progress.

these patients will fail to survive a year. Most of the rest will now gain two to four extra life-years. A small number will survive for some number of years beyond that. Again, these would be the super-responders.

A number of clinical trials with CAR T-cell therapies report reasonable levels of success (Schuster et al., 2019; Neelapu et al., 2018; Cappell et al., 2020; Chong et al., 2021). However, in contrast to these scientific reports from trials, Jacobson et al. (2020) reported results from real-world treatment situations. The results were significantly less promising than the ZUMA-1 trial. Jacobson et al. said that "the deviation from observations in the ZUMA-1 trial may be due to the inclusion of sicker patients with a poorer perfor-mance status, and/or different histologies in this patient population" (at 3102–03). The goal of clinical trials is to establish valid clinical knowledge, which is why patients are carefully chosen to avoid the risk of confounding variables. Consequently, it would be ethically problematic to use these strict clinical trial criteria to identify patients who would receive treatment in the real world at social expense. However, too liberal a loosening of trial criteria in the real world would result in poor outcomes and wasted resources in many cases. How then should such judgments be made so as to be just and balanced?

CAR T-cell therapy has not been around long enough to have ample data regarding progression-free survival and overall survival. Consequently, research regarding cost-effectiveness must often rely upon hypothetical extractions from what real-world data is available. This will be useful enough for our purposes in thinking through the relevant problems of health care justice. In the case of large B-cell lymphoma Lin et al. (2019) offer the fol-lowing extrapolations. Axi-cel, in what is described as an optimistic scenario, is assumed to yield 40% five-year progression-free survival and increased life expectancy of 8.2 years at a cost of $129,000/QALY. Given our earlier discus-sion, I would judge that our deliberators would include social funding for this therapy, whether our deliberators thought about this with egalitarian, utilitarian, or prioritarian considerations in mind. The size of the cohort and the size of the benefit would seem to justify seeing this as a matter of health care justice.

The authors (Lin et al., 2019) also looked at a tisagenlecleucel scenario. Again, the optimistic scenario assumed 35% five-year progression-free sur-vival with a relative gain in QALYs of 2.14 at a cost of $168,000/QALY (though that latter number could be as high as $414,000/QALY, depending upon various assumptions). If we assume instead 25% five-year progression-free survival, the relative gain in QALYs is 1.58 at a cost of $223,000/QALY. This might be a more challenging situation for our deliberators because you could get something close to these outcomes with chemoimmunotherapy at a fraction of the social cost, though perhaps with more quality of life–diminishing side effects. Again, these are carefully selected trial patients. If in the real world patients tended to be older with more co-morbidities than represented in the clinical trials, the results would be smaller gains in life expectancy and much higher costs per QALY gained.

Consider some other CAR scenarios. What should happen after CAR T-cell failure? Should these patients get a second CAR T-cell intervention, which would be just as costly as the first? No actual data is available, though we can imagine several possible scenarios. If there were a second infusion of CAR T cells and the vast majority of these patients gained no more than one extra year of life, our deliberators could reasonably judge that justice did not require social funding for such a second effort.[15] In another hypothetical scenario, 10%–20% of these patients gained several extra years of life. Assuming we had no way of identifying with a reliable biomarker who these patients were before the fact, our deliberators could conclude that such an effort would be a very low priority, relative to all the other unmet health care needs in our system. If some of these individuals were judged to be medically suitable for a second effort, they would have to have private health insurance to finance that effort. This would not be unjust, given the likely outcome. If anyone believed this was required as a matter of justice, this would establish a precedent that would require social funding for every terminal situation in which there was any medical option that promised the slightest chance of benefit at extraordinary cost. That would be ethically unfair and economically unreasonable. More challenging would be a situation where we could identify before the fact that relatively small number of individuals who might gain several extra years of life from a second infusion. I will postpone any analysis of that option until we discuss below various scenarios associated with ibrutinib for the treatment of chronic lymphocytic leukemia (CLL; see Section 6.8).

Another emerging research situation involves the use of CAR T-cell therapy to treat various solid organ cancers. Thus far, these research efforts have had little success. The basic biology is much more challenging in the

---

[15] See the story of Chrissy Degennaro (Chadwick, 2020), whose second CAR T-cell transplant lasted only a few months.

case of solid organ cancers. Specifically, there is the "antigen dilemma." Antigens are the targets of CAR T-cell therapy. In the case of solid organs, too many of the antigens on cancer cells are also expressed on some normal cells, which means those healthy cells would be attacked. "An 'ideal' CAR target should be highly homogeneously expressed throughout the tumor, across multiple patients, and have minimal to no expression in vital normal tissues" (Wagner et al., 2020, at 2326). The other large problem is that the tumor microenvironment tends to be immunosuppressive. In spite of these medical challenges, researchers seem to be optimistic that they will overcome these challenges. This would, however, generate another one of those situations in which we were "doing better and feeling worse" (Wildavsky, 1977).

Of the 600,000 cancer deaths each year in the United States, roughly 54,000 are from hematologic cancers; the rest are cancers involving solid tumors. If researchers were successful in devising CAR T-cell therapies that could at-tack cancers in solid tumors, that would dramatically increase the cost of cancer care, especially if each use of the therapy cost $475,000. If such an in-tervention were curative of metastatic cancer, we would have to embrace that fully. However, that is an extremely remote possibility. The more likely sce-nario would be the more modest success we see now with CAR T-cell therapy and hematologic cancers. That is, 30% or more of these patients would fail to gain an extra year of life. Another 30% might gain three to four extra years of life, and the remainder would fall somewhere in between. Recall that CAR T-cell therapy is used after other therapies have failed. In the case of solid organ cancers, we would be talking about CAR T-cell therapy after various targeted therapies and immunotherapies had failed, such as the checkpoint inhibitors. These are costs upon costs upon costs.

It is easy to imagine each metastatic cancer patient incurring costs far in excess of $1 million for whatever number of years are gained after the diag-nosis of metastatic disease. How should a just and caring society with limited resources for meeting unlimited health care needs respond to this scenario? Should we be ethically comfortable with a libertarian response? That is, indi-viduals at a relatively young age should have the opportunity to purchase health insurance that would cover the cost of CAR T-cell therapy for meta-static solid organ cancers. For a number of reasons this approach looks eth-ically problematic so far as health care justice is concerned. To begin with, we have already agreed to fund at social expense CAR T-cell therapy for he-matologic cancers. What would justify our continuing to fund those cancers needing CAR T-cell therapy but not solid organ cancers? To be sure, there would be a substantial increase in social costs, though that is not an obviously sufficient reason for making the funding distinction. We could consider no longer funding CAR T-cell therapy for hematologic cancers, though that would be politically awkward and ethically objectionable. We do defund therapies every now and then, the primary reason being that they are failing to realize the therapeutic benefit originally attributed to them. That would clearly not apply to CAR T-cell treatment of hematologic cancers.

Another consideration is that long-term survivors with HIV (more than 30 years) can easily use more than $1 million of health care. The same could prove true for patients with hemophilia and cystic fibrosis, given the extraordinarily expensive drugs recently made available. Actually, their lifetime costs could be several million dollars. Future possible patients needing CAR T-cell therapy for their solid organ cancers would have a just complaint if they were denied social funding in this context. Someone could argue for a relevant distinction by calling attention to the fact that in the examples I gave above all those patients are generally very young or somewhat young at the time of diagnosis, whereas cancer patients are generally older. However, while the latter part of that statement is generally true, many cancer patients are less than 60 years old. How could we justly and non-arbitrarily provide CAR T-cell therapy to these relatively younger patients while denying it to "somewhat older" cancer patients?

Recall that we are trying to address a wicked problem. If some patients are denied access to CAR T-cell therapy for their cancer because of the high front-end cost and less than an extra year in life expectancy, can they plausibly argue that it does not matter where the high cost occurs? In other words, the gist of their argument is: "You are willing to spend more than a million lifetime dollars on these other patients; I am only asking that you spend half that on me, which is fair and reasonable, even if I gain only one extra year of life." This is an argument with some ethical bite, at least from an egalitarian perspective. Still, this is an argument offered by individuals who are facing the end of their lives. We can all feel the emotional appeal of that argument. But we should also be able to think through the ethical implications of that argument. More specifically, individuals facing a terminal illness would be ethically justified in making unlimited demands on limited social resources, thereby skewing the availability of resources for meeting non-terminal health care needs. We would be endorsing the creation of what Daniels (1985) has referred to as "bottomless pits."

We all deserve maximal social compassion in the face of terminal illness; we do not deserve (have a just claim to) maximal social resources. Addressing this sort of wicked problem requires deliberators who are very far from being faced with a terminal illness. They are in a much better position to take a broader view of overall health care needs and available resources. In that deliberative environment it is much easier to recognize the need for trade-offs and governing criteria. Deliberators would be behind a health care veil of ignorance. They would have little, if any, idea what their own future health care needs might be or the needs of those they loved. What would likely make sense to them is that it would be more prudent to provide social resources for CAR T-cell therapy when we were reasonably confident individuals would gain several extra years of life. This would be a social agreement that our deliberators would accept as being "just enough." They would understand that if they needed CAR T-cell therapy at some point in the future, they could either benefit from its availability and extra years of life, or, alternatively, they would be denied it because it would do too little good for them, not just from a social point of view but from a point of view they autonomously endorsed at an earlier point in time.

Again, a major reason why we are faced with this problem is the extremely high front-end cost associated with CAR T-cell therapy and the mixed benefits for various cohorts of patients. Note that the company that makes the CAR T-cell therapies has nothing to lose. It gets paid whatever the outcome for any individual patient. Its incentive is to provide the therapy to as many patients as possible so long as it gets paid. We could make a policy decision that a company would only be paid if the patient survived at least one year. That would alter the economic incentives considerably. However, a pharmaceutical company would not want to take these risks unless it had control over the patients who were candidates for this therapy. The motivation of physicians under these altered circumstances would be to give patients the opportunity to be treated since, if the treatment failed in less than a year, it would cost them nothing. However, the pharmaceutical company would then be making decisions regarding who it was willing to treat. Its economic incentive would be to be conservative. A patient might have a reasonably decent chance of living somewhat more than a year. However, the economic interests of the pharmaceutical company would speak against taking that risk. Its safest bet would be patients it would judge likely to live at least two years. This would control overall costs for CAR T-cell therapies and maximize the efficient use of social resources, but it would be ethically problematic because the physicians responsible for caring for those patients and protecting their best interests would be transferring a critical care decision to another physician who was a complete stranger to that patient and whose interests were primarily corporate.

6.8. CLL, Ibrutinib, CAR T-Cell Therapy: A Case Study in Endless Needs

I now want to turn to an even more complex scenario that involves CAR T-cell therapy, namely, in the context of CLL and ibrutinib. Let me start by laying out the basic medical context. First, CLL accounts for about 25% of leukemia cases in the United States, roughly 22,000 new cases per year. The median age for CLL diagnosis is 71. CLL patients tend to be divided into two broad groups: patients with non-mutated IGHV, TP53 mutations, TP53 (del17p), and patients with mutated IGHV and no TP53 mutations. The former group will have inferior overall survival with all CLL treatments currently available. Ibrutinib is the most effective drug used to treat CLL today. It is given until progression. The cost of ibrutinib is $156,000 per year. What might be regarded as a medical oddity is that the vast majority of these patients, even those with the TP53 aberration, have many years of progression-free survival, though only a small percentage achieve either a complete response or undetectable minimal residual disease. At five years 76% of patients with CLL and the TP53 aberration will have progression-free survival compared to almost 90% of these patients without that aberration (Brander et al., 2019). However, in the ALLIANCE trial, which focused on older CLL patients (median age, 71 years), only 63% of the patients remained on ibrutinib at 3.17 years (Woyach et al., 2018). These patients tended to have more co-morbidities, which contributed to making ibrutinib more burdensome.

There are about 130,000 CLL patients in the United States today. That number is expected to grow to 200,000 by 2025. Ibrutinib has its best results when used as a first-line treatment, as opposed to patients with relapsed or refractory disease. However, from the perspective of the best (most efficient) use of social resources, that first year of costs would be $156,000 rather than $40,000. Prior to the availability of ibrutinib, most of these patients would have been on chemotherapy for several years. For example, one patient, Mike Boston, was diagnosed with CLL in 2007 (Patient Power, 2020). He went through three clinical trials with relapses at 24 months, 21 months, and

16 months. One of those trials would have involved rituximab, which costs $36,000 per year. This will work somewhat well for a limited period of time. Mr. Boston is described as having aggressive CLL, so he skipped ibrutinib and ended up jumping to CAR T-cell therapy. However, the first question to our deliberators is whether patients would be obligated to try several years of these earlier, less expensive therapies before they could receive ibrutinib at social expense. If some of these earlier, less expensive treatments yielded a durable response for a large portion of these patients, then medical, ethical, and economic considerations might all align with one another and justify not starting treatment with ibrutinib. However, the scenario with Mr. Boston is the more typical one. That is, patients who have relapsed from prior therapies will have poorer outcomes with ibrutinib, which would be a compelling reason to start with ibrutinib.

To make things as concrete as possible, we will assume that if we were to replace four years of chemotherapy with four years of ibrutinib for the 22,000 newly diagnosed CLL patients, the first-year cost would be $3.4 billion. The fourth-year cost (four cohorts of these patients) would be $13.6 billion. The net cost in Year 4 (subtracting $40,000 per patient per year) would be $10.2 billion. Here are some questions our deliberators could ask: Is ibrutinib "medically necessary"? A "yes" and a "no" answer would both be appropriate. Ibrutinib is a safe and effective treatment for CLL, which would satisfy one definition of "medically necessary." However, the same will be true for the prior chemotherapy regimens. In both cases these therapies will effectively control the disease process for those four years (though the chemotherapy will have side effects that will diminish to some degree quality of life). What justifies choosing the more expensive medication, given the "just caring" problem (i.e., limited resources to meet unlimited health care needs)?

I will inform the reader that I am on a very low dose of a very cheap blood pressure medication, hydrochlorothiazide. It is medically necessary and quite effective. The cost is less than $100 per year. Alternatively, my blood pressure could be controlled (maybe very slightly better) with azilsartan medoxomil/ chlorthalidone (Edarbyclor˚), which has a cost of $2,640 per year. In one sense, that drug is medically necessary. I need to reduce my blood pressure a bit. In another sense, it is not medically *necessary* because I have hydrochlorothiazide, which is effective enough at a fraction of the cost of Edarbyclor. No doubt, there are some patients with very high blood pressure that is very difficult to control with any of the less expensive blood pressure medications. For those patients this drug would be medically necessary in the strict sense.

These patients would have a just claim to this latter drug at social expense. How close is this analogy to our question regarding ibrutinib? That is a critical question for our deliberators. Is this a situation in which we could justly and justifiably invoke our libertarian alternatives. In other words, if individuals wanted ibrutinib for their CLL for the first four years of treatment, then they would have to have purchased supplemental health insurance that would pay for that option. I am going to leave that question partially unanswered for the time being.

Recall that patients with relapsed or refractory CLL after trying chemotherapy will have a poorer outcome on ibrutinib (i.e., a net loss of several life-years). This is not just a marginal loss, nor is the likelihood of that loss a small possibility. These considerations would speak against the libertarian option. However, the size of the additional costs with funding ibrutinib from the beginning should be concerning from the perspective of an overall just allocation scheme. Consider whether NICE in the United Kingdom would approve ibrutinib as a first-line therapy for CLL, given that the National Health Service (NHS) has a very strict budget. That $2.2 billion per year (adjusted for the British population instead of the $10.2 billion in the United States) would require giving up $2.2 billion in care for something else now provided by the NHS. Recall the Cancer Drug Fund in the United Kingdom. The demand for ibrutinib would empty that fund completely in any given year (which managers of the fund would not permit). Those managers could justify their refusal to fund any of these ibrutinib patients on the grounds that the fund is designed to provide funding for true "last chance" therapies for a limited period of time for terminal patients. Patients with newly diagnosed CLL would have these other options that would be medically effective for several years. Finally, the Brits could offer a justice-relevant egalitarian justification for their decisions: Everyone with CLL would be treated the same. Should our deliberators in the United States accept this rationale as well?

Though 30%–40% of CLL patients might be on ibrutinib for 10 years, resistance will eventually develop, and their CLL will progress. At that point CAR T-cell therapy becomes an option. Some patients will have very aggressive CLL. They will fail ibrutinib after just one or two years. Others will fail ibrutinib at Year 4 or 6 or 8 or 10. Should all of these patients have an equal just claim to CAR T-cell therapy at social expense (assuming medical suitability)? What considerations might justify a negative or partially negative response to this question? We need to put off briefly answering these latter two questions because yet another therapeutic option has emerged in the medical literature, literally within a couple of days of my writing the next few paragraphs. This should serve as a reminder of the complexity of the challenges associated with addressing these issues from the perspective of health care justice.

CLL is a fairly heterogenous hematologic cancer. The therapeutic significance of that heterogeneity is now believed to be related to the relatively early failure of ibrutinib in some patients. The newest option, after failure with ibrutinib, would be treatment with umbralisib and ublituximab (U2). This combination of drugs might have annual costs in excess of $200,000. In the Unity-CLL trial, half the patients were treatment-naïve (so this was first-line treatment for them); the rest were relapsed or refractory from earlier treatment. For the entire U2 cohort of 400 patients, median progression-free survival was 31.9 months, compared to 17.9 months for a treatment regimen that included obinutuzumab (Ingram, 2020; Lunning et al., 2019). However, for the treatment-naïve portion of the U2 cohort, median progression-free survival was 38.5 months, while the previously treated cohort had only 19.5 months of progression-free survival.

That last statistic takes us back to our discussion of using ibrutinib as a first-line therapy. The therapeutic benefit of ibrutinib would be clear and dramatic, but the cost increase would be even more dramatic. The U2 combination would be available to those patients who failed ibrutinib after anywhere from one to five years of treatment. However, for the patients in the Unity-CLL U2 clinical trial, progression-free survival was reduced by 50% if they started the U2 combination after relapse. That would suggest that they really ought to have U2 as their first-line therapy; we would not know before the fact which patients would fail ibrutinib within a few years of starting treatment. Consequently, to maximize the survival probabilities of those patients, the entire cohort of new CLL patients would have to start with the U2 combination, which would again add significantly to the overall cost of treating these CLL patients. Those patients who were most at risk from being early failures with ibrutinib would then be able to maximize the therapeutic promise of U2. In addition, assuming all of these patients would eventually fail the U2 combination, they would still have ibrutinib as an option, which could be followed by CAR T-cell therapy.

It might be the case that those patients who otherwise would have been early failures on ibrutinib would still be early failures on ibrutinib as second-line therapy. However, some researchers have proposed that second-line therapy should really be ibrutinib combined with either of the U2 drugs. This would likely be a therapeutic combination that would cost more than $200,000 per year. Moreover, this would likely be the therapeutically best option as second-line therapy for all of our CLL patients (since we would not know who would be early ibrutinib monotherapy failures). This would again add substantially to the overall annual cost of treating CLL patients. Further, if more CLL patients survived for more years as a result of the treatment option described above, that would mean larger CLL cohorts for more years (and more costs), perhaps for seven or eight years, as opposed to the four years in our original scenario.

Is this a scenario our deliberators should endorse as a matter of health care justice? Do we think NICE in the United Kingdom would endorse this scenario? Is the alternative "sacrificing" some life-years of those CLL patients who would be early ibrutinib failures, that is, denying them the extra life-years they might otherwise gain under the maximal therapy scenario I have outlined? How is this like or unlike a situation where we choose as a society not to separate all grade-level railroad crossings in the United States with the result that each year roughly 1,200 individuals will die at those grade-level crossings? We seem to accept those deaths with equanimity. That is, we do not condemn ourselves as obtuse ethical illiterates. We can raise the same issues with regard to the limits we place on access to PCSK9s. Should the logic represented by these examples be sufficient to convince our deliberators to acquiesce to the limitations on CLL treatments I have suggested? Can we in good conscience tell ourselves that these patients died of their CLL, not as a result of any socioeconomic choice?

Our deliberators must consider that CLL is mostly associated with older individuals, with a median age at diagnosis of 71. Ibrutinib does have some significant side effects. Somewhat older individuals (over 70) will tend to be less able to endure those side effects, which means they choose to go off ibrutinib. That, in turn, means they will die sooner than others who are better able to tolerate those side effects. Some of that intolerance may be related to natural aging processes; in other cases, it might be related to specific comorbidities. However, there is now an alternative for these patients in the form of ibrutinib and venetoclax as a first-line treatment for such patients (Jain et al., 2019; Brander et al., 2019). In other words, these patients would start treatment for their CLL with this combination, as opposed to any form of chemotherapy with the risk of relapse or a refractory outcome. However, the cost of this combination of drugs is about $23,000 per month, or roughly $275,000 per year. This would be an even more costly scenario than our prior scenarios. How should our deliberators respond to this option? Do these patients have a just claim to these additional social resources, as opposed to expecting these patients to find other ways of paying for access to this therapy? What is likely at risk are several extra years of life. Our deliberators seem to have agreed earlier that we ought not give up several extra years of life that can confidently be gotten by individuals through some form of life-prolonging medical care, even at significant social expense. If the ibrutinib–venetoclax combination yielded for the vast majority of older patients less than an extra year of life, I think it would be easy for our deliberators to see this as a libertarian option, not an egalitarian obligation.

Our discussion of CLL is far from being at an end. Ibrutinib is not curative, though it can yield some very long remissions for a significant portion of these patients. The remission, however, will end. The next option is CAR T-cell therapy. This has its own ethically and economically challenging features. Patients who fail ibrutinib within two years are much less likely to have a good outcome with CAR T-cell therapy. To be more precise, half of them will not survive a year after receiving CAR T-cell therapy; the rest will survive one to three years. We do not know who will be in either of these cohorts. Does that imply that a just response would require social funding for either everyone in this early failure cohort or no one in the cohort? Though the median age at diagnosis for CLL is 71, almost half of these patients will be in their 50s and 60s. Would it be just enough if we provided social funding for these early failures for CAR T-cell therapy if they were below age 72 when therapy failed but not for anyone beyond age 72? Would it be sufficient justification for this view to say that these individuals had not yet had their "fair innings," a fair opportunity to achieve a normal life expectancy? Or does this have too much of an ageist bias?

Consider an alternate scenario. We may be able in the future to identify a biomarker that will tell us with 90% confidence which individuals will be least likely to survive a year with CAR T-cell therapy (or not much beyond a year). Should our deliberators endorse this limitation as being "just enough"? Should this be another place where the libertarian option would be seen as being "just enough"? CAR T-cell therapy has been regarded as a "last chance" therapy; no other life-prolonging options were available. However, very recent research has been looking at other drugs that might offer some additional gains in life expectancy. Should these be socially funded options for those who are denied CAR T-cell therapy due to predicted survival of less than a year?[16] Is this an obligatory compassionate alternative? However, we would then have to address this challenge: The patients who were early failures on ibrutinib will likely be somewhat early failures on CAR T-cell therapy as well. That is, they might gain two or three extra years of life. Should they then have access to post-CAR T-cell therapy as well at social expense? If we had earlier provided this to the poor responders to CAR T-cell therapy, then what would justify not providing it to these somewhat later responders? Part of what challenges judgments of health care justice in this case is that these failed patients will exhibit a significant range of ages. Some of them will again be in their 50s and 60s, still short of a normal life expectancy, while others could be in their mid- to late 80s. To avoid the charge of ageism, our deliberators would have to ignore the ages of these patients.

As noted already, other patients will fail ibrutinib at Year 4 or Year 6. Presumably, they will have access to CAR T-cell therapy at social expense, though we would again have to address the one-year biomarker failure question. Likewise, would these patients be offered post–CAR T-cell therapy at social expense? And if they were offered it, would egalitarian commitments to health care justice require our deliberators to fund this therapy for all the patients who failed CAR T-cell therapy, even if they had already gained four extra years of life from the therapy?

That brings us to the patients who fail ibrutinib at Year 8 or Year 10 or beyond (Gauthier et al., 2020). These are patients who might have benefited from more than $1.5 million in treating their CLL. Should that diminish in any way their claim to social funding for their CAR T-cell therapy? Our deliberators would likely have to respond in the negative to this question, in part because we would have agreed that there would be no lifetime limits on access to needed and appropriate health care. That leaves open our two other questions regarding individuals who would not gain a full year from CAR T-cell therapy along with the issues regarding post-CAR T-cell therapies.

CAR T-cell therapy now targets CD19 on lymphomas. Still, this therapy will fail for the majority of patients by Year 4. Numerous clinical trials are ongoing that are testing variants of CAR T cells. In particular, I will mention CD19/20/22 CAR T-cell research (Fousek et al., 2021). It is described as "salvage therapy." It is intended to reinvigorate CD19 as a target, along with CD20 and CD22. It is the equivalent of using multiple drugs to attack

---

[16] One such drug in early stages of clinical research is mosunetuzumab. In this one trial 19% of the patients achieved complete remission (which is not a cure), and 83% of the patients were disease-free at a median of six months. The cost of this drug would be $240,000 per year (Skarzynski, 2019).

a cancer. However, this adds another round of $475,000 CAR T-cell therapy for the benefit of patients who failed the first round of CAR T-cell therapy. It could result in significant long-term remission. Or it could have the same range of results as CAR T-cell CD19 therapies. It would in any case add significantly to the overall cost of treating CLL patients. Is this a bridge too far so far as health care justice is concerned?

Some researchers have wondered whether patients who have been on ibrutinib for six years might take a drug holiday, maybe for a year or two. If the drug were really not necessary to sustain progression-free survival, that could save a substantial sum of social resources. The puzzle for researchers is that ibrutinib has been very successful for many patients in sustaining progression-free survival. However, only a small number of patients achieve complete remission. Drug-free holidays have been tried with HIV$^+$ patients, generally not with much success. Still, HIV$^+$ patients have some motivation for trying drug-free holidays because the side effects significantly compromise their quality of life. That motivation is lacking in the case of CLL for the most part. On the contrary, the justified anxiety would be that in going off ibrutinib the cancer might be given the opportunity to mutate (i.e., become resistant to ibrutinib). That could mean the loss of some reasonable-quality life-years. It might be emphasized that these patients could still be "rescued" by CAR T-cell therapy. However, the initiation of that therapy for a large proportion of these patients is brutal, given the frequency of neurotoxicities and cytokine release syndrome. Moreover, they could end up being among the patients denied CAR T-cell therapy because of predicted survival of less than a year. Given this overall picture, it is hard to imagine any patients wanting voluntarily to be part of a trial aimed at testing this hypothesis. Further, it should be absolutely clear that no use of inducements to motivate patients to enter such a trial would be ethically justifiable, especially if any such inducements would only be attractive to those who were financially less well off.

Imagine our deliberators looking at all of these various uses of targeted therapies, immunotherapies, and CAR T-cell therapies from the proverbial 10,000-foot level. If we consider each therapeutic effort by itself in relation to a relatively small cluster of patients, it will seem as if reasons of both justice and compassion would justify our providing access to that therapy at social expense. There are no hard choices then because we are not making any choices (other than to avert our gaze away from patients facing other life-threatening medical problems requiring very expensive interventions). Averting our gaze has nothing to justify it. It relies upon the silent assumption that cancer is somehow morally special, worthy of unlimited health care resources to fund any intervention that promises any degree of benefit. That too is not justifiable, no matter the level of social anxiety attached to cancer. I have used my lengthy discussion of CLL, ibrutinib, and CAR T-cell therapies to illustrate the problem I wish to address in the next chapter. If we need a label, we could call it the problem of "just therapeutic limits" or, alternatively, the "limits of obligatory social beneficence."

6.9. Some Preliminary Conclusions (A Resting Place)

I have reread this chapter. The level of detail is complex and exhausting but necessary. As I noted at the beginning of this chapter, the problem of health care justice in contemporary medicine is complex, difficult, and evolving as medicine itself is evolving. Medical research is an ongoing enterprise that sometimes yields unequivocal benefits but more often yields benefits that are uncertain, costly, and socially controversial. This is especially true with regard to cancer research, cancer therapies, and precision medicine. This is why simple, neat principles of justice are inadequate to address the problems of health care justice generated by precision medicine.

Cancer itself has been described as the "emperor of all maladies" (Mukherjee, 2010). This is not an honorific description. It reflects instead an ethically troubling judgment regarding the cancer enterprise. Cancer holds a privileged position in US health care, "as evidenced by significant public and private research investment in understanding and treating the disease, a powerful industry, the multitude of influential interest groups and national associations with considerable political and financial capital, and, of course the human element that almost every citizen knows of someone who has suffered from or died from cancer" (Sorenson, 2012, at 421). As Sorenson also notes, a "cancer taboo" exists with respect to making critical value judgments regarding cancer therapies. For someone to suggest that some cancer therapies yield too little benefit at too high a price is to risk being labeled a heartless, callous, unfeeling, penny-pinching bureaucrat. If Kierkegaard were alive today, he would understand that the critical task undertaken in this volume needs to be approached with "fear and trembling." Nevertheless, we shall proceed.

Let me start by reminding the reader that we are committed to the belief that every individual in our society (I deliberately avoid the word "citizen") is entitled to the same level of health care resources to meet their health care needs as every other individual in our society. This does not mean that everyone has a just claim to everything that medicine might offer with any degree of medical benefit, no matter the cost, at social expense. There are limits to what a just and caring society owes to its members as a matter of either health care justice or obligatory social beneficence. Those limits ultimately need to be determined through a fair and inclusive process of rational democratic deliberation, as opposed to pure philosophic argument and analysis. Here are the major conclusions of this chapter:

(1) A *political* conception of health care justice (following Rawls, 1996), divorced from comprehensive doctrines, is feasible and essential to the effective functioning of rational democratic deliberation in a liberal, pluralistic society. Cookson and Dolan (2000) have argued that a fair approach to health care rationing will require a pluralistic conception of health care justice. It is what Rawls refers to as an "overlapping consensus" when, for example, utility and efficiency considerations, commitment to equal respect and concern, priority to the least well off, and protecting fair equality of opportunity all converge to support the justness of a specific rationing protocol.

(2) Whatever rationing protocol we would care to legitimate regarding some specific targeted cancer therapy or immunotherapy through the process of democratic deliberation must apply equally to all in the same clinical circumstances. The deliberative process, properly conducted, represents a socially autonomous process of health care rationing that legitimately applies to all who are part of that process. No individual has the right to endorse some rationing protocol from which they would expect they would be exempted in the relevant clinical circumstances. This is one way of concretizing equal concern and respect for all as well as the Rawlsian notion of "fair terms of cooperation."

(3) What counts as a health care need, in a justice-relevant sense, will itself be a product of the deliberative process, as opposed to an individual decision. Recall our discussion of patients with headaches fearing brain tumors.

(4) Respect for patient autonomy gives patients the right to accept or refuse treatment; it does not give them the right to demand treatment to which they have no just claim. Just claims to needed health care will be a product of just social decisions, not individual demands.

(5) Unlimited access at social expense to any and all health care services, no matter the cost, no matter how marginal or uncertain the benefit,

is neither affordable nor just nor required as a matter of social beneficence. Just limits need to be created through just social agreements.
Just social agreements must be within the boundaries of the constitutional principles of health care justice and justified through reflective
equilibrium.

(6) The implication of "just limits" is that there are health care services
and interventions that are beyond those limits. Most often, those
services are beyond just limits because the likelihood of benefit or
the size of the benefit relative to social cost is too small. In the context
of metastatic cancer, that means some cancer drugs will yield relatively little benefit in the form of prolonging life, though achieving
that small benefit would be very expensive. A principle of individual
liberty would allow individuals to purchase such marginal benefits
with their own resources so long as such purchases did not undermine the just claims of others to needed health care.

(7) Metastatic cancer is extraordinarily complex from a biological perspective and capable of evading in various ways the targeted cancer
drugs and immunotherapies. This is the phenomenon of cancer
drug resistance. One response to this phenomenon has been to use
multiple cancer drugs in combination or sequentially to close down
more paths of resistance, usually increasing even more dramatically
the cost of these therapeutic efforts as well as the challenges of determining just social funding for these drugs. The primary ethical challenge becomes the extraordinary aggregated cost of funding these
complex drug interventions that will now often yield more than marginal gains in life expectancy for at least a significant portion of the
patient population so treated. This is the beginning of a number of
wicked problems.

(8) Typical efforts to solve wicked problems usually generate additional wicked problems. This is why they are wicked problems. This
is also one of the primary reasons why we will often have to be satisfied with "rough justice" or "non-ideal justice." In addition, what
Rawls (1996) refers to as the "burdens of judgment" will frustrate
our efforts to identify "perfectly just" rationing protocols. The uncertainties of medicine in practice, the plurality of reasonable values
relevant to most rationing decisions, conflicting or ambiguous empirical evidence, the vagueness of our moral and political concepts,
disagreements about how much weight to attach to competing values

in specific circumstances—all of this comprises the burdens of judgment, most especially with regard to health care justice.

(9) Probably the best illustration of a complex wicked problem and these burdens of judgment may be found in our discussion of CLL, ibrutinib, the option of CAR T-cell therapy, the option of a stem cell transplant, the option of a second version of CAR T-cell therapy, and the option of umbralisib and ublituximab (U2). It would be one thing if we had to determine which of these options might be best for a patient in specific clinical circumstances. That, however, is *not* the challenge. *All of the options could be part of the therapeutic effort for a single patient over a period of years.* Is that beyond what we owe any patient as a matter of either justice or obligatory social beneficence? What are those limits? How are they justified?

(10) We have to avoid ageism, denying older individuals needed health care because it is too costly and older individuals are less likely to gain as much for those expenditures as younger patients. Still, in our discussion of both the artificial heart and the ibrutinib scenario we suggested that some age limits could be justified through the deliberative process.

(11) Cost matters, and cost-effectiveness matters; but neither by itself should ultimately be determinative of just claims to social resources in the context of health care rationing decisions. Other social values need to be considered that will determine the limits of the use of cost-effectiveness analyses. Again, appropriate balancing judgments need to be made through a fair and inclusive democratic deliberative process informed by the best medical information, projected economic costs, and justice-relevant social consequences. Justice-relevant social consequences will require making comparisons with similar medical situations outside cancer to be certain that cancer is not given unwarranted priority for resource allocation purposes.

(12) Ragged edge judgments are a pervasive feature of contemporary medicine. Some group of patients may be in the same clinical circumstances: all have HER2$^+$ breast cancer or CLL or some form of B-cell lymphoma. Consequently, they are all treated with the same targeted therapy or immunotherapy, but the therapeutic outcomes vary dramatically along a continuum from a minimal response to a maximal response of years of high-quality survival. This happens with virtually every therapeutic intervention. Sometimes a medical

explanation might be given after the fact for a poor response or an excellent response; at other times the different responses are a complete mystery. For relatively low-cost therapies, everyone will be treated with hope for a good outcome. The cost of the marginal and minimal responses is tolerable, given the need to be responsive to the medical problems of these patients.

The challenge is very different when we are dealing with extraordinarily expensive interventions. To justify the high costs, we need substantial therapeutic benefits. This leaves us with two justice-relevant challenges: (1) We need to identify a degree of benefit we have good reason to believe a cohort of patients will achieve, or that individual patients within that cohort will achieve, that will justify the cost of achieving that benefit. This is the ragged edge, somewhere along a therapeutic continuum, below which patients will be denied that costly therapy. This is something to be determined through the deliberative process. (2) We need to fund the research that will identify biomarkers that can be used as evidence for where to establish a therapeutic cutoff, such as a minimal gain of one year in life expectancy for access to CAR T-cell therapy. Making such judgments will require our tolerating some degree of uncertainty, knowing the consequences for patients if we failed to get it right. However, if we are unwilling to make such judgments (give everyone the costly therapy or give no one the costly therapy), the result will be unwarranted economic costs or intolerable injustices. This is another wicked problem.

(13) The need for trade-offs is inescapable. The "publicity condition" is a central element in our understanding of health care justice, as Rawls has emphasized (1971, 1996). Trade-offs need to be clear and explicit, as opposed to being hidden and implicit. If we wish to save the very expensive life-years of CLL patients for a fourth-line treatment option, then we ought to know what other health needs will not be funded in order to make that possible. This allows for more fair and thoughtful assessments of the consequences of such trade-offs. Failure to do this generates greater inequities across the health care system as a whole. Again, this is part of what reflective equilibrium requires.

Making trade-offs implies that resources are saved in one part of the health care system and redirected elsewhere in order to maintain a "just enough" health care system overall. However, one of the largest justice-relevant deficiencies in the US health care system is that we have no way of "safely transporting" those savings from one marginally beneficial health care intervention to another intervention where more benefit can be provided more justly. This is because the financing of the US health care system is so fragmented, unlike the British or Canadian health care systems. Consequently, money saved through making hard choices for Medicare patients cannot be redirected to younger patients with various forms of private health insurance, as Daniels (1986) has noted. This is also why I have framed my entire discussion of these health care justice issues and wicked challenges within an assumed single-payer system.

I will add that fragmented financing means fragmented, invisible, unaccountable, inequitable efforts to control health care costs. Fragmented financing permits all manner of cost-shifting, most often toward those who are least able to defend their own health and financial interests. Moreover, in the US health care system as it is now, fragmented financing means that those with the greatest health needs will often have the least secure access to needed health care since such patients represent a threat to the profitability of private insurance firms and/or private employers. The implication of this state of affairs with regard to accessing the fruits of precision medicine (i.e., secure access and fair access to available targeted cancer therapies and immunotherapies) is clear. The rationing issues I have identified with the proliferation of all of these targeted therapies are unlikely to emerge as a problem of great magnitude because the rationing is being accomplished invisibly through our fragmented system for health care financing. Individuals without health insurance or with somewhat marginal insurance or good insurance with strict financial limitations regarding high-cost care are simply unable to pay for the medically necessary and effective cancer care they might need. No "death panel" denied them that care. Our fragmented, impersonal system for health care financing brought about that result. However, nothing about that result is either just or socially beneficent.

7

Obligatory Social Beneficence

The Sufficientarian Challenge

7.1. Obligatory Social Beneficence: Ending Endless Needs

Sufficientarianism is rooted in a reasonable core insight, namely, that there must be limits to what is required of a society by way of providing resources to meet health care needs as a matter of justice. Otherwise, everyone with any health care need for which any sort of therapy was available would have a just claim to the social resources needed to pay for that therapy. That idea is neither reasonable nor affordable nor just, given the therapeutic possibilities in society today. What is beyond justice for a sufficientarian? Either individual ability to pay or individual or social charity, freely given. However, a case can be made for saying that obligations of social beneficence exist as well, sometimes beyond justice, sometimes as part of health care justice, but prior to individual ability to pay.

All sorts of natural disasters occur with substantial costs for human welfare: hurricanes, earthquakes, massive flooding, massive forest fires, pandemics, and so on. There are also human-made disasters, such as massive unemployment or economic dislocation associated with perturbations in economic markets, which themselves might be caused by irresponsible political decisions. It would be indecent if as a society we simply turned our backs on that human misery. Personal charity can be very arbitrary and subjective. No one is open to moral criticism for donating to an African wildlife fund as opposed to a cancer fund. However, *social beneficence* cannot be that arbitrary. We have to achieve some level of social agreement through a legitimate political process for the scope of social beneficence. We typically refer to this as "social welfare policy," where "social" must be construed in the broadest sense possible to protect the legitimacy of the policy.[1] Another way to put

---

[1] Socially beneficent policies that reward political friends or social groups to which policymakers might have special attachments are inherently illegitimate.

Precision Medicine and Distributive Justice. Leonard M. Fleck, Oxford University Press. © Oxford University Press 2022.
DOI: 10.1093/oso/9780197647721.003.0007

the point is to say that our social welfare policies must aim to satisfy public interests, interests that each and every one of us has that we would be unable to satisfy through our own private initiative.

I have introduced this social beneficence digression because I want to offer as charitable a reading as possible of the sufficientarian position. Sufficientarians often try to establish the limits of health care justice with the language of "basic" or "adequate" or "minimally decent" meeting of health care needs. That is, we owe everyone in our society access to "basic" health care, as a matter of justice. We then have to argue about what health care needs and related therapies come under that rubric. This is a practically impossible challenge, primarily because of the enormous heterogeneity of health care needs and related therapeutic options. Would any of the targeted cancer therapies for metastatic disease come under the heading of "basic" health care? What about all the therapies for advanced heart disease or advanced diabetes or COVID patients in the intensive care unit (ICU)? Either we have such an amorphous understanding of the notion of "basic health care" that anything and everything medicine offers that yields any benefit at all is covered as a matter of justice (which undercuts the point of sufficientarianism), or, alternatively, we define "basic health care" in such a rigid, constrained, niggardly way that no one with an ounce of human decency and compassion could embrace that perspective as what was "just enough" or "beneficent enough" in meeting health care needs.

Allen Buchanan (2009) has offered some interesting arguments regarding commitment to a decent minimum of health care for all.[2] He is a critic of the notion of a right to health care. That notion is either too amorphous to do the serious ethical work required to address the problems of health care justice generated by precision medicine or else too expansive to be affordable. In addition, the language of a right to health care is politically divisive. What Buchanan appeals to is the political/sociological observation that the vast majority of Americans do not want to see fellow citizens suffer needlessly from some health crisis when needed health care is available but unaffordable to an individual. This is what calls forth a charitable response. However, that charitable response will be a mere inclination on the part of individuals because the needed financial assistance would be enormous. To be effective, a coordinated charitable response is necessary according to Buchanan.

---

[2] Buchanan would likely not describe himself as a sufficientarian, in part because that theoretical perspective was not part of philosophic conversations in 1984, the original date of the essay reprinted in 2009.

Government alone, as a social institution, has the authority and capacity to create and implement that coordinated response, thereby realizing the charitable wishes of the vast majority of Americans in this regard.

Buchanan describes his approach as a form of ethical pluralism because multiple justice-relevant considerations would govern that charitable response as well as considerations of beneficence and other ethically relevant values. For Buchanan no ethical theory is able to specify the content of what a decent minimum of health care is that ought to be assured to all. He writes, "Instead, there is an ineliminable role for collective choice, through legitimate political processes" (at 5). He adds, "Better theories of justice in health care can provide valuable constraints on how the right to an adequate level of care is to be fleshed out . . . but in the end what is included in the adequate level or decent minimum of care made available to all is not a fact to be discovered but rather a choice to be made" (at 5). Everything Buchanan says here seems completely congruent with my understanding of the role of rational democratic deliberation, though Buchanan believes the language of obligatory social beneficence is more palatable in public conversation than the language of health care justice. He believes that as a practical and ethical matter you can achieve the same outcome (social agreement on what health care ought to be guaranteed to everyone) with the language of social beneficence as with the language of social justice.

Social beneficence may be obligatory or non-obligatory. How should we characterize and justify the difference? The federal government funds programs in the arts and humanities. This is a reasonable and desirable use of public resources. However, if there were a serious economic crisis and that money were diverted to funding the Food Stamp program, the government would not be open to justified moral criticism because that humanities program is not obligatory. There would be no rights violations; no fundamental social values would be violated; private resources could fill the funding gaps. Alternatively, since 1972 Medicare has been funding the end-stage renal disease (ESRD) program, which pays for dialysis and kidney transplantation for patients with ESRD. That is an obligatory program. It could not be defunded without tragic consequences for the 47 million Americans who depend upon it for their very lives. We can go further and say that those 47 million Americans have a just claim to that program, given their health care needs. This is not something that could have been said just prior to the initiation of the program. The obligation came to be with the creation of the program itself.

The ESRD program came to be because dialysis had been invented, because dialysis promised many extra years of life for individuals otherwise condemned to a premature death, and because only a tiny fraction of these patients could afford the cost of dialysis. Additionally, hospitals could not provide this service on a charity care basis. A patient was dialyzed on the floor of Congress to persuade Congress to fund the program. Members of Congress would have to have had hearts of ice and brains of stone not to fund the program. This was obligatory beneficence. The situation elicits a strong sense of compassion. Members of Congress could hardly avert their eyes. They would know that they had the opportunity and authority and resources to respond positively to this situation. They could easily imagine that if they or any of their family or friends needed dialysis, they would want them to have access without any financial impediments. They would have found it difficult to muster up any compelling arguments for refusing to fund the program.[3]

Consider a little thought experiment. Imagine that members of Congress had a very clear crystal ball that showed them 100 years into the future all the costly life-prolonging medical technologies that were going to emerge that would require public funding, at least through Medicare and Medicaid, and a future possible national health insurance program. Would having that knowledge justify a decision not to fund the ESRD program under Medicare? I think a negative answer to that question would be warranted. All those future possible socially beneficent medical choices would have to be future possible choices; the choice to fund the ESRD program would remain a matter of obligatory social beneficence. This would be because tens of millions of individual lives would be at risk, each of those lives would have a number of years at risk, the vast majority of those lives would be of non-elderly individuals, no alternative therapies exist for kidney failure other than dialysis and transplantation, and no other funding mechanism would assure equitable access to this life-prolonging technology. Following Buchanan (2009), we can say that multiple justice-relevant considerations would warrant this conclusion as well as considerations related to compassion, beneficence, mutual respect, protecting freedom, and opportunity.

Recall that we are trying to determine whether various targeted cancer therapies and immunotherapies in various metastatic cancer contexts are

---

[3] Recall that the cost of dialysis in 2020 was about $88,000 per person per year. This is essentially what it cost in 1972, though that was in 1972 inflation-adjusted dollars.

matters of obligatory social beneficence as opposed to voluntary (non-obligatory) social beneficence. We are suggesting that this would be a way of cashing out what is required of a wealthy society as a matter of minimal decency with regard to providing secure access to needed health care. Put another way, we are trying to define a boundary for the sufficientarian that would distinguish what access to needed health care was a matter of justice or obligatory social beneficence and what other health care needs were a matter of private charity or ability to pay. Roger Crisp (2003) invokes the notion of an impartial compassionate spectator and writes, "when the spectator's compassion runs out, the sufficiency level is reached." This is clearly an unhelpful, paradigmatic example of vagueness, though there is a small helpful clue here.

7.2. Obligatory Social Beneficence: Application Criteria

What criteria might we use to identify health care therapies that ought to be a matter of obligatory social beneficence? First, members of Congress would have been embarrassed if they had had to explain to the persons they most respected in their lives why they voted against the ESRD amendments. "We will have to raise your taxes a little bit; we do not want to add to the national debt; people need to be more responsible and save money to pay for their future health care needs." Such statements would be callous and cruel. Crisp's compassionate spectator would be relevant here. These are patients who could be provided with many extra years of life, either with dialysis or with a kidney transplant. These are very effective interventions: Costs are reasonable; quality of life is diminished somewhat, though not to an unreasonable degree for most of these patients. Numerous medical interventions will satisfy these criteria, and consequently, they should be judged to be matters of obligatory social beneficence.

We should add the obvious: Curative medical interventions will be socially obligatory. Some individuals will suffer permanent injuries and disabilities that cannot be cured or fixed. However, if we have rehabilitative technologies that can restore functional capacities (artificial limbs, computer-assisted functioning, extensive physical therapy), these too will be socially obligatory. These are often complex interventions that would strike most of us as being far beyond "basic," which is why that term is inadequate for capturing what a just and caring society must do by way of meeting health care needs. Improving or maintaining a patient's quality of life in the face of serious or terminal illness will also be seen as a matter of obligatory social beneficence. Hospice programs would be a paradigm example of this commitment as well as palliative care generally.

What is *not* a matter of obligatory social beneficence? If an extremely costly medical intervention can yield only a small gain in life expectancy, that will not be obligatory. What counts as "too small" a gain in life expectancy? And what counts as being "too expensive"? These are matters determined through a fair and inclusive process of rational democratic deliberation. For example, it would be impossible to justify not funding the drugs needed by HIV+ patients to sustain their lives at $35,000 per year while funding dialysis for ESRD patients at $88,000 per year. Such a funding limitation would represent invidious discrimination since these drugs are more effective at sustaining life of good quality than dialysis. If a drug or intervention was slightly more effective than another drug for the same purpose but cost many times that less expensive drug, it would not be socially obligatory. The PCSK9s illustrate this point. For a small class of patients, they would make a very large therapeutic difference. Other patients with elevated low-density lipoprotein levels would have an increased risk of stroke or heart attack but could be managed at a much lower cost with statins, exercise, and dietary changes.

Obligatory social beneficence would require physicians to document that a more expensive drug was "medically necessary" in the strictest sense. A patient would have to be at great risk of serious medical consequences if this more expensive drug were not authorized. There are situations where this judgment could be very difficult to make, and potential social costs could be extraordinary. For example, roughly 400,000 women each year in the United States experience postpartum depression, one out of every seven who give birth in a year. This is a serious psychiatric disorder that too often results in suicide or harm to the children. A new drug, brexanolone (Zulresso˚), addresses the brain mechanism that triggers postpartum depression. However, the cost of this drug is $34,000. It is given as a one-time infusion (Joy, 2019). If this were thought to be a matter of obligatory social beneficence for all these women, the annual social cost would be $13.6 billion.

Might some other antidepressant relieve the depressed feelings enough to minimize the risk of suicide? These drugs would usually take a couple of weeks to elicit an effect. A bad guess could have fatal consequences for some of these women or their children. Should our democratic deliberators judge that access to this drug should be a matter of obligatory social beneficence? Could clinical guidelines be created that would restrict access to the drug at social expense to a relatively small cohort of women judged to be at highest risk of self-harm? Part of the ethical problem here is that ordinarily a commitment to equal concern and respect would require that everyone with the same medical need have access to the same effective therapeutic intervention. Are all of these women equally suicidal? How can we know that with confidence? If all these women were given Zulresso, what other care would be sacrificed to cover the cost of this drug?

Obligatory social beneficence will require giving priority to the medically least well off *but only to the extent that those individuals are capable of meaningful medical benefit*. No natural definition can identify the medically least well off. This will be a mix of medical and social judgments. Children born with a range of serious genetic disorders will be among the medically least well off. That would include sickle cell disease, cystic fibrosis, Duchenne's muscular dystrophy, spinal muscular atrophy, Pompe disease, and so on. These children are not born severely debilitated, but they will become severely debilitated and die prematurely unless very costly and very effective medical interventions available today are provided shortly after birth. These children can come close to a normal life expectancy with a reasonable quality of life. This is clearly "meaningful medical benefit."

On the flip side are children born with severe birth defects or who suffer various traumatic injuries in early life that are simply beyond the capacities of medicine to ameliorate or reverse. Gross brain deformities of various kinds, such as anencephaly or holoprosencephaly; disorders such as trisomy-13; and brain injuries resulting from tragic accidents exemplify my point. Anencephalic infants will typically die shortly after birth, though aggressive life-sustaining efforts have yielded two years of life. However, those infants derive no genuine human benefit from such efforts, and the cost of those efforts is exorbitant. This is not a matter of obligatory social beneficence. Should we think of it as a matter of *permissible* social beneficence? I would contend that considerations of health care justice would speak against this being socially permissible beneficence. Those resources would be better used (and more justly used) to meet the costly health needs of the children in the prior paragraph as well as children with very costly cancers whose lives can be saved today with the advances associated with precision medicine. These are children with hematologic cancers, 80% of whom can be cured today.

Children and adults who are in a persistent vegetative state (for whatever reason) or who might have barely emerged from such a state and are now in a minimally conscious state (which will be permanent), these too have no claim to obligatory medical beneficence. They are too far beyond being able to benefit in a meaningful human sense. The lives that are sustained in these states are "bare lives," devoid of anything we would recognize as a human experience. Given limited resources to meet virtually unlimited health care needs, these unfortunate individuals have no just claim to socially funded health care resources.

Some babies are born with extreme prematurity. They might be 22 to 24 weeks' gestation and less than 500 grams in birth weight. I will contend that infants at 22 weeks or less should be provided comfort care only and allowed to die, as opposed to being provided with $500,000 in neonatal ICU (NICU) care. Some premature infants in the 23- to 24-week range will do better than that with the highest-quality NICU care. Survivors who leave the NICU will be in the 25%–50% range, though most of those survivors will leave with either life-shortening impediments (lung and gut issues) or lifelong impediments (the result of brain bleeds). I would categorize these cases as being instances of *permissible* social beneficence, given a $750,000 cost per survivor, plus the health care costs needed to manage any lifelong deficiencies.

If we switch to adult patients who would be classified as being among the medically least well off, we would include victims of serious accidents (some only temporarily among the medically least well off, others there indefinitely), individuals living with chronic degenerative conditions that cause considerable suffering and a greatly diminished quality of life (advanced stages of amyotrophic lateral sclerosis [ALS] or Parkinson's or various types of dementia or end-stage lung disease or late-stage cancer that has gone to bone or late-stage multiple sclerosis), serious burn victims, and so on. Accident victims, even those who suffered the accident as a result of some very foolish choice, will need to be treated to the maximum extent possible to save their lives if medically possible. This is a matter of obligatory social beneficence. Likewise, if individuals have suffered spinal cord injuries that will leave them as paraplegics or quadriplegics, providing technology that will maximize their ability for social functioning will be a matter of obligatory social beneficence. For all the end-stage disease states mentioned above, providing all necessary and effective palliative care will be a matter of obligatory social beneficence. However, none of the listed disorders are curable; all such individuals are described as being in roughly the last six months of life if no aggressive life-sustaining interventions are undertaken. However, the stronger point I would make, and ask our deliberators to endorse, would be refraining from any very expensive life-prolonging efforts at this point. Such efforts would not be a matter of obligatory social beneficence. In addition, I think a case could be made for saying they should not be a matter of *permissible* social beneficence either, given the "just caring" problem. Instead, those resources should be made available for research that might result in interventions that would yield more medical good at earlier stages of these disease processes or more social good to support these patients in the very late stages of these disease processes. This would be a more just use of those limited health care resources. This is also illustrative of how at times considerations of health care justice would shape and constrain social beneficence.

7.3. Identifying the Limits of Social Beneficence

Consider some more puzzling possibilities with respect to the scope and limits of social beneficence. Some form of gene therapy may have something close to curative potential for Duchenne's muscular dystrophy (George 2021b). The cost of this intervention might be $2 million per person, though if it were to yield something close to a normal quality of life and normal life expectancy, I would contend this would be a matter of obligatory social beneficence. Muscle deterioration and muscle weakness are very often part of the aging process, which can have consequences for both length of life and quality of life. In identifying matters of obligatory social beneficence, I said above that medical interventions that yielded substantial functional benefits should be thought of as included under that rubric. I need to add an important qualifier, namely, that interventions that represent functional enhancement above normal functioning should not be regarded as matters of obligatory social beneficence. I have in mind Daniels' point (1985) that the just role of medicine is to restore individuals to the normal opportunity range of society. I believe a liberal society will have to allow individuals to purchase various medical interventions representing enhancement, at least as long as those purchases have no justice-relevant adverse consequences for those unable to afford those medical enhancements.

Consider the ambiguity that might be attached to some medical interventions that could be regarded as therapeutic or as enhancements. For example, if the gene therapy that restored normal functioning in patients with muscular dystrophy could restore something like youthful muscular strength to older individuals who have suffered muscle loss, is this something that we would have to provide to these older individuals as a matter of oblig-atory social beneficence? If this were possible with a drug that cost $100 per month, I think we would give an affirmative answer to this question. But if the gene therapy we have in mind cost $2 million, I think we would have to give a very different answer. Loss of muscle function does represent a health care need. However, millions of older individuals would have this need. As things are now, the 15% of our population over age 65 consume 35% of all health care dollars spent every year. Adding the cost of gene therapy for this pur-pose would add dramatically to the imbalance in the distribution of health care resources across the whole age spectrum. Further, the gain in quality-adjusted life-years (QALYs) would average a few years rather than the addi-tional decades gained (we assume) by individuals with muscular dystrophy. We can ask another hypothetical question. What if the cost of significantly improving muscle functioning in the elderly were $100,000 per person?[4] Sarcopenia is a problem for about 30% of those over age 65. That would be about 16 million Americans today, the cost of which would be $1.6 trillion. Even a cost of $10,000 per person would be a serious ethical and economic problem. That number would be $160 billion.

An older population will experience many sorts of functional deficits; just think of sight and hearing. Many of these problems can be addressed with relatively inexpensive interventions. However, "relatively inexpensive" can become "problematically expensive" when aggregated across millions of individuals. Roughly 30 million adult Americans have a degree of hearing loss requiring a hearing aid. Roughly 4 million hearing aids were dispensed in the United States in 2019. The cost of a hearing aid will vary from $1,000 to $10,000, depending upon the sophistication of the technology built into them. What sort of hearing aid should we think of as being a matter of oblig-atory social beneficence? Does social funding limited to the $1,000 hearing aid represent "sufficient beneficence"? That would represent $4 billion in so-cial spending annually. If the $10,000 device were available to all at social ex-pense, that would represent $40 billion. I assume that would be judged to be an inappropriate (unjust) use of social resources. Would we make that same judgment at the $3,000 or $2,000 level?

---

[4] Lest the reader think this last suggestion is pure scientific or philosophic speculation, I would call attention to a review article by Lo et al. (2020) that suggests that some form of stem cell therapy might be the key to addressing sarcopenia in the elderly. No cost is mentioned, but $100,000 would be a rea-sonable guess.

The most common intervention among the elderly with respect to sight is cataract surgery. In 2019, 3.8 million cataract surgeries were performed in the United States at a cost of roughly $3,000 each, or $9 billion. Given the importance of sight for most human functioning, I am certain our democratic deliberators would see this expenditure as a matter of obligatory social beneficence. Cataract surgery restores good vision, not perfect vision. Consider this thought experiment: Imagine an ocular surgical procedure that could restore the vision of an 80-year-old to the acuity of vision of a 40-year-old. The cost of that procedure would be $10,000, a small fraction of what any targeted therapy for metastatic cancer would cost. If that surgery were provided for 3.8 million Americans each year, the aggregated social cost would be $38 billion. Again, I would not see that as a matter of obligatory social beneficence, though the procedure can be described as correcting a visual deficit and restoring vision to its normal state (at an earlier point in life).

Dementia is feared by most Americans almost as much as cancer. There is scientific controversy regarding the primary causes of Alzheimer's dementia, either β-amyloid or tau in the brain. Numerous drugs have failed to modify the downhill course of Alzheimer's dementia. However, two new drugs have shown some promise in clinical trials, donanemab (George, 2021a) and aducanumab (Belluck, 2020). Neither one represents a cure. Both suggest some marginal ability to slow disease progression in the early stages of the disease. The cost of either drug is put at $56,000 per year, given as a monthly infusion (Belluck, 2020). In 2020 six million Americans had been diagnosed with various stages of Alzheimer's disease (AD). Roughly one million will be in late-stage AD, and 3.1 million will be in early-stage AD. The average length of time in early-stage AD is two to four years.

Evidence of effectiveness for either drug is limited. Consequently, consider this hypothetical scenario. Assume that either drug would maintain these patients in a mild state of AD for three additional years. Over three years we would have a cohort of five million AD patients receiving one of these drugs. The annual cost would be $250 billion. Should socially funded access to this drug be a matter of obligatory social beneficence? AD is a progressive disease. Hence, I would imagine that any newly diagnosed patient would much prefer to be in that early, mild stage rather than any later stage. Would such a universal preference justify that $250 billion additional expenditure as a matter of obligatory social beneficence and/or health care justice (also keeping in mind the proposed additional expenditures associated with sarcopenia, hearing issues, and seeing issues)? To be clear, that "universal preference" refers to newly diagnosed AD patients, as opposed to younger patients who would likely have to bear these costs in the form of higher taxes or insurance premiums and who themselves might never be faced with AD. Roughly 14% of our population over age 70 will develop AD, 5% of those below age 80 but 37% of those over age 90. In other words, the "universal preference" is in reality a very self-interested preference. That diminishes considerably any justificatory weight that preference might have.

Note that there would be no offsetting savings, such as fewer years in a long-term care facility. These drugs would simply prolong the length of time that individuals would live as an AD patient; long-term care costs would remain essentially the same. How should our democratic deliberators respond? Would the libertarian option be ethically acceptable? In other words, individuals would have to choose at a relatively young age to purchase private add-on insurance for these AD drugs or else absorb these costs as an older individual. If the chances of being diagnosed with AD are one in seven, that will not be strongly motivating to a younger individual with many other personal expenses and limited income. Our democratic deliberators might endorse this same conclusion, also with respect to both our very expensive hearing aids and some future form of eye surgery that would restore ocular keenness to that of a 40-year-old person. The same will be true for our gene therapy for sarcopenia, even if the price of that intervention could be brought down to either the $100,000 level or the $50,000 level. Funding any of these interventions would skew social resources very heavily into the upper age ranges at the expense of the just claims to other forms of needed health care in a somewhat younger population. Our democratic deliberators are not being ageist because they would be making these prudent trade-offs for their future possible selves. They would want to minimize the suffering and limitations associated with the physiological decline of aging but less expensively. Such an outcome would, all things considered, be just and reasonably socially beneficent. To answer one of our original questions—"What is enough?"—we are saying that these interventions are "beyond sufficiency," beyond what a decent society owes each and every one of its members.

One more complication: Some researchers are working on some drugs that would attack these tau tangles. More relevant is research on two biomarkers used to identify the earliest stages of AD: p-tau181 and p-tau217 (Moscoso et al., 2021). Most researchers believe that the earliest stages of AD begin two decades before clinical manifestations. These biomarkers, identified through a simple blood test, would have diagnostic and prognostic value.

This would be personally frightening for many people. However, it would be ethically and economically frightening from a social point of view if we had a tau-relevant drug that could slow (but not stop or reverse) the process of cognitive decline and that could be given, say, 10 years in advance of when symptoms would be clinically detectable. Such a drug would not be as cheap as aspirin. It would be very problematic, ethically and economically, if the drug were as expensive as PCSK9s ($6,000 per patient per year). It would be impossibly problematic if the drug were as expensive as aducanumab ($56,000 per year). I mention this emerging technology as a reminder of the allocation challenges on the health care horizon, most especially with regard to an aging population and expanding health care needs.

7.4. Seeking Sufficiency by Setting Priorities

Each increment of medical technology that has life-prolonging potential is regarded as obligatory and "affordable enough" when taken in a perfectly isolated way by most compassionate persons but wickedly problematic when aggregated and the focus of comparative judgments across the entire health care spectrum. Recall our discussion of chronic lymphocytic leukemia (CLL) and ibrutinib. Try this thought experiment. Imagine a continuum of medical interventions that were matters of obligatory social beneficence. At one end would be an enormous number of routine medical interventions but note especially those that are very expensive and intended to be significantly life-prolonging. Renal dialysis, kidney transplantation, and all other major organ transplantations would be at this end of the continuum as well as treatments for HIV. These latter individuals are mostly younger patients who can gain 30 years or more from time of infection with the protease inhibitors, fusion inhibitors, and so on, though at a cost of about $35,000 per year. As we move across the continuum, we try to figure out which interventions should be matters of obligatory social beneficence.

Start with CRISPR-based gene editing for sickle cell disease as well as hemophilia and several other single-gene disorders that manifest themselves very early in life. Considerable medical excitement has been generated by these gene-editing therapeutic trials for sickle cell disease (Frangoul et al., 2020; Marcus, 2020; Stein, 2020a). Sickle cell is a truly awful disease that causes excruciating pain for its victims as a result of the sickling of red blood cells that clog up tiny blood vessels. Some of these individuals will die by age

20; others might survive to age 40 or beyond, though they will be terribly crippled by the disease and its effects on joints all over the body. All of them will require multiple hospitalizations and transfusions over the course of a year. Roughly 100,000 Americans have sickle cell disease, most of whom are African American. This just cries out for a compassionate response. Several individuals have been treated with a form of gene editing more than a year ago. The painful experiences seem to have all disappeared. No one can say with medical confidence at this point that these individuals have been cured. Failure could occur three years from now or 10 years or 20 years.

For our purposes, however, we are going to assume that this therapy has proven to be completely successful. It costs $2 million per person. If we were going to offer this technology to all sickle cell patients, the aggregated cost would be $200 billion. Is this a matter of obligatory social beneficence? That figure is startling and clearly unaffordable if borne in a single year. Imagine instead that this cost is spread out over 10 years. Of course, that would raise another ethics issue: What criteria would be used to determine which 10% received the CRISPR therapy in any given year? That might be less problematic than we would first imagine. Recall two new sickle cell drugs which dramatically reduce the symptoms of sickle cell disease: voxelotor and crizanlizumab-tmca. Each of these drugs has an annual cost of $100,000, which would add $9 billion to aggregated health costs for the first year in which CRISPR gene editing was used for the sickle cell patients (to be reduced by $1 billion each year thereafter). I will suggest that our deliberators would see this as a matter of obligatory social beneficence.

If this CRISPR gene-editing technology is extremely successful with sickle cell disease, it might be equally successful in curing hemophilia, cystic fibrosis, muscular dystrophy, fragile X syndrome, and lysosomal storage disorders, all of which are single-gene disorders.[5] CRISPR gene editing might not be able to correct damage already done, which is unfortunate. The number of potential births in the United States with these disorders would be in the 8,000–12,000 range. The key considerations that would justify treating all these individuals with CRISPR gene editing as a matter of obligatory social beneficence would be: (1) the numerous loss of life-years that would be prevented with this technology; (2) the enormous amount of suffering that would be prevented; (3) the lack of any alternative medical interventions that

---

[5] Lysosomal storage disorders are a group of approximately 50 inherited disorders that occur when a missing enzyme results in the body's inability to recycle cellular waste.

would be less expensive and roughly equally effective; and (4) a reasonable cost per life-year saved relative, for example, to the costs of targeted cancer therapies. As noted, the $2 million front-end cost is startling. This is four times the cost of front-end chimeric antigen receptor (CAR) T-cell therapy. However, if these infants and children each gain 60 years of normal quality of life, each of those life-years gained would have a cost of $35,000.

I am mindful of the fact that the scenario I have constructed may be on the optimistic side. For the sake of discussion, we can imagine that the therapy begins to fail after five years. Patients would then require another $2 million infusion of the CRISPR-edited cells. This would be necessary at five-year intervals to sustain the initial cure and prevent disease progression. Under this scenario, it would be much harder to argue that this remained a matter of obligatory social beneficence. This would have become a truly wicked problem. How would we imagine justifying to ourselves withholding this life-prolonging care from these children, allowing them to suffer "unnecessarily" the ravages of one or another of these disorders, then die very prematurely? On the ethical surface, this looks very much like the introduction of dialysis as a life-prolonging technology, except the cost would be four times greater per life-year gained in this five-year scenario, or 25 times greater per patient if we imagine a 60-year scenario. If some terrible side effects were emerging at five years, we would have good reason (regrettably) for withholding its further use. Or if we had evidence that a second infusion would only be marginally effective, petering out in a year or two, then too we would have good reason for withholding further use. But if these pessimistic possibilities are not there and if we have every reason to believe these patients would get another five very good years, we (caring citizens) would likely "feel compelled" to continue to provide this therapy, though this might not be a choice that was ethically obligatory.

To pursue this scenario one step further, imagine that we have a relatively fixed budget. That is, we cannot imagine adding another $20 billion into the health care budget every year to cover this contingency.[6] We would have to find that money elsewhere. We might aim to reduce waste and inefficiency in the health care system. However, one person's waste and inefficiency are often another person's livelihood or life-prolonging medical care. In addition, even if we could identify all the waste and inefficiency in the health care

---

[6] In case it is not clear, each year each cohort of infants available for CRISPR editing would cost $20 billion, assuming 10,000 infants or children comprised that cohort.

system with the economic equivalent of fluorescent dye, the practical challenge would be aggregating all those enormously disaggregated dollars to meet the very costly health care needs of these children. Perhaps someone would care to argue that finding another $20 billion every year in a $4 trillion health economy and a $22 trillion national economy should not be that great a challenge. However, the CRISPR gene-editing challenge is only one of numerous costly medical technologies being introduced into the health care system each year. Where is the funding for all these other technologies supposed to come from if we have to live with a relatively fixed budget, either hard dollars or a fixed percentage of gross domestic product? Remember that we are trying to determine the scope and limits of obligatory social beneficence as a way of specifying what would count as the "minimally decent" level of health care owed to all in our society.

7.5. How Many Artificial Hearts Will Be Sufficient? Age-Based Rationing Redivivus

Let us move away from children to the other end of the age spectrum. Let us consider again the totally implantable artificial heart (TIAH) (Morshuis et al., 2020; Cohn et al., 2015). This is still an experimental item, but perfection is expected. This device would completely replace the natural heart of patients in end-stage heart failure. It would be entirely powered from within, no external battery pack. The total cost of the device plus surgery and hospitalization is estimated to be $500,000. Roughly 350,000 Americans would be candidates for this device each year. At this writing (late 2021), roughly 5.5 million Americans are in various stages of congestive heart failure (CHF), with about 550,000 newly diagnosed patients each year. The vast majority of these patients are older than 65. About 1.4 million Americans with CHF will be under age 60. Roughly 2% of Americans from age 40 to 59 will be in some stage of heart failure. More than 70% of Americans with end-stage heart failure will be over age 70. If the TIAH were a therapeutic option for 350,000 Americans each year, the total additional health care cost would be $175 billion per year. Is providing the TIAH to all who could medically benefit from it with an average gain in life expectancy of five years a matter of obligatory social beneficence?

To be clear, the TIAH is not thought of as a device that will wear out after five or eight or 10 years. If it is implanted in an older population, they will have a high likelihood of death from other causes in that five-year window, whereas a 50-year-old could get 20 extra years of life from that device. This generates a number of wicked problems. In theory, all those problems would disappear if we decided as a society that we would not make the TIAH clinically available. However, it is difficult imagining our deliberators embracing that option.

Failure to provide the TIAH as a clinical option for patients with advanced CHF who were in their 40s or 50s would be a potential loss of salvageable, reasonable quality of life of 10 or more years. If each of these individuals gained only 10 extra years of life, the cost per life-year saved would be $50,000. In other words, this was a cost-effective investment. Of course, we would also be spending much more per year for ALS patients at $100,000 or for rheumatoid arthritis patients requiring biologics at $65,000 per year or more than $100,000 per year for almost all of our metastatic cancer patients. That would provide additional support for the claim that these individuals should have access to the TIAH at social expense as a matter of obligatory social beneficence. What about the rest of the individuals who will need access to the TIAH?

If we are reluctant to fund that full $175 billion each year so that all these patients with late-stage heart failure would have access to a TIAH, then where should we draw the line? Age 70? Patients in their 60s would still be short of a normal life expectancy, which might be a reason why our deliberators should endorse this idea as a matter of obligatory social beneficence. This argument will be compelling with regard to patients in their early 60s. Will it be equally compelling for a patient who is 69 years old? It seems that it should be. They are less than 70 years old. However, that means the patient who is 69 might gain five to 10 extra years of life. The patient who is 71 years old would be equally capable of gaining those five to 10 extra years of life. However, they will be denied that opportunity if we use age 70 as a bright cutoff line.[7]

Our deliberators are unlikely to be ethically comfortable with such a rule. Too many life-years would be sacrificed with too little justification. Further, it would feel even more ethically uncomfortable if we suggested

[7] This is a perfect example of Callahan's "ragged edge" (1990). Callahan writes, "We should be prepared to make such decisions, knowing perfectly well that some lives will be lost at that ragged edge we decide to accept and not to overcome . . . we know that, once a ragged edge is defeated, we will then simply move on to still another ragged edge, with new victims—and there will always be new victims. It is a struggle we cannot win. . . . We can ask . . . how to make life tolerable on the ragged edges; for we will all one day be on such an edge, sooner or later" (at 65). This is a critical insight for our democratic deliberators.

that individuals over age 70 could always pay for the TIAH themselves. We noted earlier a range of circumstances in which various very costly targeted cancer drugs would not be socially funded. Instead, individuals would have to decide whether they would pay for those drugs from their own resources. However, that situation is radically different from the situation with the TIAH. The cancer drugs we discussed yielded only marginal benefit for the vast majority of patients, and even that marginal benefit was very uncertain to obtain. The TIAH would promise these extra five or more years of life of good quality with a high degree of confidence. From an ethical point of view, that would represent a more substantial loss which would require some compelling ethical justification. This is not a matter of marginal benefits.

What other options are available for reducing the potential costs of having TIAHs available? Canada, as well as some European countries, restrict the number of magnetic resonance imaging and positron emission tomographic (PET) scanners that are available, thereby compelling physicians to make their best judgments regarding which patients will benefit the most from having access to these diagnostic technologies. Should we limit public funding to no more than 50,000 TIAHs per year at a social cost of $25 billion. Physicians would be required to make their best medical judgment regarding who would benefit the most. Such judgments could be too subjective, too likely to incorporate in subtle ways prevailing social prejudices described as objective medical judgment. If we endorsed that idea, what criteria would our democratic deliberators employ for making these decisions, from the perspective of either health care justice or obligatory social beneficence?

In natural organ transplantation there is a clear bias toward younger patients; few patients over age 70 would be preferred as a transplant recipient if a younger patient were available and a good match. We accept that as fair and reasonable, especially if we imagine choosing this policy from behind a health status veil of ignorance. If we have 50,000 TIAHs, half of those might go to patients under age 70. The remainder would likely be available for patients in their 70s with no life-threatening co-morbid conditions. They would likely all have more or less the same number of life-years at risk.

Maybe our deliberators would be ethically comfortable with picking age 80 as a sharp cutoff. Unfortunately, medical circumstances will provide an environment where gamesmanship could threaten the legitimacy of that age 80 cutoff. Consider: When should someone in the early stages of heart failure consider seeking access to a TIAH if they are 78 years old? Heart failure is a progressive disorder. They know they will advance from Stage I to Stage IV over a period of years. Stage III might last for three years. If this individual is very early in Stage III, they would not "need," in a strong medical sense, the TIAH. But if they waited until later in Stage III, they would be beyond age 80 and ineligible. Strict medical/surgical criteria would have to be used to prevent any such gamesmanship. We (citizens intending to be just and caring) might feel badly for patients in this gray area very close to a sharp cutoff point that presumably would have been democratically legitimated. However, what this illustrates is the need for our sense of obligatory social beneficence to be constrained by relevant considerations of health care justice.

Consider another hypothetical scenario. We have winnowed down the pool of potential candidates. At the end of that process, we still have two viable surgical candidates beyond age 70 for every available TIAH democratically agreed upon. Should personal responsibility be used as a tiebreaker? In other words, if a patient had been a smoker for three decades or if that patient had a diet very heavy on fatty foods or if that patient had been poorly compliant with the medications that were supposed to control the advance of their heart disease, then such a patient would be denied a TIAH. I have argued elsewhere that such a policy would be neither just nor socially beneficent (Fleck, 2012). In brief, such a policy would likely reflect prevailing social biases. So-called Type A personalities are typically the recipients of social praise, though their intense, stressful behavior will often contribute to heart disease. They would be regarded as worthy recipients of a TIAH, unlike the alcoholic. Likewise, the factors that generate unhealthy behavior are typically medically, psychologically, and socially complex such that making simple attributions of personal responsibility for unhealthy health status are likely to be uninformed and, hence, unfair.[8]

Several other factors should also be ruled out as a basis for denying someone access to a TIAH. For example, someone may have required extensive use of the health care system at some early stage in their life, perhaps racking up health care costs of more than $1 million. Our deliberators should see this as completely irrelevant to the current situation of the patient now in heart failure. Health care needs are not distributed fairly or equally by nature, which is why appealing to such a factor to limit access to a TIAH would violate both our sense of fairness and beneficence. Likewise, if an individual had expensive ongoing health needs that would not diminish the likely effectiveness of the TIAH which they also needed, then that too should not be used as

---

[8] For further discussion of this issue, see also Eyal (2013), Levy (2019), and Friesen (2018).

a factor that would disqualify the individual from access to a TIAH at social expense. In other words, the fact that giving this individual a TIAH would mean that the social costs of sustaining each year of their life into the future would be greater than the social cost of each additional life-year for someone without those additional expensive health needs is not a sufficient basis for justly denying that individual a chance for equal access to a TIAH.

Consider some additional situations where we would limit access to a TIAH. If we have the capacity to predict with 90% confidence that an individual would likely not survive at least two years with a TIAH, perhaps because of some co-morbid medical condition, then that individual would not be a candidate for a TIAH. This might offend the sensibilities of a strict egalitarian, but there are legitimate and reasonable competing values at issue. This is not a matter of an egalitarian tribe competing to get their way with a utilitarian or prioritarian tribe. These competing value considerations would be within each of our democratic deliberators. From behind our health status veil of ignorance, our deliberators could reasonably judge that their future possible self could be either the individual who would gain one or two extra years of life with a TIAH or the individual who could gain five or 10 extra years of life. They could reasonably judge that they would not want to give up the chance for those five or 10 years. Consequently, they would agree to give up that extra year or two if it turned out that that were their future possible self. This would be neither unjust nor uncaring. This would not violate our sense of obligatory social beneficence.

I want to return to the issue of age-based rationing and our sense of obligatory social beneficence as well as our commitment to equal concern and respect. Imagine a 90-year-old who has heart failure that would likely result in their death by age 92 but who is otherwise in reasonably good health (no other chronic degenerative condition). This individual will get at least five extra years of life with a TIAH. How could we, just and caring citizens, allow such an individual to die when we have the capacity to prolong their life significantly? We have already decided (though we can make exceptions) that we will provide only 25,000 TIAHs for those judged to be medically suitable candidates who are over age 70 but under age 80. We feel ethically uncomfortable with simply allowing this individual to die from their heart disease. What options are available to us that would be "just enough" and "caring enough" *and that would yield a reasonable reflective equilibrium?*

I remind my readers that our democratic deliberations are constrained in several ways, one of which is the need to preserve a stable reflective equilibrium among relevant competing social values. We might imagine "making an exception" for this 90-year-old. However, how could we justly make an exception for this one individual? There would be thousands or tens of thousands of such individuals beyond age 80 who would be somewhat equally reasonable candidates for being given an exception. If we stuck with our 25,000 TIAH limit, that would mean that each of these exceptions would be taken somehow from individuals in their 70s who might have equally good prospects for those five extra years of life. That would not strike most of us as either fair or socially beneficent, in part because all of these individuals would have already exceeded a normal life expectancy, maybe because of an excellent genetic endowment or maybe because an individual was especially scrupulous regarding maintaining a healthy lifestyle. In either case, responding positively to these individuals and giving them a TIAH would disturb for the worse an otherwise just reflective equilibrium.

Recall that the focus of our discussion is heart failure. However, in many other areas of medicine (costly targeted cancer therapies or immunotherapies) we might have to consider some sort of age-related limit to very costly life-prolonging therapies. In other words, we could hardly permit generous exceptions to our age-based limits with respect to TIAHs and heart failure but maintain those rigid limits in every other area of medicine. What would we imagine the justice-based or social beneficence–based justification would be for such a constrained policy of exceptions? The basic problem is that, apart from major organ transplants, no natural limits exist with respect to how many TIAHs are implanted or immunotherapies are made available or diagnostic PET scans are performed. If there are limits, those limits will be a product of social choices.

One response available to us for addressing the "exceptions issue" is to expand the number of TIAHs we are willing to fund publicly. However, that would likely result in a different version of social disequilibrium. Again, we would be faced with the question of what would justify expanded social funding for TIAHs, as opposed to any other costly life-prolonging technology. We could readily admit that no such justification existed for that constrained limitation, and consequently, we would increase social funding in every area of medicine that was directly connected with providing life-prolonging technology. In many respects this might appear to satisfy our commitment to social beneficence, though our concern is with *obligatory* social beneficence, as opposed to *supererogatory* social beneficence. If no limits exist with regard to social resources for meeting health care needs, then such supererogatory social beneficence would not be ethically problematic. However, if we must accept limits, then supererogatory social beneficence is achieved at the expense of obligatory social beneficence in other non-life-prolonging areas of health care. Most often, those other areas will include mental health care, home health care, long-term care, and some range of services for persons with various disabilities. Meeting adequately these other health care needs will never yield a Nobel Prize or any other scientific plaudits. These are mundane, non-dramatic needs that nevertheless are likely to be the needs of the vast majority of our population in their advanced years since only a minority of our population is likely to die suddenly without having experienced the need for such services. Failure to meet these needs adequately would result in another sort of unjustified disequilibrium so far as health care justice and social beneficence are concerned.

One practical conclusion to draw from this analysis is that some form of age-based and effectiveness-based limitations will have to be identified and legitimated through our democratic deliberative process with regard to all forms of expensive life-prolonging care. We might still feel ethically distressed with regard to our paradigmatic, mostly healthy 90-year-old patient. What can be said to relieve that sense of distress? First, we do make social choices on occasion that are biased in favor of the elderly at the potential expense of younger portions of the population. The clearest current example pertains to the distribution of the COVID vaccines. In the first distributional tier were patients (mostly older) in long-term care facilities, and in the second distributional tier were patients over the age of 75. Eventually there would be enough vaccine for everyone, though that required nine more months. The ethical justification for giving priority to these older individuals is that they are at greatly increased risk for more serious illness and death from COVID than the *generally* younger population.

I want to call special attention to that word "generally." Quite clearly, some number of younger individuals, including children, suffered serious health consequences (some lifelong) as well as death from COVID during that interval before a vaccine became available to them. In other words, as a society we accepted a trade-off of some relatively small number of younger lives for a much greater number of older lives we hoped to save. We were not treating those older lives as socially expendable because no longer economically productive. The loss of those younger lives is random and unfortunate, not unjust. In addition, those younger individuals are out and about in the world and have the capacity to protect themselves from COVID by following all the public health recommendations. This is exactly the option not available to patients in long-term care facilities or assisted living facilities.

A second consideration concerns the trade-offs that future possible elderly individuals would make with regard to their future possible selves. Again, imagine that our deliberators are on the younger side of middle age, which is to say that each deliberator could imagine themselves as many different future possible elderly selves. Consequently, that makes possible a significant degree of impartiality with respect to these future possible selves. They might imagine themselves as our 90-year-old, and they might imagine wanting for that future possible self those five extra years promised by a TIAH. However, our deliberators are rational and reasonable. As rational individuals, they would realize that the likelihood of their being that future 90-year-old is at best a remote possibility, though a family genetic endowment might improve those odds. Still, they are a reasonable person capable of a more expansive range of concern for the well-being of others within their family and circle of friends and acquaintances. As deliberators their role would be to choose social policies regarding the allocation of health care resources across a broad and diverse range of health care needs. Consequently, they would be mindful of the future needs of friends and family who would become older, suffer various chronic degenerative diseases, and need home care or long-term care. They would want those services adequately funded for all, again mindful of the current deficiencies regarding those services. This is what would motivate them to trade off some very expensive life-prolonging interventions for individuals over age 80, for example, that would then ensure adequate funding for those services that would more likely be needed by older members of the population, including several future possible versions of themselves.

If what I have described is a reasonable scenario, then such a scenario would involve age-based allocation of health care sources that would be regarded as both just and socially beneficent. There would be no violation of our commitment to equal concern and respect. The deliberative process itself would make such trade-offs legitimate. The outcome would be a reasonable reflective equilibrium, something that could be socially and politically stable for the right reasons. To illustrate that last point, we can imagine 50 years into the future one of the members of this deliberative group has become our 90-year-old in heart failure. They are not ready to die. They very much want that TIAH and the extra five years of life that would represent. This expectation cannot be honored. They might complain that they have been exceptionally attentive in protecting their own health. They conclude that this should give them a right to that TIAH at social expense.

At that point we would concede that they might not have already benefited from the policy choices made 50 years earlier. In fact, they could have died suddenly from a heart attack and never benefited from the choices they endorsed at the time. However, a number of other family members and friends would have benefited from their choices. That was an outcome that was very much part of the reason why they endorsed those policy trade-offs in the first place. They also had the option at the time to purchase some form of add-on health insurance that would have paid for a variety of very expensive life-prolonging options, including the TIAH and various cancer therapies in various clinical circumstances that were not going to be socially funded. This add-on policy was going to be somewhat expensive, still affordable by them, but they judged at the time that all these possibilities were too remote and too likely to yield only marginal benefits for them. They had better things to do with that money. This same reasoning would have been collectively endorsed through the deliberative process. Society would have no right to renege on the promise it made to provide adequate funding for home care and long-term care services for all with the relevant need. The same would be true for this person. They cannot renege on the policies and trade-offs to which they had agreed and from which they might have benefited and from which many of their friends and family did benefit. Further, their cardiac problems, including a future possible heart attack, will be managed with the best medical care available that is guaranteed to all in society in similar circumstances. In that regard they cannot complain that they are not being treated with equal concern and respect or that they are being treated unjustly. They have no just claim to a TIAH in these circumstances.

7.6. Being the National Institute for Clinical Excellence: Health Care Justice and the Terminally Ill

The National Institute for Clinical Excellence (NICE) has defended the claim that when we are doing cost-effectiveness analysis, we ought to be more generous in allowing less cost-effective care to be available at social expense to terminally ill individuals. This claim has a socially beneficent halo around it. It feels as if it would be indecent to question this claim, much less to reject it. This has baked into it the rhetoric of a "last chance" therapy with a smidgen of the rescue analogy and seasoned with sprinkles of compassion. To be precise, NICE's current position is that, in general, it will only approve new health care interventions that have a cost per QALY of £20,000–£30,000 (roughly $30,000–$50,000). However, if a drug is used for patients who have less than a two-year life expectancy and if that drug *has the potential to provide at least three extra months of life*, then that drug may be approved by NICE with a cost per QALY as high as £50,000 (roughly $70,000). In addition, NICE emphasizes that these cost-effectiveness numbers are not rigid, that in special circumstances drugs might be approved that exceed these cost-effectiveness criteria.[9] This refers to cancer drugs for which the Cancer Drug Fund is an option that exceed that £50,000 criterion.

Charlton (2020) notes that NICE has become especially permissive with regard to these cancer drugs (compared to its rigorous practices prior to 2010), generally being satisfied that a cancer drug has the "mere potential" to provide an additional three months of life, as opposed to "consistently providing" those extra months of life, as demonstrated in clinical trials. This is a very low bar for approval. Charlton feels that NICE is bowing to political pressure generated by public expectations for greater access to these cancer drugs. However, these public expectations are of a non-deliberative nature; they are largely generated through the clever use of the media by pharmaceutical companies. Successful treatment of some patients is hyped in the media; think of the super-responders introduced in Chapter 1. In the minds of many people, this will generate the thought: "How could those bureaucrats at NICE deny these patients those extra years of life? That is cruel and inhumane." What is not considered are the injustices and inefficiencies that are a necessary consequence of these more lenient approvals of these cancer drugs. Again, the National Health Service (NHS) has a fixed budget, as do the Commissioning Groups responsible for allocating health care resources at a more local level. The money spent through the NHS to fund these very expensive cancer drugs requires not funding something else, often something that would generate more QALYs at a much lower cost. The patients who are, in essence, the victims of these rationing decisions are invisible and diffuse. They may have no sense at all that they were denied needed and effective health care. They are not a coherent constituency in the way that cancer

---

[9] A third criterion was that the patient had to be part of a "small population group." I am not sure what that was supposed to mean. I do not know how "small" a group was supposed to be. In any case, it is far from obvious that such a limitation would be just.

patients are a coherent constituency. The harm done to them may be unjust, and the overall result will be societally inefficient. Both, however, will be invisible for purposes of social correction.

With regard to the Cancer Drug Fund, it seems patently unjust to make cancer a social favorite for special funding. Other patients will be faced with terminal illness and need very expensive drugs or other therapeutic interventions that might yield extra months or years of life for them, but no fund exists to meet that need. Epanomeritakis (2019) endorses that judgment without a moment's hesitation. However, having said that, he argues that it would be unjust to discontinue the Cancer Drug Fund once established. This strikes me as an ethically problematic claim, as a matter of both justice and social beneficence.

We might consider a comparison with the ESRD amendments to the Medicare program in 1972. After a decade or so of operation, some critics wondered whether this program was a good idea. It was much more expensive than anticipated. It was ethically flawed in that it paid for kidney transplants (which most patients could not afford) but not heart or pancreas or liver transplants (which few patients could afford as well). Still, no one would think it would be ethically permissible to cancel the program outright as a way of "correcting" for its economic or ethical challenges. Is the Cancer Drug Fund just like that? No! One obvious difference is that both dialysis and kidney transplantation are very effective therapeutic interventions yielding many extra years of life for the vast majority of these patients. However, the major criticism of the Cancer Drug Fund is that it was funding all these marginally beneficial cancer drugs and at very great cost. These were all drugs that NICE had failed to approve for general NHS funding for these very reasons. These were drugs that generally failed to yield "clinically meaningful benefit" (Cohen, 2017). In addition, no effort was made by managers of the fund to gather actual data regarding the survival benefit associated with these drugs.

In the research that was done to determine survival benefit (Aggarwal et al., 2017), the researchers looked at 29 cancer drugs used for 47 indications. What they found was that only 38% of these indications were supported by clinical trials and that these clinical trials showed a median overall survival benefit of only 3.2 months, just a hair above the minimal expectations established for use of the fund. In addition, another 36% were approved for use despite "no statistically significant overall survival benefit" (i.e., wasteful health care, which considerations of both justice and social beneficence would condemn).

What then would justify the continued existence of the Cancer Drug Fund? The short answer is political considerations alone. It was created to address public dissatisfaction with the perception that NICE was too stringent in its non-approvals, that cancer patients were dying unnecessarily and prematurely because these life-prolonging drugs were being denied them for monetary reasons alone. Of course, given a fixed budget, the money to underwrite the Cancer Drug Fund would have to come from somewhere else in the health budgets (Collins and Latimer, 2013). Where was "elsewhere"? Were patients seriously affected? If patients were adversely affected, would that show up on political radar? In fact, the effects would be politically invisible and, therefore, politically inconsequential. Abolishing the Cancer Drug Fund as a poor use of health care dollars would be very visible and very politically consequential. However, this does not represent any sort of moral justification for maintaining the fund.

One of the key arguments in support of the fund is that the public places greater value on funding end-of-life QALYs than non-end-of-life QALYs. If we are committed to supporting democratic preferences, the argument goes, then we ought to alter our policies to reflect those preferences. This, of course, is an empirical claim. However, this claim does not seem to be well supported by actual social science research. Collins and Latimer (2013) cite research by Linley and Hughes (2013), who found that "only 34% of the 4118 respondents, with all else being equal, would prioritize patients with a reduced life expectancy." Those same researchers also found "no evidence to support the claim that, all else being equal, society places a higher value on health benefits to patients with cancer." See also research in the Netherlands (Wouters et al., 2017).[10]

Are there powerful moral considerations that would justify giving greater weight for priority-setting purposes to interventions that are aimed at prolonging the lives of terminally ill individuals, especially if that means sacrificing funding for non-terminal health care needs? Start with making a sharp distinction between a "broad" and a "narrow" sense of being terminally ill. Patients diagnosed with ESRD are terminally ill in that broad sense

---

[10] Other research in England and Wales supports this same conclusion: "Overall, we find little evidence that members of the general public prefer to give higher priority to life-extending end-of-life treatments than to other types of treatment. When asked to make decisions about the treatment of hypothetical patients with relatively short life expectancies, most people's choices are driven by the size of the health gains offered by treatment" (Shah et al., 2015, at 48).

since they typically have several extra years of life as long as they have access to dialysis. Patients diagnosed with metastatic cancer will generally have a two-year life expectancy, which is still the broad sense of being terminally ill. When the disease process has progressed to the point that a patient has less than a six-month life expectancy, they are terminally ill in the narrow sense. That is, death is relatively imminent and unavoidable.

Cookson (2013) has argued that no coherent ethical justification can be given for NICE's end-of-life premium. Is the rule of rescue relevant? We spend grossly disproportionate sums to rescue individuals who are at risk of dying in some unfortunate circumstance, such as the Chilean miners. What Cookson notes is that the rescued individuals will have "the rest of their lives" (many years) to look forward to. But in the case of terminal illness we know before the fact that we might be successful in giving individuals only a couple extra months of life of diminished quality at very great social expense. Note also that invoking the rule of rescue is something very rare. Having 600,000 terminally ill cancer patients in the United States each year is not a rare event, not to mention individuals who are terminally ill with non-cancer diagnoses.

A second argument Cookson considers is the "fair chances" argument. However, this argument only applies to distributing absolutely scarce resources. Hypothetically, we could constrain CAR T-cell therapies. Cookson would then suggest that what "fair chances" would require is the use of a lottery to determine which patients would receive CAR T-cell therapy. However, that undercuts the reason NICE exists. NICE exists to provide NICE-like rational guidance for the best use of limited health care resources (something not achievable with a lottery). Also, we do not use a lottery for organ transplantation. If an individual is unlikely to gain an extra year of life with a transplanted organ, that individual will simply be denied the transplant. This is neither unjust nor unkind. Both utilitarian and egalitarian perspectives on health care justice clearly warrant this conclusion. Most often, it will be an "impartial nature" (a sort of natural lottery) that will determine survival possibilities for individuals. The same will be true with respect to the terminal stages of cancer, that is, who will survive less than a year with CAR T-cell therapy and who will survive for several years. Moreover, I am certain this is the outcome that our democratic deliberators would endorse for themselves as being "just enough" and "beneficent enough" from behind a future health status veil of ignorance. Again, individuals denied very expensive, marginally beneficial cancer therapies and those extra months of life would still be provided with excellent palliative care.

The other argument Cookson assesses is what he calls the "*ex post* willingness to pay" argument. In other words, what are those individuals willing to pay to have a chance for those extra months of life when they are already afflicted with a terminal cancer? Survey research suggests that they would be willing to pay very much more in order to secure those extra months of life compared to extra months of life with a non-terminal illness. That makes it sound as if NICE got it right; people do attach a premium to gaining extra months of life. However, this conclusion only holds if individuals believe they are spending *social resources* to achieve these extra months of life as opposed to their personal resources. This would reflect very much a self-interested perspective; there is nothing just or socially beneficent about such a choice.

If we want to know what sort of just or socially beneficent choices people were willing to make, then we have to elicit those choices *before the fact*, that is, before individuals find themselves afflicted with a potentially fatal cancer. In that situation individuals would have to decide, presumably through a democratic deliberative process, how much more they were willing to spend in the form of taxes or insurance premiums to assure access to these very costly, marginally beneficial cancer therapies near the end of life. Further, these are decisions that would apply to everyone in that society, thereby demonstrating equal concern and respect for all. The more relevant question our deliberators would have to ask themselves would be whether to use those same resources to fund research aimed at more effectively treating various cancers before they get to the metastatic stage.

Readers will notice that I did not include prioritarians in the list of justice-relevant perspectives that would concur with opposition to NICE's end-of-life premium. Actually, they *ought* to concur. Cookson considers one last basis for endorsing NICE's position, the "severity of illness" criterion. These terminally ill patients are clearly among the "medically least well off." That suggests that they are more worthy of more resources to address their profound health care needs. However, we should distinguish severe health care needs for which an effective therapy is available, even if very costly, from severe health care needs for which we have only extremely costly interventions that will yield very limited benefits, extra months of life, for example.

We saw in Section 7.4 how new, very costly forms of gene therapy may improve dramatically (possibly cure) the fate of children with sickle cell disease or hemophilia or cystic fibrosis. Here is where the prioritarian perspective is most helpful and most relevant, so far as health care justice is concerned. This is where the severity of illness criterion has been met and can be most effectively addressed. Our end-stage cancer patients are severely ill; unfortunately, they are beyond being effectively treated. These very costly cancer drugs will yield some marginal benefit, far outside any reasonable understanding of cost-effectiveness. Unless prioritarians believe society has unlimited resources for meeting unlimited health care needs, they *ought* to accept the need to establish just priorities congruent with our sense of social beneficence among severely ill patients. If they insist that all patients who are severely ill have an equal claim to any health resources that will possibly yield any degree of benefit for them, then in a world with limited health care resources the serious health needs of the non-severely ill would be unjustly compromised because an excess quantity of those resources will have been directed uncritically to all the severely ill.

We return to our original question: What is enough? What does a just and caring society owe in the way of socially funded access to needed and effective health care for all its members as a matter of justice or obligatory social beneficence, including metastatic cancer patients? NICE does provide us with an answer. If NICE approves one of these cancer drugs, that means that considerable expertise (medical, financial, and ethical) has gone into assessing that drug for specific indications. The experts must judge that the drug is reliably effective in yielding additional life-prolonging benefits with tolerable side effects. What "reliably effective" means is that its predicted ability to manage metastatic cancer for a sufficient period of time will come to be for a large part of the defined patient population as opposed to 10% to 20% of that population. If the drug cost $30 per month, then that low level of effectiveness might be irrelevant since we might reasonably judge (ethically speaking) that it was very important (as a matter of compassion) to at least help that 10% or 20% of patients. However, the drugs we are actually talking about generally have costs of more than $12,000 per month, which would stretch the limits of affordable compassion if only 10% or 20% of the relevant patients benefited with an extra year of life or less. Further, another virtue of NICE is the use of citizen panels to review their initial recommendations from the perspective of social values such as justice and social beneficence.

We emphasize that the need for trade-offs is inescapable. However, NICE does not make any trade-offs. Each approval or rejection is isolated from every other approval or rejection. What NICE assumes is that the NHS would request additional funding for approved cancer drugs from the British government. However, that funding from the British government does not happen routinely. Consequently, real trade-offs need to occur at the local level of the Commissioning Groups, which are now faced with increased demands to be paid for by a flat budget. Further, these groups lack the expertise that NICE has available. Nor is there any effort to engage with broad democratic deliberative groups. Consequently, trade-offs occur in a somewhat haphazard way without much effort to explain or justify such trade-offs to those most directly affected. In brief, this is invisible rationing, which is essentially flawed as a matter of justice. Patients with a very specific cancer may have a just claim to a cancer drug that NICE has approved. However, nothing requires that that claim is honored if a local clinical practice lacks the funds to cover the drug costs. Moreover, the Cancer Drug Fund is irrelevant. That fund was created for individuals with a very short life expectancy needing a cancer drug that NICE had *not* approved. Consequently, if a cancer patient needed an approved drug for a couple of years, that would be a very large expense for a clinical group with a very fixed budget. That clinical group might not see the necessary trade-offs to fund that drug as being either reasonable or just, though in practice they would not explain that judgment to anyone. The net result would be inconsistency in the making of these judgments across the NHS. In other words, the formal equity promised by the NHS did not necessarily translate into equity in practice.

7.7. NICE Alternatives: Canada

NICE represents one approach to answering the question: What is enough? NICE has its limitations. Canada has the Agency for Drugs and Technologies, which would be the analogue of NICE. Within that agency is the pan-Canadian Oncology Drug Review program. That very specialized program exists because drug costs have been increasing at more than 10% per year (Peacock et al., 2019). Canada is much more committed to a citizen-based process of rational democratic deliberation, a process that sees the public "in the role of 'value consultants' in helping to define policy issues and advise on the social and normative aspects of scientific or technical issues" (Peacock et al., 2019, at 294).

In one of these deliberative events, participants recommended that there should be a re-review of already approved cancer drugs based upon "real-world" evidence of effectiveness and cost-effectiveness. They were aware of the highly selective nature of experimental trials in terms of participants and the idealized data that resulted. The deliberators concluded that if there were a very substantial deviation in real-world cost or cost-effectiveness of some cancer drug for some specific condition, then that drug should be withdrawn from publicly funded coverage.[11] That seems a reasonable conclusion. However, I would expect some pushback from physicians treating these patients.

The problem will be that each physician will have had a small number of these patients who will have gotten significant clinical benefit. They will understand intellectually that most of these patients will have gotten only a small benefit from that drug and that it is not cost-effective to continue providing that drug to all these patients. Still, if they have nothing else to offer these patients with a specific genetic mutation, they will want to protect the interests of that small number of patients who might well benefit significantly from that drug. They will take no comfort in being told about the money saved because those savings will not redound to the benefit of their cancer patients with this specific mutation. How does this happen? Can anything be done to correct this situation?

One recent report is perfectly illustrative of this allocation problem. One new drug, tiragolumab, was combined with atezolizumab, to treat patients with non-small cell lung cancer and high PD-L1 expression (Slater, 2021). As a result of only a Phase 2 clinical trial this combination was given "breakthrough therapy designation." That means this combination can be brought into the clinic. The basis for this designation was median progression-free survival: 5.4 months for patients who received the combination compared to 3.6 months for those who received atezolizumab alone. Each of these drugs costs $12,500 per month. In theory, a Phase 3 trial ought to be done to gain greater confidence that this very modest level of benefit is preserved. However, the drug is already "in the clinic," which would mean that if the results were even more marginal, it would make both ethical and economic sense to withdraw the drug, regardless of clinician objections. If a robust enough Phase 3 clinical trial were done, then it might be possible to identify a small cohort of patients before the fact who would gain substantial benefit without incurring all the costs of patients with very small benefit.[12] That would mean a delay in having this "breakthrough" combination available for

---

[11] I must mention that coverage of cancer drugs taken orally can vary from province to province. Cancer drugs provided in a hospital context (infusion) are paid for completely across the provinces. There are obvious inequities that result (Sorin et al., 2019).

[12] We will note that NICE did not approve atezolizumab for small cell lung cancer or non-small cell lung cancer, primarily because the benefit was too small (less than two months median gain in progression-free survival) compared to available chemotherapy regimens (Columbus, 2020).

at least two years, which in turn would mean the loss of marginal gains in life expectancy (assumed) for patients who would otherwise be candidates for that combination.

This brings us back to Canada. Both drugs are given by infusion. Costs would be paid for entirely in every province by the provincial governments. However, Canada has this more robust form of democratic deliberation. Their deliberators accepted the need for trade-offs and tough funding decisions. They also insisted on cost data and cost-effectiveness data that reflected the real world. Moreover, if a new drug cost twice as much as current drug therapy in the case of cancer, then Canadian deliberators wanted to see a gain in life expectancy with a reasonable quality of life of at least a year. For Canadian researchers (Bentley et al., 2019) the goal of the deliberative process is to produce advice for policymakers that is thoroughly informed and that "considers different social perspectives and reflects collective priorities rather than aggregating individual preferences or highlighting diverse stakeholder perspectives." In other words, the emphasis on "collective priorities" means that what is reported to policymakers are considered judgments regarding a specific allocation issue along with the reasons and reasoning that supported that judgment. Further, that reasoning will have considered a diversity of perspectives as a way of conveying the overall fairness and comprehensiveness of thought in the deliberative process, which is to say that what is being conveyed to policymakers is not some form of special pleading that represents the interests of cancer patients.

The deliberative process would have little added value for policymakers if it simply offered an array of perspectives, which they would likely already have from a diversity of special interest groups seeking to exert whatever political pressure was available to them. What the deliberative process must offer is an assessment of the relevant public values for any particular allocation from the perspective of public reason (to use Rawls' language, 1996), which is to say that those public values would be separated from any comprehensive doctrine. To illustrate this point, Canadian deliberators strongly endorsed a pan-Canadian policy regarding payment for cancer drugs, whether given by infusion or given orally. The province of Ontario did not automatically cover oral cancer drugs, requiring instead a somewhat complex appeal process with no guarantee of an affirmative response. What that meant for its residents is that if they wished to avoid financial catastrophe, they would have to purchase a private insurance policy that would cover those costs. Needless to say, those plans would likely not be available at all or at an affordable price for anyone with cancer or a family history of cancer. Consequently, the financially well off would be able to afford these oral cancer medications, but the less well off would likely have to deny themselves these drugs or impoverish their families.

If the drugs under discussion were only very marginally beneficial and very expensive, then this outcome would not be inequitable. On the other hand, if the drugs yield significant benefit in life prolongation, even if somewhat expensive, Ontario would need a compelling justification for failing to publicly fund these oral cancer drugs. Taxes would have to be raised to cover these costs, but that would be a less than compelling justification for refusing to fund these drugs publicly, given that other provinces were able to accomplish this. If Ontario is less wealthy than the western provinces, then perhaps the federal government needs to step in to equalize resources to eliminate what is otherwise a significant inequity among its citizens. I have to assume that Canada does not automatically finance all cancer drugs given by infusion, no matter their cost, no matter their marginal benefit. Consequently, I take it that Canadian deliberators who endorse a pan-Canada pharmaceutical policy would also endorse the idea of rejecting cancer drugs given by infusion that were excessively costly and only marginally beneficial for all Canadian provinces. To illustrate, the combination therapy of atezolizumab and tiragolumab for non-small cell lung cancer at $25,000 per month, with a median gain in progression-free survival of less than two months over atezolizumab alone, should be rejected across all the provinces. That these drugs are given by infusion would be ethically irrelevant. The resources thereby saved could be redirected to funding other cancer drugs for everyone with a specific cancer who could gain more health benefits at a lower cost.

As I see it, and as I think Canadian deliberators would see it, egalitarians, utilitarians, and prioritarians could readily endorse this last conclusion as being just and beneficent from their respective perspectives. These are judgments that are (or should be) of much greater value to policymakers, who might ultimately be responsible for making these trade-offs, than the self-serving messages delivered by various disease-related interest groups. The ultimate value of democratic deliberation, suitably informed by the relevant expertise and suitably conducted, is that it can deliver considered judgments to policymakers that are fair, reasonable, thoughtfully reasoned, and inclusive of the diversity of perspectives that must be heard. Ultimately, this is the best answer that can be given to the question "What is enough?" This will never be a perfect answer; the world of health care and the plurality of values that must govern it are too complex for any perfect answers. This is why we must accept "rough justice," "limited social beneficence," and "wicked uncertainty."

7.8. Two-Tiered or Not Two-Tiered? That Is the Problem

In concluding this chapter, I want to return to the most difficult challenges offered by precision medicine. I have in mind CAR T-cell immunotherapy and the use of multiple targeted therapies or immunotherapies sequentially or conjointly. My goal is to make clear why, with regard to these examples, the democratic deliberative process cannot get beyond rough justice, limited social beneficence, and wicked uncertainty.

Must these two broad therapeutic interventions be included in a basic benefit package guaranteed to all, either as a matter of health care justice or as a matter of obligatory social beneficence? In both cases we are talking about extremely expensive interventions. If, for example, either of these interventions cost $1 million but were needed to treat a few hundred people, this would be socially affordable. However, in the case of CAR T-cell therapies, their success has been limited to hematologic cancers. Still, 130,000 individuals will die each year in the United States of their hematologic cancers. With a front-end cost of at least $475,000 and a basic fairness requirement that a life-prolonging technology available to anyone with a hematologic cancer ought to be available to all with that cancer, this is not sustainably affordable. In addition, research is ongoing that would find ways to use CAR T-cell therapy (in novel variants) to treat solid organ metastatic cancers. If successful, it would not be socially affordable.

It would be politically illegitimate in a liberal society, of course, if we were to ban access to CAR T-cell therapy or comparable technologies for everyone because they could not be included in a health benefit package guaranteed to all. Private health insurance would be an option for individuals with the financial resources needed. This does create a two-tiered health care system, which some would regard as essentially unjust but that others would regard as being an instance of rough justice (Krohmal and Emanuel, 2007; Hunt, 2015). An outcome such as this will often be "just enough," so long as those in the basic, socially funded health care system are made no worse off and so long as the benefits of these very costly life-prolonging technologies are very marginal at best, that is, extra months of life at a cost judged by our democratic deliberators to be unreasonable, given other health needs that had to be met with the limited resources available. However, this last qualification is what generates some wicked uncertainty.[13]

CAR T-cell therapies are now generating a few extra years of life for at least 40% of the patients who have been fortunate enough to have access to the technology. Roughly 30% of these patients will fail to gain an extra year of life. I am part of a research project in Norway (Blanchard and Strand, 2017) seeking various sorts of biomarkers that were either prognostic or predictive, in part so that limited costly resources could be distributed more justly and so that the medical harms associated with many of these technologies, such as cytokine release syndrome, would not be visited upon patients whose gains in life expectancy would be very marginal. I believe our democratic deliberators would be ethically comfortable with denying access to CAR T-cell therapy for those patients for whom a 90% reliable biomarker predicted they would fail to gain a year from the therapy. However, we do not now have such biomarkers. This is wickedly problematic.

I doubt that our democratic deliberators would quickly endorse the idea of relegating CAR T-cell therapy to second-tier, privately funded health care primarily because a significant number of these patients would gain extra years of life. In other words, if this became a second-tier funded technology, the financially well off could afford to purchase this insurance, which would likely be very expensive because numerous costly, marginally beneficial technologies would be included in that tier along with some very expensive technologies that yielded substantial medical benefit. Both egalitarians and prioritarians would be very ill at ease with this idea; it just seems unfair to those who are financially less well off. The benefit is not trivial or marginal. The same problem is emerging with regard to the targeted cancer therapies used sequentially and conjointly. If these therapies are used singly, they only yield marginal benefits due to the resistance problem. However, as with CAR T-cell therapy, using these drugs in combination or sequentially has yielded for many patients several extra years of life. This is still not curative, and less than a majority of patients with any specific cancer will gain those extra years of life. Still, given the number of patients benefited and the magnitude of the

[13] CAR T-cell therapy as well as the use of multiple targeted therapies sequentially can be included in the benefit package guaranteed to all, but with *clinical restrictions related to the likelihood of sufficient effectiveness, given the clinical circumstances of certain types of patients.* This would require the use of biomarkers with sufficient predictive reliability of effectiveness that these interventions could be justly provided or denied to patients.

benefit, we should not allocate these therapies to second-tier status where only the relatively wealthy would benefit.

What complicates this situation with wicked uncertainty is that at least half of metastatic cancer patients at present do not have one of these complicated therapeutic options available to them, though paying increased taxes for the more fortunate other half. They might be tempted to relegate these combination therapies to the second tier, though that would be imprudent, given the likely success of future research. However, such success would add to the wicked uncertainty of what would be the most ethically appropriate response, given increasing numbers of metastatic cancer patients who would benefit (i.e., 500,000 instead of 300,000). The cost could be anywhere from $100,000 to $200,000 per life-year saved. This is less than the front-end cost of CAR T-cell therapy, but the cost per patient could exceed that CAR T-cell therapy cost if these medical advances yielded multiple years of life with very high costs for each year of life saved.

This last possibility is most clearly illustrated with our CLL example in Chapter 6 that involved ibrutinib, CAR T-cell therapy, potential stem cell transplants, obinutuzumab, umbralisib, and ublituximab. The ethical challenge here is twofold. Egalitarians and prioritarians would ethically object to denying access to these combination therapies that are quite effective for a substantial number of patients by placing access to these therapies in that second tier. On the other hand, at the aggregated social level, insisting that all these metastatic cancer therapies be included in the basic benefit package guaranteed to everyone would involve a disproportionate share of health care dollars flowing into cancer care. This too should raise concerns regarding health care justice and obligatory social beneficence among egalitarians and prioritarians since their concerns must extend beyond the health care needs of metastatic cancer patients.

Here is another perplexing example. A new option is available for HIV⁺ patients who were on three-drug or four-drug options to manage their HIV (Mandavilli, 2021). Instead of taking these drugs on a daily basis and doing this somewhat religiously to prevent mutated strains of HIV from emerging, they could get a monthly injection of Cabenuva˚, a combination of cabotegravir and rilpivirine. From a patient perspective, this is enormously easier than managing the drug combinations and their various requirements. However, the annual cost of these injections is $48,000, compared to the $20,000–$35,000 annual costs associated with the prescription medications. Does this belong in the second tier of private health insurance for funding?

Or is this something that ought to be part of the socially funded benefit package guaranteed to all?

To be clear, the injections are not *intrinsically* more effective in managing HIV than the prescription medications. In practice, they are more therapeutically effective because they correct for various human deficiencies associated with missing doses, etc. Does that provide sufficient justification for including Cabenuva in the socially financed benefit package? Approximately one million Americans are living with HIV. If the average cost of their current therapy is $25,000 per year, then offering them Cabenuva instead would double the social costs per year from $25 billion to $48 billion. How should our democratic deliberators respond? Should they endorse a policy of permitting individuals who were poor compliers with HIV drugs to switch to Cabenuva at social expense? Would it be too easy for HIV+ individuals to present themselves as poor compliers so that they could manage their disease more conveniently? This is another wickedly difficult challenge. Clearly, no private insurance would underwrite the cost of Cabenuva for individuals who sought such insurance after becoming HIV-infected.

What are the moral risks associated with having a two-tiered health care system? A two-tiered system is unavoidable in a liberal society, given too many marginally beneficial costly interventions. Consequently, the real ethical challenge is to identify a very limited range of health care interventions for that second tier that do not corrupt the societal commitment to health care justice and social beneficence. This is a matter for democratic deliberation.

How should our basic package of health care benefits be financed? Should that be through a progressive income tax with no financial barriers to accessing health care judged to be medically necessary by a physician (i.e., no co-pays, no deductibles, no coinsurance)? How comprehensive a benefit package would those in the lower half of the income spectrum want under those circumstances? Keep in mind that these individuals would be paying through taxes far less of their income for this benefit package than individuals in the top quintile of the income spectrum, *but they would be paying something that would be a significant enough portion of their income.*

Menzel (1983, chap. 4) has raised the question with regard to the Medicaid benefit package of whether the poor might regard that package as being "too generous." Might the poor prefer other welfare benefits? If so, must a liberal society respect their autonomous choice? Menzel asks, why impose some of these benefits on the poor if the poor themselves do not value the benefit in the way the middle class might value that benefit? Are we being too paternalistic? Should we ask a similar question? Is the comprehensive benefit package I have in mind too comprehensive for those who are financially less well off?

We might be tempted to say, "How could the relatively poor refuse this very generous benefit package when they are getting it for free?" However, that is a mistake. The package is not free to them. They are paying from their income some portion of the cost of that package. Consequently, if our democratic deliberators agree that CAR T-cell therapy ought to be available within that comprehensive package for both hematologic cancers as well as solid organ cancers, that will add substantially to the overall cost of that package. The same will be true if we add coverage for all of the very expensive therapies used to treat CLL. That additional cost will also have to include all of the other targeted therapies and immunotherapies that are out there (and that *will be* out there) that yield a net benefit for enough patients. That might add 1% to the tax burden of the working poor in the fourth quintile and a fraction of 1% to the income of those in the bottom quintile. For these individuals, that takes away a portion of their personal purchasing power, which they would prefer to allocate to something they value more than these (to them) exotic therapies.

Next, consider the top quintile of the income spectrum. Recall that they are paying a much greater portion of their income to support this comprehensive health plan guaranteed to all. They might resent subsidizing access to needed health care for those who are financially less well off. They would contend that they are not getting value for their money. As beneficent individuals, they would agree that they should pay for the *basic* health care needs of the financially less well off. However, that should be for a much less comprehensive benefit package. More specifically, they would want all of these elegant, targeted cancer therapies and immunotherapies shifted to this second tier, along with the artificial hearts and other such very costly interventions. They would have to purchase private health insurance that would be costly but less costly than their taxes through a progressive tax system. Should a just and caring society allow this to happen, given the perspectives I have outlined from both ends of the income spectrum?

Our democratic deliberators ought to consider both of these perspectives in determining what the content of the benefit package assured to everyone should be. However, the middle-income perspective must be considered. Those are individuals who, if the basic benefit package were stripped of all the costly but effective cancer therapies, would find it impossible to afford the cost of a second-tier insurance policy. These individuals would clearly be less well off in such a system, compared to a system that offered a more comprehensive benefit package. I would not describe that situation as representing "rough justice." It would be unjust. I would invoke a Rawlsian perspective to justify this claim. Society is this broad system of social cooperation in which we agree to share fairly the benefits and burdens of that cooperation. Everyone will have paid through the tax system for the basic science research that has made possible this enormous wealth of medical innovation. However, the real beneficiaries of that investment will be those individuals in the upper quintiles of the income spectrum who can afford to purchase that insurance that will give them access to therapies available only through that second tier. That hardly represents a "fair share" of the product of those complex forms of social cooperation that have yielded the health care system we have today.

Some might argue that the second tier could include a variety of insurance products with different degrees of affordability (i.e., $5,000 front-end deductibles or 30% co-pays). This would essentially duplicate the current US health insurance market, which is neither just nor beneficent, given its tight connection to ability to pay, as opposed to the urgency and severity of the need and the effectiveness of the available therapy. Nothing would justify reproducing that as a "reform" of our health care system. What then are the alternatives?

Our democratic deliberators would be faced with two challenges. First, they have to identify a comprehensive set of health care benefits that are judged to be matters of obligatory social beneficence. Second, that benefit package must be affordable through the tax system. In particular, deliberators must be mindful of the financial burden for those less well off. Without getting too mathematical, the answer to this latter challenge would be having a progressive tax system that roughly generated an *equally felt* tax burden for each income class with respect to the cost of the health care benefit package. To illustrate, 1% for someone earning $20,000 per year might be "equally burdensome" to 4% for someone earning $100,000 per year.

In fairness to those who are financially less well off, who may have serious doubts about the costworthiness of either CAR T-cell therapy or the sequential use of these very expensive targeted therapies, two things ought to be done. First, access to all of the life-prolonging technologies for patients faced with a terminal prognosis ought to be limited by reliable medical criteria that can predict likely effectiveness for patients in specific clinical circumstances.

Constraining the overall use of these technologies would reduce overall social costs and corresponding tax burden. That might be sufficient to assure access to these technologies for the financially less well off who would derive substantial clinical benefit. Second, some of these individuals may still not see access to such technologies as being "worth it" from their point of view, even as they vividly imagine themselves or their loved ones faced with a terminal illness. We could reduce their tax burden corresponding to the value of these technologies in exchange for their forgoing access to these technologies should they have that need. This respects the autonomy of all; it is roughly just and socially beneficent; it minimizes wicked uncertainty, whether moral or clinical. In effect, this creates some moral and political space below that second tier. This is sufficient.

8

Precision Medicine, Precision Health

Finding Just and Reasonable Trade-offs

It is easy to see "precision medicine" and "precision health" complementing one another. We want precision medicine available to us when we are unfortunate enough to be faced with a life-threatening cancer that could be cured or managed with a targeted cancer therapy. At the same time, we would rationally prefer to take advantage of whatever medicine might offer us that would prevent the emergence of that cancer in the first place or treat it in its earliest stages, which is the goal of precision health. However, precision medicine and precision health can just as easily and realistically be seen as competing for resources with one another. The technology that will create some justice-relevant conflicts is that of the "liquid biopsy," a non-invasive way of identifying circulating tumor cells in the blood, often at the earliest stages in the evolution of cancer (Alix-Panabieres, 2020; Shohdy and West, 2020; Serrano et al., 2020). The obvious utility of liquid biopsies (if they had near perfect sensitivity and specificity) would be to treat a cancer so early that a cure would be achieved, and a premature death would be averted. The additional implication is that the economic and ethical costs associated with using targeted therapies and immunotherapies would be avoided as well. However, the proposed uses of these liquid biopsies are very likely to generate their own wicked ethical and economic challenges.

8.1. Just Caring: Cancer, Targeted Therapies, and Cost Control

These targeted therapies have strained social budgets in both the United States and the European Union (Vokinger et al., 2020; Wilking et al., 2017; Hofmarcher et al., 2020; Peppercorn, 2017; Yabroff et al., 2019; Leopold et al., 2018).[1] Relieving that strain means controlling health care costs by

---

[1] The primary messages from these articles would be the following: (1) The very high prices of these drugs do not reflect the very marginal clinical value produced in most cases; (2) the projected

controlling need for and access to these very expensive life-prolonging technologies.[2] Prevention is aimed at reducing need (and cost).

Prevention is supposed to be quite inexpensive: Do not smoke, consume alcohol in moderation, use sunscreen, get a reasonable amount of exercise, eat a healthy diet. However, in spite of adhering with saintly devotion to these health directives, some individuals will still find themselves faced with a cancer diagnosis. This could be for genetic reasons or for environmental reasons or just the random breakdown of cellular machinery. Roughly 40% of Americans will develop a cancer over the course of their life. The projections in the United States for 2022 are that 1.9 million individuals will be diagnosed with cancer; cancer deaths will be 610,000 (National Cancer Institute: Surveillance, Epidemiology, and End Results Program, 2020). Projections to 2050 put the annual incidence of cancer in the United States at 2.3 million cases. Comparable figures for Europe are 3.9 million cancer diagnoses in 2018 and 1.9 million deaths (Ferlay et al., 2018). These statistics tell us the magnitude of the problems we face, medical, economic, and ethical. Projections to 2040 for the EU expect a 21% increase in cancer cases and deaths.

8.2. Cancer: Finding the First Cell/Preventing Future Cells

If cancer cannot be completely prevented by good health behavior and if metastatic disease is essentially incurable, then the next best preventive strategy would be to identify and attack cancer at its earliest possible stages. This is the perspective embraced by Dr. Azra Raza in her recent book *The First Cell* (2019). Raza is an oncologist who has been in practice for more than 30 years. Her cancer research has been focused on myelodysplastic syndromes (MDS), a pre-leukemic condition. Her husband's research was in the same area, though, ironically, he died of acute myelogenous leukemia, which happens in about 33% of patients with MDS. The basic thesis of her

---

aggregated social costs of these targeted therapies are not sustainable; (3) if nothing is done to control these escalating prices and costs, both social equity and solidarity will be unjustly compromised.

[2] Price controls represent another option. That is another book. However, even if the price of these targeted therapies and immunotherapies were reduced by 50%, the justice issues would remain.

book is that we are wasting tens of billions of dollars every year on cancer therapies that are extraordinarily costly and that yield only marginal gains in life expectancy and maximal increases in suffering (physiological, psychological, financial, and social). She believes that these same resources should be redirected to destroying cancer in its earliest stages, those "first cells." On one level, this is an eminently reasonable position. On another level, this is an ethically radical proposal, given that she wishes to redirect tens of billions of dollars from aggressive life-prolonging care to a preventive strategy that would reduce the need for such aggressive life-prolonging care. This generates our key questions: Is this strategy ultimately ethically defensible? Is this a strategy that ought to be embraced by a "just and caring" society, given that the consequence of embracing such a strategy would be the "premature" death of hundreds of thousands of metastatic cancer patients each year, most of whom would be denied extra months of life?

Do these questions represent a false choice? We should be doing whatever is possible to prevent cancer or to attack it in its earliest stages, but if those efforts fail, then we certainly ought to pursue therapeutic life-prolonging options for those unfortunate patients who are faced with metastatic disease, even if those efforts might never be curative. Why would Raza not endorse that view? Here is one scenario Raza has in mind. She suggests that "everyone from birth to death is regularly screened for the first appearance of cancer cells in the body." Once those cancer cells had been identified, "protein markers would be identified, providing a zip code for the cancer cells. A tube of blood from the individuals would be obtained, and T cells would be isolated, activated, and armed with the address for the cancer based upon the unique protein bar code and the RNA signature it expressed" (Raza, 2019, at 238). This scenario has something of a futuristic quality to it. However, what we do have in reality is a new "liquid biopsy" test introduced by a company named GRAIL (Oxnard, 2019). The original test could detect 20 different cancers in their earliest stages by examining cell-free DNA in the blood. More recent news reports suggest that the upgraded test is capable of detecting 50 different cancers as well as the source of that cancer in 89% of cases. This is not a perfect test. Dana-Farber reports that the test has a sensitivity of 32% for a Stage I cancer, 76% for Stage II, 85% for Stage III, and 93% for Stage IV (Oxnard, 2019). The test became available for clinical deployment in late 2021. News reports a give the price at $950. Recall in the quotation how Raza imagined that individuals would be "regularly screened" with such a test. What might that mean?

Though cancer is much more of a threat to older individuals, a significant number of young adults are diagnosed with a cancer, and some will die from that cancer. Approximately 10% of individuals between age 21 and age 49 in the United States will be given a cancer diagnosis. Given that everyone has a 40% lifetime risk of a cancer diagnosis, annual screening would not be unreasonable. To save money, should we limit annual access to these screening liquid biopsy tests to those with a family history of cancer? However, only 5% to 10% of cancers are hereditary. The other 90%+ arise spontaneously, sometimes for behavioral or environmental reasons (smoking, failure to use sunscreen), at other times for reasons entirely unknown. This is reason enough for many adults to have concerns about their vulnerability to cancer. If the test is only offered to adults over age 21, that would be 200 million individuals in the United States. At a cost of $950 per test, the potential cost to "society" would be $190 billion per year.[3] That figure brings into sharp focus Raza's imperative that funding this preventive effort ought to come from what she regards as wasteful and marginally effective spending on these targeted cancer therapies for metastatic disease. This raises multiple ethics issues.

Raza deserves to be ethically commended for requiring that this preventive effort come from *within* current cancer spending, as opposed to taking that money from heart disease or resources dedicated to treating addictions or mental illness or some other disease category. Her basic argument is that most of the targeted cancer therapies represent low-value care. Clearly, it would be unjust to take resources from high-value health care to purchase in its place low-value cancer care. Let's focus on ethics issues related to Raza's proposal.

Start with some additional background. The test that GRAIL introduced in 2021 is named "Galleri." This test can accurately detect 50 different cancers by assessing circulating DNA that has its origins in cancer cells that have been shed by a tumor into the bloodstream. Researchers at GRAIL point out that 45 of those 50 cancers lack recommended screening tests today. That means that in those 45 cases the cancer is first diagnosed with the presentation of symptoms, which, in some cases, will mean the cancer is well established and more difficult to treat. In the case of pancreatic cancer, symptoms

---

[3] The population of the European Union (still counting the United Kingdom, just for sentimental reasons) is about 520 million, of which 334 million would be adults over age 21. For that population the hypothetical cost of annual testing with the GRAIL liquid biopsy would be $310 billion per year.

will typically not occur until the cancer is Stage IV (terminal in less than a year). Avoiding that outcome represents both an ethical and a medical good. An obvious benefit of this intervention is that it is a non-invasive "liquid" biopsy, as opposed to the normal invasive biopsy. It is a relatively simple blood test. An invasive biopsy will always carry risks. A liquid biopsy will be less expensive than an invasive biopsy. A liquid biopsy will provide useful medical information about a cancer without the dangers of an invasive biopsy, as in the brain. Further, results are available in days from a liquid biopsy, as opposed to two weeks. What might be most medically and ethically important is that representatives of GRAIL claim that use of Galleri will reduce cancer deaths in the future by about 100,000 per year (Taylor, 2020).

One of the more interesting responses to the use of liquid biopsies came from an oncologist in Boston, Dr. Ryan Corcoran. He said, "There was a mutation known to cause resistance to that drug, which wasn't present in the tissue biopsy but was fairly abundant in the blood sample. If we had just biopsied a different lesion, we might've picked an entirely different therapy" (Eisenstein, 2020). Recall Chapter 1. We noted there that metastatic cancer is genetically heterogeneous, both within a single tumor and across multiple tumors in a single patient. This is why Dr. Corcoran said that a tissue biopsy from a single spot in a single tumor may yield information that would cause an oncologist to choose the wrong targeted therapy with a result of either no benefit or actual harm. The liquid biopsy can yield a more complete picture of the complexity of the cancer for purposes of guiding therapy. Corcoran observes, "In 78% of the people tested, circulating tumor DNA revealed mutations associated with drug resistance that were absent from tissue biopsies" (Eisenstein, 2020, at S7). Part of the reason Corcoran sees the GRAIL test as being so useful is that it not only sequences the DNA of the tumor but also captures patterns of DNA modification called "methylation," which strongly affects gene expression. This is essentially a screening tool. However, Galleri has therapeutic potential when a resistance process has begun. It would be used to monitor either the effects of therapy or the specifics of disease progression. In the latter case, a different drug could be introduced in a timelier fashion in the hope of sustaining a therapeutic response by preventing the tumor burden from becoming excessive or incurable (Alix-Panabieres, 2020).

Having presented this very positive picture of Galleri, some caveats are in order. One researcher commented that circulating DNA may contain many mutations, some of which are clearly related to the emergence or progression of a cancer, others of which are ambiguous regarding their relevance. Another researcher again called attention to the heterogeneity of cancer but drew a very different conclusion. He concluded that because of the heterogeneity of cancer, a liquid biopsy might miss some of the complexity and that, therefore, it was necessary to do an invasive biopsy as well (Levenson, 2020).

8.3. Trading off Identified Lives and Statistical Lives: Ethical Issues

Perhaps the most salient ethical concern would pertain to the implied trade-off between the *identified* lives of patients with metastatic cancer and the *statistical* lives that we would hope to save through annual preventive liquid biopsies. The defining feature of statistical lives is that they are nameless and faceless. This is typically true both before the fact and after the fact when considering preventive measures. If we install guardrails at dangerous curves on state highways, we might save 50 lives per year. One year later we might see a decline in fatal slides off the highway of 45 lives. We would have no idea who those 45 individuals might have been whose lives were saved or if the guardrails were necessarily what made that difference. By way of contrast, we know with perfect clarity the identities of individuals with metastatic cancer whose lives were extended (if only for months) as a consequence of their having received one of these targeted cancer therapies. GRAIL's liquid biopsy may correctly identify individuals with a very early-stage cancer (no clinically evident symptoms). That cancer may eventually manifest itself symptomatically, at which point it will most likely be effectively treated (minimal likelihood of recurrence). This is why we currently have 17 million cancer survivors in the United States today (Simon, 2019). Projections put that survival figure at 21.7 million by 2029. This projection would not include any assumption about the successful clinical deployment of GRAIL's liquid biopsy.

We need to emphasize that the vast majority of these cancer survivors will ultimately die of something other than their cancer. Why does this matter? It matters because GRAIL cannot claim that its liquid biopsy would have saved all these lives. Most of these lives would have been saved by current cancer therapies provided at the appearance of clinical symptoms. This point is important for judging whether GRAIL's liquid biopsy represents high-value care. If GRAIL's liquid biopsy reduced the number of metastatic cancer deaths by 70%, that would constitute significant evidence for thinking of the test as representing high-value care. However, that will still leave us with both ethical and economic concerns.

Keep in mind that we are assessing Raza's proposal (as I have constructed it). The hypothetical I am proposing says that we would reduce the number of metastatic cancer deaths in the United States by 400,000 annually.[4] That would still leave 200,000 individuals with a terminal metastatic condition. Dr. Raza would provide those individuals with comfort care, but they would be denied these extraordinarily expensive targeted cancer therapies. These are clearly *identified* individuals who might desperately wish to gain whatever additional life these targeted therapies promised.[5] We are trading off for their sacrifice of that additional life indefinite gains in life expectancy for these 400,000 other individuals who also would otherwise have died prematurely from their metastatic disease. From a purely rational, utilitarian maximization perspective, this looks like an eminently reasonable trade-off. However, those 400,000 individuals are *statistical* lives.

It may sound odd to say that these are statistical lives, but we cannot identify who those 400,000 individuals might be. Consequently, they have something of an abstract, ghostly status. This is certainly true from a psychological perspective, compared to those patients with metastatic cancer who want to live longer. To clarify, 1.8 million individuals in the United States are diagnosed with cancer each year. Some of them are diagnosed with metastatic disease. However, the vast majority of those cancer diagnoses will be treated with current therapies. Some portion of those individuals, despite treatment with curative intent, will go on to have metastatic disease. Most of those metastatic cases will not be predictable at the time of initial treatment, even though that treatment was timely. Others might have gone on to have metastatic disease, except that they were treated early and effectively. At this point in time these are all statistical lives. Eventually, however, in this hypothetical example we end up with 200,000 identifiable individuals with metastatic disease. Is it just and justified that we would deny these individuals our very expensive targeted therapies, as proposed by Raza, because that $190 billion was allocated to the preventive effort which (by hypothesis) saved 400,000 lives that otherwise would have died prematurely? How much ethical weight

---

[4] This is a generous hypothetical example that likely takes us into a somewhat distant future (more than 10 years). A more realistic number is that we might be able to save 100,000 lives per year with liquid biopsy technology closer to clinical implementation, along with related support technology.

[5] Of course, it is worth recalling that some of these individuals would have been significant responders (losing two years of life) and that others might have been super-responders (losing several years of life).

ought to be attached to statistical lives versus identifiable lives when we are allocating resources for purposes of saving/prolonging lives?

Should identifiable lives (patients with metastatic cancer) have more moral weight (greater just claims to health care resources) than statistical lives (patients at risk of a premature death from cancer)? Brock (2015) would answer this question negatively.[6] He considers and rejects a number of arguments in support of the opposite conclusion. He first calls attention to the rule of rescue. The rule of rescue might seem to require prolonging the lives of the identifiable metastatic cancer patients, in part because we have at hand the capacity to do so readily with these targeted cancer therapies. By way of contrast, 99% of the liquid biopsies performed annually would have saved no one since the results would be negative for any cancer cells. However, the typical application of the rule of rescue involves huge societal expense to rescue trapped miners deep underground (or others in various dire circumstances, such as the cave rescue in Thailand [see Cheung and Wong, 2018]). It would be tragic if we (society) were aware of these situations but could not prevent that loss of life. However, it would be unconscionable if we had the ability to intervene but simply ignored the plight of those desperate individuals and allowed them to die. This is the moral logic that says we must do what we can to prolong the lives of those metastatic cancer patients. Notice that I did correctly describe this latter situation by saying that our goal would be to *prolong*, not *save*, the lives of these patients. In the typical successful rescue situation individuals have their lives saved; they have an indefinite life expectancy. That is precisely what is not true with regard to our metastatic cancer patients. Consequently, the moral logic embedded in the rule of rescue does not apply in this situation.

A second objection addressed by Brock concerns the uncertainty associated with preventive efforts.[7] We might invest $100 million in an anti-smoking campaign, hoping to save 100,000 lives from lung cancer. The campaign might fail abysmally because smoking is addictive and woven in complex ways into the lives of individuals. Lots of uncertainty seems integral to many preventive efforts. By way of contrast, we are certain to get some benefit in the form of additional life when we provide various targeted therapies

---

[6] See also Paul Menzel (2012). He will defend a position similar to Brock's view. Menzel writes, "If any of us loses our life from lack of adequate prevention, surely, it seems, we lose something *just as valuable* as we do if we lose our life from lack of effective treatment" (at 194). This too seems to support Raza's view.

[7] To be clear, Brock's ultimate conclusion is that identified lives are not intrinsically more ethically valuable (and worthy of costly life-prolonging resources) than statistical lives.

to individuals with metastatic lung cancer. However, making an analogy with an anti-smoking campaign would be misleading. By hypothesis, we are certain that 400,000 lives will be saved from a cancer death through reliance on annual screening with this liquid biopsy. We are uncertain which particular lives will have been saved, but those statistical lives are not *merely* statistical lives. Those are real lives (Menzel, 2012) that should have substantial moral weight in allocating life-saving resources, as Raza would insist. In addition, very few lives are *saved* by these targeted therapies among metastatic cancer patients. Only a marginal gain in life expectancy is achieved compared to the 400,000 lives correctly described as being saved in our hypothetical example.

A third ethically relevant consideration that comes into play is *urgency of need*. Metastatic cancer patients who have failed several therapeutic regimens surely have an urgent need for one of these targeted cancer therapies since they have exhausted all other therapeutic possibilities. In contrast, those individuals who would be discovered to have a relatively early-stage cancer through the liquid biopsy would have a substantially less urgent need because they would have many other options for treating their cancer. The conclusion we are supposed to accept, contrary to Raza, is that these metastatic cancer patients have a stronger just claim to costly targeted therapies than the statistically possible metastatic cancer patients have a claim to an annual liquid biopsy.

Daniels (2015) offers a supporting argument to this last conclusion. He refers to this as the "concentration of risk" argument. He asks us to imagine Alice, who has a life-threatening infectious disease certain to kill her unless she receives five life-saving tablets of some drug. Five other women have been exposed to Alice. There are only these five tablets. If each of these women receives one preventive tablet, their lives are certain to be saved. If all the tablets are given to Alice, then one of these five women will end up dying as a result of the exposure. It appears we have one death either way. Should we just flip a coin? Daniels opposes that idea and asserts that 100% of the risk of death is concentrated in Alice, whereas only a 20% risk of death is associated with each of the five women. Therefore, Alice has the strongest just claim to the five tablets. Again, there is a disanalogy between the Alice example and our 200,000 metastatic cancer patients.

Alice has her life saved, but our 200,000 metastatic cancer patients are still doomed to die (with few exceptions) in a relatively brief period of time. We might be tempted to call attention to that small cadre of super-responders among those 200,000 metastatic patients. Those individuals can be correctly regarded as being Alice-like; their lives will be saved. However, returning to Raza's main point, if saving the Alice-like super-responders required reallocating that $190 billion to these targeted cancer therapies for metastatic cancer patients, then we would be sacrificing the 400,000 Alice-like lives that (by hypothesis) would be saved by investing in population-wide screening with our liquid biopsy for the sake of that small cadre of super-responders. Those may well be statistical lives, but they are not *merely* statistical lives. They have as much moral worth as the lives of any of those metastatic cancer patients.

Brock next calls our attention to the "aggregation" problem as the basis for (in our case) preferring to allocate resources to the metastatic cancer patients as opposed to screening with the liquid biopsy for preventive purposes. In brief, the aggregation problem involves giving very high priority to a small number of patients who will derive very substantial benefits over a very large number of other patients who will only receive a small benefit with some limited budget. For example, we can spend $5 million to save 10 patients by implanting in each of them an artificial heart (without which they would all have died in six months), or we can use that same money to stabilize 10,000 sprained ankles. We will stipulate that treating the sprained ankles will yield many times the health benefits (by whatever measure) than saving the lives of those 10 patients needing the artificial heart. Still, our fundamental moral intuition would be that such a trade-off would be unconscionable. Once again, however, it can be argued that there is a disanalogy here. It is a relatively small benefit that accrues to our metastatic cancer patients and an enormously greater benefit that would be denied to those 400,000 individuals whose cancer will go undetected without the liquid biopsy and result in their premature deaths. We may not know the identity of those individuals, either before the fact or after the fact. Nevertheless, that fact does not alter the moral equation.

Finally, there is the argument that the "medically least well off" ought to have priority for limited life-prolonging resources over those who are relatively healthy but at risk for serious illness. When stated in this very abstract form, this argument would strike many as being eminently reasonable. However, specification regarding patients who are among the medically least well off will yield results that are far from being either fair or reasonable. The assumption must be that the medically least well off have some capacity for significant benefit if society makes available the necessary resources. Patients in a persistent vegetative state or in the late stages of dementia are clearly among the medically least well off. Just as clearly, they are incapable of significant benefit beyond bare life maintenance at costs in excess of $100,000 per year. Daniels (1985) has argued that what health care justice requires is protecting fair access for all to the normal opportunity range of a society. These are patients who are entirely outside that opportunity range. They have no capacity to participate in life.

Our metastatic cancer patients are also rightly thought to be among the medically least well off. Most would still have some access to the opportunity range of a society, though that access will be limited. They are not like patients with very advanced dementia. In most cases they will have had access to multiple cancer therapies that had already provided them with extra years of life. In that respect they have not been unjustly ignored. Their just claims to needed health care have been met. If these targeted cancer therapies yielded, say, five extra years of life on average at a cost of $150,000 per life-year gained, we would have a much more difficult problem in determining whether that $190 billion should not be spent on them or should be spent instead on cancer screening with the liquid biopsy. However, given the factual scenario that is current cancer care, as Raza would attest, the benefits for the vast majority of these patients are marginal. If we were to forbid allocating that $190 billion to liquid biopsy screening, we would be sustaining an annual population of 600,000 or more individuals with metastatic cancer who would be for that last year of life among the medically least well off, instead of reducing that population to 200,000 per year by using the liquid biopsy screening technology. On the face of it, that outcome would not be either reasonable or just, whether we were egalitarians or utilitarians or prioritarians in our understanding of health care justice.

8.4. Can We Just Abandon Metastatic Cancer Patients to Save Money?

I have presented the most compelling arguments in support of Raza's position. However, ethically problematic features of her position remain. It still feels ethically awkward to deny social funding for targeted cancer therapies or immunotherapies for 200,000 (hypothetical) metastatic cancer patients who did not benefit from our annual liquid biopsy screening protocol. Though I have emphasized marginal gains in life expectancy along with a small cadre of super-responders who would gain multiple extra years

of life, that is ultimately an inaccurate characterization. There will be a continuum of gains in life expectancy. The most unfortunate patients will gain
nothing; others will gain a few months or a year or maybe two years. This
makes it harder to endorse with ethical equanimity redistributing all our
life-prolonging cancer resources to the preventive liquid biopsy strategy.
A simple solution would be to just pour more money into cancer treatment.
However, that means failing to take seriously the "just caring" problem. In
addition, no arguments would justify spending unlimited sums of money
to meet the needs of cancer patients, as opposed to patients with any of a
number of other life-threatening medical conditions.

Cancer is not ethically special. Raza is clearly correct. We currently spend
vast sums of money on low-value care for metastatic cancer patients. The
problem is that we only know after the fact that what we provided was low-
value care. Does our liquid biopsy strategy also represent low-value care?
This might sound odd since the scenario I sketched suggested that 400,000
lives annually would be spared by such a strategy from progressing to a terminal metastatic disease state. Recall that this was an arbitrary number, not
based upon any empirical evidence at all. The objective was simply to establish an initial framework for ethical analysis.

My critic will point out that if we are doing 200 million liquid biopsies each
year, more than 99% of them will be negative at a cost of $190 billion. That
sounds like low-value care. In addition, it is far from clear that simply calling
attention to the 400,000 lives annually spared from a premature cancer death
because of this preventive effort would sufficiently justify this massive expenditure of resources.[8] Should we be far more selective in the population
screened with our liquid biopsy strategy? Here are some possible options: (1)
Screen only those individuals and first-degree family members where there
has been a family history of cancer. (2) Add to (1) individuals with established behaviors likely to result in increased risk for various cancers, such
as smokers or individuals with significant sun exposure. Roughly 40% of all
cancers are attributed to behavioral choices by individuals (Mendes, 2017).
(3) Add to (1) and (2) individuals who have been diagnosed with a cancer and
successfully treated (likely at increased risk of cancer recurrence). (4) Add to
(1), (2), and (3) individuals who have compromised immune systems that

[8] Louise Russell has critically assessed the widespread belief that preventive care always saves
money. She has argued that, in many circumstances, prevention is just not cost-effective. She would
likely conclude that with regard to our annual liquid biopsy screening proposal. See her book *Is
Prevention Better Than Cure?* (2010).

might increase their risk of cancer. (5) Add to all the previous categories individuals above the age of 50, the assumption being that cancer is most often a disease for which older individuals are at risk. Note: In all these cases we are assuming that the cost of this testing would be a social expense. Individuals outside these categories would be free to obtain this testing at their own personal expense.

Trying to identify categories of individuals who would have the most reasonable and strongest just claims to this annual liquid biopsy screening would likely have a strong arbitrary component. Maybe the need to draw these lines could be avoided if we could show that our initial proposal made economic sense. If we are saving 400,000 lives from a premature death from metastatic cancer each year, then we are also saving the cost of treating those metastatic cancers. That cost might be $100,000 per metastatic cancer patient saved. If so, that savings would amount to $40 billion. That would still leave $150 billion in screening costs each year for which there were no offsetting economic gains.

Though ethicists would likely not endorse this next point, economists would note that those 400,000 individuals are still going to die, and not cheaply, likely from other chronic degenerative conditions with multiple years of high health costs. A substantial number will develop dementia and require at least a couple of years of long-term care at $100,000 per year. Consequently, if our concern with controlling health care costs is about *all* health care costs, then the bottom-line savings would be substantially less than $40 billion. For the sake of argument, let us say that the net savings would be $20 billion.[9]

Someone might then argue that that $20 billion in savings ought to be used to provide $100,000 worth of targeted cancer treatments for the 200,000 individuals each year who would still end up with metastatic cancer. However, our erstwhile economist will again call our attention to an awkward economic fact, namely, that the savings we would expect to achieve by not having to pay for targeted cancer therapy for 400,000 individuals will only be realized more than two decades into the future. The costs of doing the screening will all be incurred in the present and represent additions to current health care costs. The assumption behind this conclusion is that it

---

[9] To be clear, few moral philosophers would endorse the idea of denying a patient life-saving care today because we were confident that they would incur very substantial health care costs in the future. Those future health care needs and related costs are entirely irrelevant to the justice requirements of meeting present life-threatening health needs.

would be unethical for reasons of both justice and compassion to deny the current 600,000 patients who will die this year from their metastatic cancer the targeted cancer therapies and immunotherapies that can give them additional months (sometimes years) of life in order to offset the current costs of the proposed liquid biopsy screening program. In other words, transitioning from our current metastatic cancer therapeutic protocols to the biopsy screening protocol proposed by Raza would be ethically, economically, and politically problematic. Is there a just and reasonable way of addressing the "transition" challenge?

8.5. The Transition Challenge: Efficiency versus Compassion

Menzel (2012) has addressed the transition challenge. Menzel asked: "*Should we provide relatively inefficient treatment to identifiable individuals at relatively high risk for relatively immediate harms rather than more efficient preventive care to equally identifiable individuals at lower risk for more distant harms*" (at 214, his italics). He defends what he calls the equivalence thesis, namely, that the lives on either side of the equation are equally worthy of being saved through the allocation of social resources. However, the identifiable individuals at high risk can only have their needs met *inefficiently*. In other words, this is an unwise use of social resources, which is what Raza would argue. Society, he contends, in the form of future generations, would be much better off if the resources now being used inefficiently to purchase marginal gains in life expectancy were to be used instead in the preventive mode to prevent the need for the future inefficient uses of those resources. However, he argues, we cannot afford to do both things during some sort of transition period. This has the ethically problematic consequence of sacrificing the lives of a whole generation (in our case) of metastatic cancer patients who would all be denied access to these expensive targeted therapies in order to eliminate the need for such therapies for future generations. This does not appear to be either fair or compassionate.

Menzel asks us to consider the alternative. If we agree that it would be wrong to sacrifice this generation for the sake of future generations, then how would we ever make the transition that he would argue is rationally, ethically, and economically required? We would be stuck in the present circumstances. We would be compassionate to the current generation of metastatic cancer patients, but we would be sustaining the pain and suffering and costs associated with metastatic cancer for numerous future generations who would not otherwise need that compassion because they would not have to endure this suffering if we now made a different decision aimed at preventing the need for such care in the future. Menzel (2012) writes: "By spending at a lower health productivity rate for that prevention than we do for treatment, we would fail to decrease the incidence of these very diseases for future generations, condemning more people than necessary to never being situated where they can find it in their rational self-interest to vote for a more limited priority for treatment, with all the benefits of such a policy" (at 214). Menzel sees the "long run" perspective associated with prevention as justifying the "unfairness" objection raised in connection with denying life-prolonging care to a current generation of seriously ill patients. This is essentially a utilitarian perspective.

One way of reading Menzel is to imagine a very costly preventive intervention that is completely successful in eliminating that disease from future generations. This reading makes sense since Menzel thinks of this situation as requiring tragic sacrifice from just one generation of patients. However, that is not the scenario that we have sketched with regard to our annual liquid biopsy protocol. In our scenario we do save 400,000 individuals every year from dying as a result of metastatic cancer. That would still leave those 200,000 individuals each year who will die from their metastatic cancer. Consequently, what we would have to be willing to sacrifice are those 200,000 individuals *every year* far into the indefinite future, as opposed to "just" one generation of metastatic cancer patients. That seems to require much more in the way of ethical justification than the scenario Menzel has in mind. We can readily imagine the situation Menzel envisions as being tragic, ethically necessary to effect a greater life-saving result but still regrettable. However, it is much more difficult to justify as a "regrettable tragedy" a situation that occurs repeatedly and persists far into the indefinite future without any obvious effort to end it.[10]

If we consider the situation from a very "raw" utilitarian perspective, then the argument can be made that we *save* 400,000 lives with our liquid biopsy protocol while "only" giving up 200,000. In addition, the 400,000 lives are

---

[10] To see this point more readily, imagine a bank robber who robs a bank, then posts media messages expressing profound contrition for robbing that bank, followed by another bank robbery and profound contrition, and another bank robbery with profound contrition, into the indefinite future.

restored to having an indefinite life expectancy, while the vast majority of the 200,000 will have lost less than a year of potential life if provided with some targeted cancer therapy. Still, perhaps 20% of those 200,000 individuals would end up losing prematurely anywhere from one to 10 extra years of life (the higher numbers pertaining to the super-responders). Of course, as things are now, we would not know who those individuals were who would lose so much. However, to tolerate this outcome as a society, we would have to harden our hearts, close our eyes, and numb the compassion-generating portion of our brains. That, by itself, suggests the need for more critical and creative thinking. How, then, can we effect the transition Raza recommends in a way that is congruent with what a just and caring society ought to be?

8.6. Whole Genome Sequencing: Another Precision Health Ethical Challenge

Can we slim down the liquid biopsy screening protocol in a way that is at least "roughly just"? One group of patients who would seem to have top priority for access to these liquid biopsies would be those identified as being at risk for hereditary cancers. That represents no more than 10% of all cancers (National Cancer Institute, 2017). How would we imagine identifying them? We could do whole genome sequencing (WGS) of almost all Americans alive today and every child born each year. Such sequencing with professional analysis and interpretation and counseling would cost about $5,000 per person, or $1.6 trillion for 330 million Americans today. In addition, it would cost $20 billion per year to do WGS of each birth cohort. In the real world we do not have the technological capacity or personnel needed to accomplish this task, never mind the huge economic costs. As with our liquid biopsy screening protocol, we would have to slim down and prioritize who would have access to such WGS at social expense. How can that be done fairly?

I would certainly not endorse as "just enough" the libertarian view that it should be up to individuals with their own resources to determine whether such WGS was "worth it" to them. This would clearly disadvantage the financially less well off. What about an egalitarian perspective? There are several varieties of egalitarianism. Broadly speaking, egalitarians are committed to equal concern and respect for all. Would that mean everyone has an equal claim to WGS to establish their vulnerability to cancer? That would be a practical impossibility and ethically indefensible, given limited resources for meeting unlimited health care needs, not just cancer-related needs. Egalitarians will generally accept the view that serious health needs justly command more social resources (appendicitis commands more resources than a sprained ankle). How serious or urgent is the need for WGS to establish lifetime cancer risk relative to managing heart disease or Parkinson's or multiple sclerosis or dozens of other chronic degenerative conditions? This would not be an easy or obvious answer for an egalitarian.

If the whole US population underwent WGS, 60% of those individuals would never develop cancer over their entire lifetime. Another 30% would get a cancer diagnosis for non-hereditary reasons. Given those statistics, utilitarians would not endorse WGS for the population as a matter of social justice. Prioritarians want to ensure that a society meets the just claims for needed health care for those who are "medically least well off." We might imagine that the 10% of the population at risk for some hereditary cancer would fit that criterion. However, this is where prioritarians might find themselves internally conflicted. There are the metastatic cancer patients who desperately need the targeted cancer therapies for some additional gain in life expectancy (sometimes a significant gain in life expectancy), not to mention all the other patients at substantial risk for premature death because they are in the advanced stages of some chronic degenerative condition. These are all patients with *urgent, imminent, actual* health care needs, as opposed to the *potential* health care needs of individuals with a hereditary risk of cancer. In the debate over the moral weight that should be attached to identified lives as opposed to statistical lives for purposes of allocating life-prolonging resources, prioritarians would generally strongly endorse giving more weight to those identified lives. What we need to keep in mind is that having a hereditary risk for cancer does not necessarily mean that one will actually have cancer during one's lifetime. Women with a BRCA1 mutation will have a lifetime risk of breast cancer in the 40% to 85% range, depending upon which of several hundred mutations in the gene they might have.

Consider another complicating factor. We have the capacity to determine a polygenic cancer risk score for virtually everyone. Such a score would be the product of literally hundreds of genetic variants in an individual, each of which might increase very slightly their lifetime risk of cancer. Their lifetime risk would likely not be as great as someone at risk for a hereditary cancer. They might be told that their lifetime risk was "just average," that is, at 40%. Would they have a just claim to our annual liquid biopsy? An enormous number of people would get a result like that, which would defeat the need to reduce the use of annual liquid biopsies at social expense. Many individuals would also be told that their lifetime risk of cancer was below average, say at 20% or 30%. That is not zero. Some of these individuals will develop a cancer. Most of them will have that cancer caught at an early and treatable stage. Others will be less fortunate. They will progress to metastatic cancer and a premature death. So, we need to keep in mind, whether for the average or below average cancer risk patients, that the fewer annual liquid biopsies we do, the greater (statistically) will be the increase in patients with metastatic disease. Should we see this as being unjust, ethically problematic? This is again the "ragged edge" problem (Callahan, 1990, chap. 2) or the "cutoff" problem (Rosoff, 2017). No perfectly rational or perfectly just rationale can be offered for drawing a line at one point rather than another point. A line has to be drawn because we have only limited resources for meeting unlimited health care needs. There will always be patients with health needs or health risks just below that line who could make a reasonable just claim for the resources being provided to those above the line. The most we can reasonably hope for is rough justice.[11]

We noted earlier that roughly 40% of cancers are linked to individual behavioral decisions. Luck egalitarians, who are committed to a responsibility-sensitive conception of justice, would note this. We might imagine luck egalitarians would endorse WGS that provided a polygenic cancer risk score, primarily as a way of educating everyone regarding their cancer risk. Unfortunately, most humans do not seem to be open to educational efforts to alter pleasurable behavior that represents a threat to health. What we might imagine instead as being more likely is that individuals with average or above average or somewhat below average cancer risk scores would be the first to demand annual liquid biopsy screening with the hope that this would catch an early treatable cancer without having to change the behavior that might have generated that cancer. Given this scenario, luck egalitarians would likely oppose WGS for a population at social expense as both wasteful (unjust) and irresponsible.

Economists again contribute to mucking up our intuitions regarding preventive efforts to reduce the incidence of fatal cancers in our society. We want efficiency, justice and compassion reflected in our efforts to prevent

---

[11] If a line were drawn that systematically resulted in individuals who were already among society's least well off (health-wise and economically) being further discriminated against, then that would be an unacceptable form of rough justice. An acceptable form of rough justice would put all identifiable social groups at roughly equal risk of being on the "wrong side" of that resource allocation line.

(reduce) the incidence of fatal cancers. We noted that the total annual cost of providing access to a liquid biopsy as a screening tool in the United States would be $190 billion. We hypothesized (for the sake of argument) that this effort would save 400,000 individuals annually from a premature death from cancer. That yields a cost-per-life-saved of about $250,000. This is not an unreasonable figure. What makes that even more reasonable is if the average gain in life expectancy for those 400,000 individuals is 20 years. That means the cost-per-life-year-saved is $12,500. Compare that to the 200,000 individuals per year who would die from metastatic disease but whose lives could be extended (mostly briefly) if they were provided with some of these targeted cancer therapies. If each of those individuals were given a $100,000 targeted cancer therapy, then for those individuals who gained only three extra months of life, the cost-per-life-year-saved would be $400,000. This number would support Raza's proposal for shifting resources away from treating these patients toward the preventive efforts represented by the liquid biopsy screening protocol. However, a significant number (at least 20%) of those 200,000 metastatic cancer patients would gain at least an extra year of life for that $100,000. This is very close to what we spend per year for end-stage renal patients needing dialysis. From the perspective of health care justice and compassion, that makes it more difficult to justify sacrificing these lives for the sake of the proposed preventive effort. What makes it even more difficult to justify such sacrifice would be the 5% to 10% of patients in this category who would gain multiple extra years of life from access to one or more targeted therapies (albeit at a cost of at least $100,000 for each of those extra life-years gained). What is the right thing to do, all things considered?

Again, we do not know before the fact who might survive an extra year or more with targeted therapy. However, research regarding cancer biomarkers to answer this question is ongoing. Recall our discussion of checkpoint inhibitors. These drugs target PD-1 and PD-L1, whose job it is to regulate the immune system. However, cancer cells can use these proteins to hide themselves from the immune system. The checkpoint inhibitors are intended make the cancer cells more visible to the immune system. Higher levels of PD-1 expression are often a good biomarker of a more effective response to these checkpoint inhibitors. The actual literature in this regard is mixed (Dudley et al., 2016; Ugurel et al., 2020; Yi et al., 2018). What if, however, a slight majority of cancer patients with these higher levels of expression gain one or two extra years of life, not just seven months? Do all these patients then have a just claim to have access to these checkpoint inhibitors at social expense?

High levels of tumor mutational burden are also a good (not perfect) bio-marker for a more effective response to these drugs (Chan et al., 2018).

These are just illustrative examples. The core ethics question is this: Should we use these biomarkers to separate moderate and strong responders from marginal responders for purposes of allocating these therapies at social expense? In other words, would considerations of justice and compassion justify this rationing practice as part of an effort to balance providing limited resources to both prevention (our liquid biopsy protocol) and treatment?

Consider one more possible scenario. Because the vast majority of metastatic cancer patients achieve only marginal gains in life expectancy Raza believes we ought to pursue aggressive cancer prevention rather than aggressive treatment. However, using multiple targeted therapies in combination has yielded increased life expectancy for many cancer patients (along with significant increased costs). Workman et al. (2017) note that the cost of combining nivolumab and ipilimumab would be about $252,000 per year for the treatment of advanced melanoma. More recently, Larkin et al. (2019) show a five-year overall survival rate of 52% for these same patients with this same combination of targeted therapies. Again, these examples are illustrative of the direction of advances in cancer care at present.

Imagine future research that is successful in yielding three to five additional years of life for 75% of that batch of 200,000 metastatic cancer patients. How should that alter the balance in the distribution of social resources between our liquid biopsy prevention strategy and the effective treatment needs of these 150,000 metastatic cancer patients? That would amount to $30 billion for that first cohort of patients, $60 billion for that second cohort, and $90 billion for that third cohort and every year thereafter. To be clear, that $90 billion is *only* for the care of *these metastatic cancer patients*. This is roughly half the amount of our liquid biopsy screening proposal.

As a matter of health care justice, would we be ethically obligated to increase by $90 billion per year what we spend on cancer, again keeping in mind other areas of medicine where lives could be prolonged at a similarly high cost? That would represent a rejection of the limited resources premise behind the "just caring" problem. Alternatively, we could trim the costs of our liquid biopsy protocol. Let us say that we would screen annually only half the American population, thereby saving $80 billion per year.[12] Unless

---

[12] Alternatively, we could screen everyone every two years. That would save the same amount of money. However, that would be neither just nor rational, given that we would know in many cases before the fact that certain identifiable population groups were at greater risk for cancer in the future.

we somehow managed to choose the exactly correct 50% who were at the highest risk for metastatic cancer, we would increase the number of patients who would eventually have metastatic disease.

Simple math (under this scenario) would suggest that we would increase the number of annual metastatic cancer cases by 200,000. We will assume instead that we are cleverer than that, and consequently, the increase would be 125,000 (for the sake of argument); 25,000 of that annual cohort would be added to the 50,000 who would receive comfort care only: no targeted therapies or immunotherapies at social expense. The other 100,000 would receive the advanced targeted therapies described above at an annual cost of $20 billion for the first cohort, $40 billion for the second cohort, and $60 billion for the third cohort and every year beyond that, which would really amount to $150 billion for each of the out years under this scenario for treatment and $50 billion for the ongoing preventive screening effort. Again, this would be in addition to the $160 billion (2020) current annual costs for cancer treatment. What choices should a "just" and "caring" society make that has only limited resources for meeting virtually unlimited health care needs? A companion question might be: What choices should be relegated to individual willingness and ability to pay?

8.7. Rational Democratic Deliberation: Not Precision Ethics But "Roughly Just"

Note that there is no "most just" or "most reasonable" response to the above questions. Many trade-offs are possible that would be "just enough" and "reasonable enough." To be clear, unjust and unreasonable trade-offs are possible as well. The trade-offs are among the core values that define competing conceptions of distributive justice, as well as with other fundamental social values. These are policy choices, not choices made by individuals. Consequently, a sufficient level of social agreement is necessary for these policies to be both fair and legitimate. I have argued elsewhere (Fleck, 2009, chap. 5) that this agreement should be achieved through fair and inclusive processes of rational democratic deliberation governed by what I refer to as "constitutional principles of health care justice." Before elaborating on that, let us review our key questions in this chapter for democratic deliberation.

- Should resources currently used to treat metastatic cancer patients be redirected to efforts at either preventing the emergence of cancer or identifying and treating it in its earliest stages?
- Should identified lives of patients with metastatic cancer be given equal moral weight for the distribution of life-prolonging resources as the statistical lives (future possible patients) whose early cancer can be prevented from progressing to metastatic disease?
- Should resources be allocated in a more balanced way between treating metastatic cancer patients and minimizing through prevention the number of cancer patients who progress to metastatic disease? If so, what justice-relevant criteria should be used to limit our screening efforts and to limit our treatment efforts?
- What is the fairest, reasonably cost-effective way of meeting the "transition challenge" as we sought to shift resources from aggressive treatment of metastatic disease to prevention aimed at reducing the number of future patients with metastatic disease?
- Should we do WGS of every American early in life to establish a lifetime cancer risk score that would then be used to identify individuals most likely to benefit from more targeted preventive efforts?
- Should we as a society invest in more research aimed at identifying biomarkers that would allow us to identify and predict more reliably which individuals with metastatic cancer would gain the most in life expectancy if provided with the relevant targeted therapies at social expense?
- If we were successful at improving the survival of 75% of metastatic cancer patients for an average gain in life expectancy of three years at a cost per patient of $600,000 for those three years, should the resources needed to cover that expense come from the preventive screening efforts we have described?

Why do we need rational democratic deliberation to address these issues? All of these questions are about public goods whose fair distribution or resolution cannot be fairly or adequately addressed through any private decisional mechanism. Does the GRAIL protocol that I described represent high-value care that would justify a very high level of social investment? This is not a question that can be answered fully by asking the relevant experts to work out the cost-effectiveness equations. Multiple other social values would need to be considered and trade-offs assessed that are not in the realm of any particular area of expertise. To be sure, lots of relevant expertise needs to be introduced into the social conversation, but the conversation itself should be a matter of inclusive rational democratic deliberation.

In the European context we would be asking the question whether a commitment to solidarity required public funding for the GRAIL protocol *and permitted reducing or eliminating funding for targeted cancer therapies for patients with metastatic cancer.* In the American context we would be asking whether a commitment to individual liberty meant that individuals should make the decisions for themselves whether it was worth it to them to pay for annual cancer screening with GRAIL's liquid biopsy. Alternatively, should annual liquid biopsy screening be seen as a public health measure, a dramatic measure to reduce premature deaths from cancer, for much the same reasons that we carefully assess the processing of our food supply or the introduction of pharmaceuticals to protect the health of all. This is a matter of equal concern and respect for all. However, this would be an additional $190 billion in the United States.

Where should that money come from? Should that money come from additional taxes or increased insurance costs? This is one option. However, it would raise the political and ethical question of whether giving cancer this "special" or "supreme" health status would be justified relative to many other possible health investments in other disease areas where we might be able to save more lives at a lower cost (what is referred to as "onco-exceptionalism"). The alternative proposed by Raza would have us simply take those funds from these targeted cancer therapies and immunotherapies for metastatic cancer patients. Imagine the reluctance (maybe horror) many would experience in contemplating that option. Of course, nothing requires us to do annual screening with our liquid biopsy for everyone. We could limit that screening to some range of high-risk cancer groups in order to protect funds for treating metastatic cancer patients. However, we could then imagine the anxiety that would provoke in many Americans, knowing that their lifetime risk of cancer was 40% (maybe higher) and that the cancer that might afflict them did not present symptoms until a very advanced stage, such as pancreatic cancer. Finally, we might ask, given the emotional overtones expressed in these last few sentences, how could we possibly have a *rational, civil, mutually respectful* conversation about such controversial and emotionally charged issues. How could self-interest not corrupt and disrupt the possibility of such a conversation?

John Rawls (1971) introduced into discussions of political philosophy the notion of a "veil of ignorance." Many see the veil of ignorance as unrealistic, though at any point in our life we are largely behind a health status veil of ignorance. Even at my advanced age, I have no idea what my most likely health risks are or the most likely cause of my future death. Alternatively, imagine that in my early 20s I underwent a genetic test that indicated I had a 70% chance of dying of some specific cancer before age 60. Would I then want all sorts of social resources allocated for research and treatment of my specific cancer?

In purely private moments I might answer that last question affirmatively. But if I am part of a social policy conversation regarding the allocation of health dollars for social health insurance, as well as prevention and research, my fellow citizens would remind me that, if I seemed too single-minded an advocate for my cancer, many members of my family, as well as friends and co-workers, were vulnerable to many other health problems that could result in their succumbing to a premature death. I would also be reminded that I likely had 40 years ahead of me and that I was vulnerable to lots of other diseases or serious injury related to accidents for which social resources would need to be allocated. It would be irrational for me to focus exclusively on my risk for that cancer. In addition, it would be unkind for me to ignore the health risks to which all whom I cared about were vulnerable.

I would also be reminded that I was engaged in this very broad social conversation regarding the allocation of health care resources. We could allocate as much money as we wished to meeting health care needs, not just my health care needs but everyone else's health care needs as well. However, if we wanted to increase the size of the health care budget to cover anything and everything in the way of contemporary treatment, then I would have to be willing to pay unlimited sums as taxes or insurance premiums. On the other hand, if I want limits on that budget and my wallet, then I would have to work with everyone else who was part of this social conversation to establish what sort of health needs will justify accessing that social budget to meet those needs.

I do understand what health needs are and how unmet health needs can greatly disrupt or shorten a life. Consequently, I want allocation policies that are fair and compassionate and that represent a wise use of limited resources. I want those policies to reflect the best medical and scientific knowledge available so that we are funding effective therapies. I am mindful of the health care needs of my friends and family and acquaintances. It is more difficult to be very mindful of the health needs of numerous faceless strangers; however, I will be reminded that I am a complete stranger to all of them as well. I do endorse the view that every member of our society is entitled to equal concern and respect. I can imagine a situation in which at age 60 I am afflicted with the cancer that I feared. I am not ready to die. I can imagine a targeted cancer therapy that would cost $200,000 and offer me only a 25% chance of six extra months of life. I would want that paid for from this insurance pool. Given a commitment to equal concern and respect, that would mean that I would have to be willing to absorb those same costs for all the other metastatic cancer patients who would want that costly treatment for a very uncertain marginal gain in life expectancy. If I thought that was a poor expenditure of my money for those others who are strangers to me, then they would have the right to make the same judgment regarding the cancer treatment I want for myself since I am just as much a stranger to them.

What this last paragraph illustrates is how, in reality, we can begin to achieve social agreement regarding health care priorities and corresponding limits. Individuals must be willing to be reasonable. If I want to be treated justly, then I must be willing to treat others justly as well. What counts as being "just enough" will have to be articulated through this process of rational democratic deliberation.

What keeps this deliberative process from becoming biased, dominated by special interests that skew the results unfairly? First, the relevant medical and scientific facts (such as they are at any point in time) must be rationally respected. Some facts are mushy, such as survival curves with most of these targeted cancer therapies, which adds to the complexity of social decision-making through democratic deliberation. Second, what I (Fleck, 2009, chap. 5) refer to metaphorically as "constitutional principles of health care justice" are intended to prevent majoritarian abuse and tyranny. For example, in the United States today with employer-based insurance, many of these policies include very high deductibles and co-pays, especially with regard to these targeted cancer therapies. What that means in practice is that well-paid managers and executives can afford those co-pays and deductibles. Hence, they have effective access to these therapies. Ordinary workers would find it impossible to meet those requirements. Hence, they have no practical access to these therapies, though a portion of the cost of that insurance will be paid by them. In other words, they will be subsidizing access for the very well off. That would violate "equal concern and respect" as a constitutional principle of health care justice, which is to say that such a policy would not be an option for democratic deliberation, much less legitimation. It represents a form of exploitation.

Third, Rawls' (1971, 1996) notion of "wide reflective equilibrium" constrains democratic deliberation as well. Complex policy choices typically have wide-ranging dispersed consequences. What needs to be avoided are policy choices that generate a more unjust situation than the situation a policy change was intended to correct. If enormous social resources flow into cancer treatment, research, and prevention and yield mostly marginally beneficial results, other areas of medicine can justly inquire why comparable resources are not available for treatment, research, and prevention where there is a greater likelihood of more substantial health outcomes. This is the sort of "imbalance" that must be avoided or corrected in order to maintain overall a wide reflective equilibrium with respect to the just allocation of health care resources. In the earlier portions of this chapter, I have tried to illustrate the sort of imbalances between our liquid biopsy protocol (precision prevention) and targeted cancer therapies (precision medicine) that must be addressed.

Let me conclude with an illustration of how a deliberative question might be talked through. I assume we cannot afford to do that annual liquid biopsy for all adult Americans at social expense. I also assume we would not endorse providing only comfort care for metastatic cancer patients in order to afford the liquid biopsy protocol (given that some patients might gain several extra years of life from one or another targeted therapy). I also assume we would not endorse providing unlimited access to all cancer therapies, no matter how high the cost, no matter how marginal the benefit. All of these assumptions are ethical and economic; all (I believe) are reasonable (even if not self-evident). That means we need limits and compromise in all three regards.

Can we come to agreement regarding when it is ethically permissible to allow access to either advanced cancer therapies or our preventive liquid biopsy on the basis of an individual's willingness and ability to pay from their own resources? I think we could agree that if we can identify individuals at reasonable cost who are at significantly elevated risk for cancer, then those individuals ought to have access at social expense to our liquid biopsy annually. We will recall that any random American has a 40% lifetime risk of cancer. That is a significant number. However, if that is a number that triggers anxiety in a large portion of the population who demand annual liquid biopsy testing for a potential cancer at social expense, then we would be compelled to spend (wastefully) that $190 billion per year. What can be pointed out in the deliberative process is that 70% of individuals diagnosed with cancer will have it treated successfully and will not die of their cancer. We noted earlier that 40% of cancers are linked to behavioral choices by individuals. Increased efforts at public health education in this regard would be much less expensive than funding annual liquid biopsies for the entire population.

Given this background, it would be neither unreasonable nor unjust to expect that individuals with very high anxiety levels regarding cancer could pay from their own resources the cost of annual liquid biopsy screening. Somewhat wealthier individuals would make this choice. Somewhat poorer individuals could not make that choice. Does that represent an injustice? NO! This is a very low-value intervention relative to all the other health care needs poorer members of our population might have, to which they would have just claims, such as effective treatments for early-stage cancers. In addition, the poor are not made worse off by the purchase of these liquid biopsy tests by the financially well off. Of course, we have to consider the fact that not providing this test at social expense will increase the number of individuals with metastatic disease relative to the 400,000 hypothetical individuals saved from metastatic disease in my scenario. What does a just and caring society owe those unfortunate individuals?

We owe these unfortunate individuals effective and cost-effective cancer treatments that yield significant benefit. At present, we have somewhat costly and somewhat effective treatments for many forms of metastatic disease. The very costly targeted therapies and immunotherapies are typically offered after these prior lines of treatment have been used, though many researchers and oncologists would like to see these targeted therapies become first-line treatment for metastatic disease. This might make medical, ethical, and financial sense in some range of cases. This can then be seen as the trade-off for individuals who would have given up on endorsing social payment for the liquid biopsy option. Still, not everyone diagnosed with metastatic cancer will have access to these very expensive targeted cancer therapies at social expense. To preserve fairness and objectivity, we ought to fund research aimed at identifying reliable predictive biomarkers that would identify before the fact patients most likely to achieve substantial benefit from one or more targeted therapies, the precise definition of "substantial benefit" being left to the deliberative process. Again, the wealthy could buy access to targeted cancer therapies likely to be only very marginally beneficial. This does not represent an injustice to the non-wealthy, who are no worse off as a result of permitting such purchases.

The limits we would collectively place on accessing targeted cancer therapies at social expense should be congruent with comparable limits we place on accessing comparable life-prolonging therapies in many other areas of medicine. This is what would be required for maintaining a just reflective equilibrium in the deliberative process. Finally, creative options are possible. We could endorse a policy of permitting individuals who were hyper-anxious about their cancer risks (without any objective basis for that anxiety) to have annual liquid biopsies at social expense with the understanding that they would give up their right to expensive targeted therapies should they still be unfortunate enough to end up with metastatic disease. Speaking personally, I would not see this as a wise trade-off. However, in a liberal, pluralistic society that places a high value on maximizing individual liberty, so long as that liberty is not used to violate the equal rights of others or public interests, this might be an option that should be permitted.[13]

In conclusion, it is reasonable for us, future possible cancer patients, to want both precision medicine and precision health. However, if we want both to the maximal degree that is technologically possible, we will create ethical, economic, and political challenges that would be ethically disruptive, economically unsustainable, and politically divisive. If we want a society that is just and caring, given limited resources and unlimited health care needs, we will need to define limits and legitimate trade-offs that are reasonable and "just enough." Competing theories of justice, as articulated by philosophers, will be too abstract for the inherent complexities associated with health care rationing and priority-setting in the real world. What we require instead are fair, well-structured, and inclusive processes of rational democratic deliberation to address these issues. Such processes are most congruent with what a liberal, pluralistic, tolerant democratic society aspires to be. The role of philosophers in this process is to guide the construction of public reason, that is, the rational capacities and value commitments necessary for sustaining effective civil discourse regarding the most controversial social problems a democratic society must address. Precision medicine, unguided by just public reason, will yield unhealthy public policy and noxious injustices in our health care system.

---

[13] This can get complicated. What should a just and caring society do if an individual has chosen this option at age 21 but at age 45 realizes this was not a wise choice? This individual no longer wants society to pay for these annual liquid biopsies. Do they then have a just claim to social payment for these targeted cancer therapies, should they end up with a metastatic cancer? What if they have this awakening at age 60? These are complexities that would have to be considered as part of the deliberative process.

9

Public Reason, Precision Medicine

Future Hopes

No one should read what I have written in this book as a screed against precision medicine. The research that is occurring under the rubric of precision medicine is elegant and profoundly fascinating as scientific research. However, that work is being implemented in a medical, economic, and political system that is generating wicked problems of health care justice. This is most evident in the United States, though the deployment of precision medicine in the European Union is straining the bonds of solidarity there as well (Fleck, 2022). Why is this the case? Let us review our main themes.

(1) Cancer has proven to be extraordinarily wily in its ability to evade everything that the medical armamentarium has thrown against it. We see this most clearly in the case of cancer drug resistance. Cancer is extraordinarily complex as a biological phenomenon with multiple defenses against our best efforts to defeat it. This is especially true once cancer has metastasized. It is dispersed in the form of genetically heterogeneous tumors, which makes it virtually impossible to defeat with any single targeted therapy, or even combinations of targeted therapies.

(2) Wicked ethical problems have been generated by precision medicine because of both the wiliness of cancer and the fragmentation of the financing of health care in the United States (Cole et al., 2020). The wiliness of cancer has resulted in these targeted cancer therapies yielding only very marginal gains in life expectancy for the vast majority of patients. Those marginal gains might be seen as being regrettable, except that these drugs are so expensive that they threaten to unjustly alter the allocation of health care resources within our health care system. Metastatic cancer does represent an unfortunate, genuine medical need. However, there is nothing morally special about cancer as a life-threatening phenomenon that would justify according

Precision Medicine and Distributive Justice. Leonard M. Fleck, Oxford University Press. © Oxford University Press 2022.
DOI: 10.1093/oso/9780197647721.003.0009

it some sort of preeminent moral status for purposes of justly allocating health care resources.

(3) Philosophers tend to have high hopes for the utility of their various theories of justice. Those theories might work well in a limited range of contexts. However, metastatic cancer and very costly precision medicine generate extremely complex problems of health care justice that none of these theories can address adequately. Should it matter, for purposes of the just allocation of limited health care resources, that the most common cancers (lung and melanoma) are mostly a result of bad health choices by individuals? Luck egalitarians would offer one response to this question, but other egalitarians and prioritarians would offer a very different answer. Should we be investing vast sums of research dollars into identifying biomarkers that would predict which patients would be very expensive marginal responders to these targeted therapies so that we would deny them those resources in order to reallocate those resources to other medical needs where more life-prolonging good would be accomplished? Utilitarians would give one sort of answer to this question, while egalitarians and prioritarians would give very different answers. How much weight, from which perspective of health care justice, should be attached to the fact that these metastatic cancer patients are terminally ill, are among the medically least well off, tend to be elderly, see these targeted therapies as their "last chance" for prolonged survival, and desperately want to live? Such patients command compassion. Should that be limited to just compassion? In brief, wicked problems do not lend themselves readily to being effectively addressed by any of these theories of justice.

(4) What we need to recall is that these wicked problems need to be addressed in a liberal, pluralistic, democratic society. Rawls (1996) provides us with a strategy for addressing these wicked problems, starting with his notion of political liberalism. Political liberalism is not a comprehensive philosophic theory in the way that utilitarianism or egalitarianism might be seen as comprehensive moral or political theories. We need to make the same move with regard to our understanding of health care justice. That is, we need a *political* conception of justice, suitably detached from all the prevailing comprehensive theories of justice. That political conception of justice will be liberal and pluralistic, open to adapting and integrating the core

values of alternative comprehensive theories of justice as needed to address specific wicked problems linked to precision medicine. That political conception of justice will be an integral part of *public reason*, which will govern the public deliberations of *citizens as citizens* (suitably detached from their own comprehensive commitments), as well as public leaders and legislators. A political conception of justice will serve as a focal point for creating an overlapping consensus regarding how to address specific wicked problems of health care justice generated by the deployment of precision medicine in meeting the needs of metastatic cancer patients.

(5) Public reason needs to be embodied in processes of rational democratic deliberation. Public reason needs to be practical or pragmatic, as John Dewey might say. Public reason must involve developing the capacity to address political problems respectfully and reasonably (no matter how initially controversial the issue might be), most especially problems of justice at the foundations of any well-ordered political society. The primary ethical and political virtue of rational democratic deliberation is that it allows citizens as citizens to fashion autonomously shared understandings of how to address fairly the complex problems of health care justice generated by precision medicine. A just democratic deliberative process must be inclusive of all who could be affected by the outcomes of that deliberative process. In addition, all within that process must be treated as persons deserving equal concern and respect with the equal right to voice their views. The deliberative process will need to be constrained in various ways to assure that the outcomes are "just enough" or "roughly just." In a pluralistic world, ideally just outcomes are a moral and political impossibility. Constraints on the deliberative process will include relevant medical and scientific facts related to precision medicine, stable considered judgments of health care justice from elsewhere in the health care system, constitutional principles of health care justice, and the need for what Rawls would describe as wide reflective equilibrium among all these factors.[1]

---

[1] As Cristina Lafont (2020) notes, there are no shortcuts to addressing these problems through democratic deliberation. "Taking shortcuts that bypass public deliberation about political decisions would further erode the fundamental commitment of the democratic ideal of self-government,

(6) Wicked problems themselves can have something of a metastatic character. They can spill out to infect the entire health care system or, worse, to infect the entire political climate of a society, sowing distrust, deceit, disputes, and derogatory and destructive political rhetoric. We see that most clearly with the so-called culture wars regarding abortion, euthanasia, embryonic stem cells, pre-implantation genetic diagnosis, alternative reproductive technologies, gene editing, uses of whole genome sequencing, and so on. These also become issues of health care justice to the extent that just access to these technologies requires public funding. Worst of all, if these wicked problems are allowed to metastasize, they represent a threat to our capacity as a society for rational democratic deliberation. With respect to the problems of health care justice generated by precision medicine, if we are tempted to permit rationing decisions to be made invisibly, in ways that are effectively hidden from those affected by those decisions, then we are facilitating the metastasis of these wicked problems and undermining our capacity for fair and inclusive rational democratic deliberation.

(7) Near the end of the *Critique of Pure Reason* Kant raises the three most fundamental questions that must be safeguarded by philosophers: "What can I know? What should I do? What may I hope?" I would argue (along with Socrates, the philosophers of the Enlightenment, Dewey, and Rawls) that the primary role of philosophers is to serve as advocates, architects, and critical analysts of public reason and rational democratic deliberation. It is the integrity of the deliberative process for which philosophers must be most solicitous and most attentive. This is the role of Locke's under-laborer in his *Essay Concerning Human Understanding*. As Locke says, this would be "ambition enough." Philosophers do not need to be the master builders of precision medicine. Philosophers should be content to nourish the hopes for more just access to the fruits of precision medicine through fostering our social capacities for rational and respectful democratic deliberation regarding contentious problems

---

namely, that all citizens can equally own and identify with the institutions, laws, and policies to which they are subject. In pluralist societies this is a fragile and quite burdensome commitment" (at 3). I would just add that this is a burden we must undertake.

of health care justice. There is no metaphysical imperative that contentious problems must become wicked problems. Immunizing that political conversation from the ideologies, irrationalities, and absurdities that threaten the integrity of that conversation is ambition that is worthy enough for philosophers.

Appendices

Selected Examples of Ongoing Large Genotype–Drug Matching Precision Cancer Medicine Trials

Mutations matched	Targeted drugs used
EGFR/HER2-activating mutation	Afatinib
MET, ALK, ROS1	Crizotinib
EGFR T790M or other activating mutation	Osimertinib
BRAF V600E/R/K/D, BRAF fusion, non-BRAF V600 mutations	Dabrafenib + trametinib
NF1, GNAQ, GNA11	Trametinib
PIK3CA	Taselisib
HER-2 amplification	Trastuzumab + pertuzumab
FGFR mutation or fusion	Erdafitinib
mTOR, TSC1, TSC2	Sapanisertib
PTEN mutation	GSK2636771 (PI3K-beta inhibitor)
HER-2 amplification	Trastuzumab, emtansine
SMO, PTCH1	Vismodegib
NF2 inactivating mutation	Defactinib
cKIT mutation	Sunitinib
FGFR1, FGFR2, FGFR3 mutation	AZD4547 (FGFR inhibitor)
Certain DDR2 mutations	Dasatinib
AKT mutation	Capivasertib
NRAS mutations	Binimetinib
CDK4, CDK6	Palbociclib
Mismatch repair deficiency	Nivolumab
NTRK1, NTRK2, NTRK3 fusions	Larotrectinib
PIK3CA, PTEN mutations	Copanlisib
BRCA1, BRCA2 mutation	Adavosertib

Mutations matched	Targeted drugs used
AKT mutation	Ipatasertib
BRAF non-V600 mutation or BRAF fusion	Ulixertinib
ALK, ROS1, MET	Crizotinib
CDKN2A, CDK4, CDK6	Palbociclib
CSF1R, PDGFR, VEGFR	Sunitinib
mTOR, TSC	Temsirolimus
ERBB2	Trastuzumab + pertuzumab
BRAFV600E/D/K/R	Vemurafenib + cobimetinib
NRAS, KRAS, NRAF	Cetuximab
BCR-ABL, SRC, KIT, PDGFRB,	Imatinib
EPHA2, FYN, LCK, YES1	Dasatinib
RET, VEGFR1/2/3, KIT, PDGFRB, RAF-1, BRAF	Regorafenib
BRCA1, BRCA2, ATM	Olaparib
POLE, POLD1, high mutational load	Pembrolizumab
MSI-high, high mutational load, and others	Nivolumab + ipilimumab

Taken from Malone ER et al., 2020, Molecular profiling for precision cancer therapies. *Genome Medicine* 12 (8). https://doi.org/10.1186/s13073-019-0703-1) [Open Access]

Cancer Drugs, 2021

Type of cancer	Drug name	Monthly cost	Annual cost
Acute lymphocytic leukemia			
	Ponatinib	$16,561	$198,732
	Blinitumomab	$	$178,000
	Inotuzumab	$	$168,300
Acute myeloid leukemia			
	Midostaurin	$27,324	$327,888
Basal cell carcinoma			
	Vismodegib	$11,883	$142,596
Bladder cancer			
	Atezolizumab	$13,231	$158,772
Breast cancer			
	Pertuzumab	$7,350	$88,200
	Trastuzumab emtansine	$11,263	$135,156
	Palbociclib	$12,703	$152,436
	Ribociclib	$13,450	$161,400
	Neratinib	$12,578	$150,936
	Abemaciclib	$12,570	$150,840
Chronic lymphocytic leukemia			
	Ofatumumab	$20,411	$244,932
	Obinutuzumab	$9,048	$108,576
	Idelalisib	$10,717	$128,604
	Venetoclax	$11,474	$137,688
Chronic myeloid leukemia			
	Bosutinib	$14,927	$179,124
	Ponatinib	$16,561	$198,732
Colorectal cancer			
	Aflibercept	$5,053	$60,636
	Regorafenib	$18,606	$223,272
Hodgkin lymphoma			
	Brentuximab vedotin	$29,352	$352,224

Type of cancer	Drug name	Monthly cost	Annual cost
Melanoma			
	Ipilimumab	$	$120,000
	Vemurafenib	$10,851	$130,212
	Trametinib	$11,321	$135,852
	Dabrafenib	$10,427	$125,124
	Pembrolizumab	$14,167	$170,004
	Nivolumab	$14,299	$171,588
	Talimogene laherparepvec	$20,439	$245,268
	Cobimetinib	$7,505	$90,060
Multiple myeloma			
	Pomalidomide	$18,436	$221,232
	Panobinostat	$12,733	$152,796
	Daratumumab	$8,600	$103,200
	Ixazomib	$10,652	$127,834
	Elotuzumab	$9,737	$116,844
Non-small cell lung cancer			
	Crizotinib	$16,859	$202,308
	Afatinib	$8,807	$105,684
	Ceritinib	$10,554	$126,648
	Osimertinib	$14,763	$177,156
	Necitumumab	$13,127	$157,524
	Alectinib	$14,947	$179,364
	Brigatinib	$15,964	$191,568
Ovarian cancer			
	Olaparib	$14,025	$168,300
	Rucaparib	$15,922	$191,064
	Niraparib	$16,727	$200,724
Prostate cancer			
	Cabazitaxel	$10,531	$126,372
	Abiraterone	$10,887	$130,644
	Enzalutamide	$11,549	$138,588
Renal cell carcinoma			
	Everolimus	$10,686	$128,232
	Pazopanib	$13,079	$156,948
	Axitinib	$15,082	$180,984
Stomach cancer			
	Ramucirumab	$14,015	$168,180

20 Most Expensive Drugs in the United States, 2021

Drug name	Disease treated	Cost monthly
Zokinvy	Progeria	$86,040
Myalept	Leptin deficiency	$74,159
Mavenclad	Multiple sclerosis	$60,371
Ravicti	Urea cycle disorders	$57,998
Actimmune	Chronic granulomatous disease	$55,310
Oxervate	Neurotrophic keratitis	$48,498
Takhzyro	Hereditary angioedema	$46,828
Juxtapid	Homozygous familial hypercholesterolemia	$46,502
Cinryze	Hereditary angioedema	$45,465
Chenodal	Dissolves gallstones	$42,570
Gattex	Short bowel syndrome	$41,664
H.P. Acthar	Rheumatoid arthritis, multiple sclerosis, etc.	$39,864
Orladeyo	Hereditary angioedema	$37,308
Tegsedi	Hereditary transthyretin amyloidosis	$35,638
Ayvakit	Gastrointestinal stromal tumor	$33,568
Vitrakvi	NTRK fusion cancers	$32,800
Qinlock	Gastrointestinal stromal tumor	$32,000
Korlym	Cushing's syndrome	$31,440
Cerdelga	Gaucher disease type 1	$28,599
Idhifa	Acute myeloid leukemia	$28,246

20 Most Expensive Drugs in the United States, 2021

Drug name	Disease treated	Cost a month

References

Abola MV, Prasad V. 2016. The use of superlatives in cancer research. *JAMA Oncology* 2: 139–41.

Abrams EM, Szefler SJ. 2020. COVID-19 and the impact of social determinants of health. *Lancet Respiratory Medicine* 8: 659–61.

Abramson Cancer Center. 2018. Hope, faith, and second chances: how Barbara beat cancer with CAR T-cell therapy. Accessed 2/2/2019. https://www.pennmedicine.org/cancer/about/patient-stories/non-hodgkin-lymphoma-barbara

Acuna SA, Fernandes KA, Daly C, Hicks LK, Sutradhar R, Kim SJ, et al. 2016. Cancer mortality among recipients of solid-organ transplantation in Ontario, Canada. *JAMA Oncology* 2: 463–69.

Aggarwal A, Fojo T, Chamberlain C, Davis C, Sullivan R. 2017. Do patient access schemes for high-cost cancer drugs deliver value to society?—lessons from the NHS Cancer Drugs Fund. *Annals of Oncology* 28: 1738–50.

Alexander S. 1962. They decide who lives, who dies. *Life Magazine* (Nov. 9). Accessed 3/22/2018. http://ihatedialysis.com/forum/index.php?topic=23860.0. This website reproduces the original article.

Alix-Panabieres C. 2020. The future of liquid biopsy. *Nature* 579 (March 26): S9.

Al-Lazikani B, Banerji U, Workman P. 2012. Combinatorial drug therapy for cancer in the post-genomic era. *Nature Biotechnology* 30: 679–92.

ALS Association. 2016. Who gets ALS? Facts you should know. Accessed 11/24/2018. http://www.alsa.org/about-als/facts-you-should-know.html

Alzheimer's Association Report. 2020. 2020 Alzheimer's disease facts and figures. *Alzheimer's & Dementia* 16: 391–460.

Arneson RJ. 2000. Luck egalitarianism and prioritarianism. *Ethics* 110: 339–49.

Arneson RJ. 2011. Luck egalitarianism—a primer. In *Responsibility and Distributive Justice*, edited by C Knight and Z Stemplowska. New York: Oxford University Press, 24–50.

Asher N, Ben-Betzalel G, Lev-Ari S, Shapira-Frommer R, Steinberg-Silman Y, Gochman N, et al. 2020. Real world outcomes of ipilimumab and nivolumab in patients with metastatic melanoma. *Cancers* 12: 2329. doi: 10.3390/cancers12082329

Axelsen DV, Nielsen L. 2017. Essentially enough: elements of a plausible account of sufficientarianism. In *What Is Enough? Sufficiency, Justice, and Health*, edited by C Fourie and A Rid. New York: Oxford University Press, 101–18.

Azvolinsky A. 2020. Despite generic imatinib, cost of treating CML remains high. *Cancer Today* (Feb. 24). Accessed 6/18/2020. https://www.cancertodaymag.org/Pages/cancer-talk/Despite-Generic-Imatinib-Cost-of-Treating-CML-Remains-High.aspx

Bach PB. 2019. Insights into the increasing costs of cancer drugs. *Clinical Advances in Hematology & Oncology* 17: 287–88, 298.

Bach BP. 2018. National coverage analysis of CAR-T therapies—policy, evidence, and payment. *New England Journal of Medicine* 379: 1396–98.

Bach BP. 2015. Walking the tightrope between treatment efficacy and price. *Journal of Clinical Oncology* 34: 889–90.

Bach PB, Giralt SA, Saltz LB. 2017. FDA approval of tisagenlecleucel: promise and complexities of a $475,000 cancer drug. *JAMA* 318: 1861–62.

Bachtiger A, Dryzek JS, Mansbridge J, Warren ME. (eds). 2018. *The Oxford Handbook of Deliberative Democracy*. New York: Oxford University Press.

Baker R, Mason H, McHugh N. 2018. UK spends generously to extend the lives of people with terminal illnesses—against the public's wishes. *The Conversation* (May 31). Accessed 10/3/2020. https://theconversation.com/uk-spends-generously-to-extend-lives-of-people-with-terminal-illnesses-against-the-publics-wishes-96562

Bankhead C. 2016. ASCO: more good news for PD-1 Tx of melanoma. *MedPage Today* (May 19). Accessed 5/22/2016. http://www.medpagetoday.com/meetingcoverage/asco/58007

Bansal A, Radich J. 2016. Is cure for chronic myeloid leukemia possible in the tyrosine kinase inhibitors era? *Current Opinions in Hematology* 23: 115–20.

Bardia A, Mayer IA, Vahdat LT, Tolaney SM, Isakoff SJ, Diamond JR, et al. 2019. Sacituzumab govitecan-hziy in refractory metastatic triple-negative breast cancer. *New England Journal of Medicine* 380: 741–51.

Basett M. 2018. Survey: cancer patients will pay anything for treatment. *MedPage Today* (Aug. 29). Accessed 12/2/2018. https://www.medpagetoday.com/hematologyoncology/othercancers/74820

Batlle E, Clevers H. 2017. Cancer stem cells revisited. *Nature Medicine* 23: 1124–34.

Belluck P. 2020. FDA panel declines to endorse controversial Alzheimer's drug. *New York Times* (Nov. 6). Accessed 1/12/2021. https://www.nytimes.com/2020/11/06/health/aducanumab-alzheimers-drug-fda-panel.html

Benbaji Y. 2006. Sufficiency or priority. *European Journal of Philosophy* 14: 327–48.

Bentley C, Peacock S, Abelson J, Burgess MM, Demers-Payette O, Longstaff H, et al. 2019. Addressing the affordability of cancer drugs: using deliberative public engagement to inform health policy. *Health Research Policy and Systems* 17:17. doi: 10.1186/s12961-019-0411-8

Bentley TS, Phillips SJ. 2017. 2017 U.S. organ and tissue transplant cost estimates and discussion. *Milliman Research Report*. Accessed 4/2/2018. https://www.milliman.com/en/Insight/2017-US-organ-and-tissue-transplant-cost-estimates-and-discussion

Berg M, Grinten T, Klazinga N. 2004. Technology assessment, priority setting, and appropriate care in Dutch health care. *International Journal of Technology Assessment in Health Care* 20: 35–43.

Bifulco CB, Urba WJ. 2016. Unmasking PD-1 resistance to next-generation sequencing. *New England Journal of Medicine* 375: 888–89.

Biomarkers Definitions Working Group. 2001. Biomarkers and surrogate endpoints: preferred definitions and conceptual framework. *Clinical Pharmacology and Therapeutics* 69(3): 89–95.

Blanchard A, Strand R. (eds). 2017. *Cancer Biomarkers: Ethics, Economics, and Society*. Kokstad, Norway: Megaloceros Press.

Blanchard A, Wik E. 2018. What is a good (enough) biomarker? In *Cancer Biomarkers: Ethics, Economics, and Society*, edited by A Blanchard and R Strand. Kokstod, Norway: Megaloceros Press, 7–24.

Board C, Kelly MS, Shapiro MD, Dixon DL. 2020. PCSK9 inhibitors in secondary prevention—an opportunity for personalized therapy. *Journal of Cardiovascular Pharmacology* 75: 410–20.

Bohman J. 1996. *Public Deliberation: Pluralism, Complexity, and Democracy*. Cambridge, MA: MIT Press.

Bohman J, Rehg W. (eds). 1997. *Deliberative Democracy: Essays on Reason and Politics*. Cambridge, MA: MIT Press.

Boku N. 2014. HER2-positive gastric cancer. *Gastric Cancer* 17: 1–17.

Bradley C, Clement J, Lin C. 2008. Absence of cancer diagnosis and treatment in elderly Medicaid-insured nursing home residents. *Journal of the National Cancer Institute* 100(1): 21–30.

Brahmer J, Reckamp KL, Baas P, Crino L, Eberhardt WE, Puddubskaya E, et al. 2015. Nivolumab versus docetaxel in advanced squamous-cell non-small-cell lung cancer. *New England Journal of Medicine* 373: 123–35.

Brander D, Islam P, Barrientos JC. 2019. Tailored treatment strategies for chronic lymphocytic leukemia in a rapidly changing era. *ASCO Educational Book* 39: 487–98. https://doi.org/10.1200/EDBK_238735

Brill S. 2015. *America's Bitter Pill: Money, Politics, Backroom Deals, and the Fight to Fix Our Broken Healthcare System*. New York: Random House.

Brock D. 2015. Identified versus statistical lives: some introductory issues and arguments. In *Identified Versus Statistical Lives: An Interdisciplinary Perspective*, edited by IG Cohen, N Daniels, N Eyal. New York: Oxford University Press, 43–52.

Brock D. 2002. Priority to the worse off in health-care resource prioritization. In *Medicine and Social Justice: Essays on the Distribution of Health Care*, edited by R Rhodes, M Battin, A Silvers. Oxford: Oxford University Press, 362–72.

Buchanan A. 1998. Managed care: rationing without justice, but not unjustly. *Journal of Health Care Politics, Policy, and Law* 23: 617–34.

Buchanan A. 2009. Introduction and the right to a decent minimum of health care. In *Justice and Health Care: Selected Essays*. New York: Oxford University Press, 3–36.

Bulik BS. 2017. Bristol-Myers' new Opdivo ad asks, "who wouldn't want a chance to live longer?" *Fierce Pharma* (June 7). Accessed 12/11/2018. https://www.fiercepharma.com/marketing/bristol-myers-squibb-new-ad-for-opdivo-asks-who-wouldn-t-want-a-chance-to-live-longer

Burstein HJ, Krilov L, Aragon-Ching JB, Baxter NN, Chiorean EG, Chow WA, et al. 2017. Clinical cancer advances 2017: annual report on progress against cancer from the American Society of Clinical Oncology. *Journal of Clinical Oncology* 35: 1341–67.

Butler J. 1999. *The Ethics of Health Care Rationing: Principles and Practices*. London: Cassell.

Buyx AM, Friedrich DR, Schöne-Seifert B. 2011. Ethics and effectiveness: rationing healthcare by thresholds of minimum effectiveness. *BMJ* 342, d54. Accessed 6/18/2020. https://www.bmj.com/content/342/bmj.d54

Caceres M, Cheng W, De Robertis M, Mirocha JM, Czer L, Esmailian F, et al. 2013. Survival and quality of life for nonagenarians after cardiac surgery. *Annals of Thoracic Surgery* 95: 1598–1602.

Calabresi G, Bobbitt P. 1978. *Tragic Choices: The Conflicts Society Confronts in the Allocation of Tragically Scarce Resources*. New York: W.W. Norton.

Callahan D. 1990. *What Kind of Life: The Limits of Medical Progress*. New York: Simon and Schuster.

Calltorp J. 1999. Priority setting in health policy in Sweden and a comparison with Norway. *Health Policy* 50: 1–22. doi: 10.1016/s0168-8510(99)00061-5

Canary LA, Klevens M, Holmberg SD. 2015. Limited access to new hepatitis C virus treatment under state Medicaid programs. *Annals of Internal Medicine* 163: 226–28.

Caplan A. 2011. Will evidence ever be sufficient to resolve the challenge of cost containment? *Journal of Clinical Oncology* 29: 1946–48.

Cappell KM, Sherry RM, Yang JC, Goff SL, Vanasse DA, McIntyre L, et al. 2020. Long-term follow-up of anti-CD19 chimeric antigen receptor T-cell therapy. *Journal of Clinical Oncology* 38: 3805–15.

Carbone DP, Reck M, Paz-Ares L, Creelan B, Horn L, Steins M, et al. 2017. First-line nivolumab in stage IV or recurrent non-small-cell lung cancer. *New England Journal of Medicine* 376: 2415–26.

Casal P. 2007. Why sufficiency is not enough. *Ethics* 117: 296–326.

Castro DG, Clarke PA, Al-Lazikani B, Workman P. 2013. Personalized cancer medicine: molecular diagnostics, predictive biomarkers, drug resistance. *Clinical Pharmacology and Therapeutics* 93: 252–59.

Centers for Medicare & Medicaid Services. 2012. Accessed 4/24/2022. https://www.cms.gov/Research-Statistics-Data-and-Systems/Statistics-Trends-and-Reports/MedicareMedicaidStatSupp/2012.

Cha AE. 2015. Healthy people can now order a $299 "liquid biopsy" blood test for cancer. Should you get it? *Washington Post* (Oct. 15). Accessed 1/25/2019. https://www.washingtonpost.com/news/to-your-health/wp/2015/10/15/you-can-now-order-a-299-liquid-biopsy-blood-test-for-cancer-should-you-get-it/?utm_term=.65107bae8b7a

Chadwick D. 2020. The price of hope: weighing the cost of CAR T-cell therapy in treating blood cancers. *CURE, Hematology* (Sept. 23). Accessed 1/10/2021. https://www.curetoday.com/view/the-price-of-hope-weighing-the-cost-of-car-t-cell-therapy-in-treating-blood-cancers

Champiat S, Dercle L, Ammari S, Massard C, Hollebecque A, Postel-Vinay S, et al. 2017. Hyperprogressive disease is a new pattern of progression in cancer patients treated by anti-PD-1/ PD-L1. *Clinical Cancer Research* 23: 1920–28.

Chan TA, Yarchoan M, Jaffee E, Swanton C, Quezada SA, Stenzinger A, Peters S. 2018. Development of tumor mutation burden as an immunotherapy biomarker: utility for the oncology clinic. *Annals of Oncology* 30: 44–46.

Charlton V. 2020. NICE and fair? Health technology assessment policy under the UK's National Institute for Health and Care Excellence. *Health Care Analysis* 28: 193–227.

Charlton V, Rid A. 2019. Innovation as a value in healthcare priority setting: the UK experience. *Social Justice Research* 32: 208–38.

Chen S. 2016. Economic costs of hemophilia and the impact of prophylactic treatment on patient management. *American Journal of Managed Care* 22: S126–33.

Chernew ME. 2020. The role of market forces in U.S. health care. *New England Journal of Medicine* 383: 1401–04.

Cheung H, Wong T. 2018. The full story of Thailand's extraordinary cave rescue. BBC News. Accessed 5/23/2020. https://www.bbc.com/news/world-asia-44791998

Chong EA, Ruella M, Schuster SJ. 2021. Five-year outcomes for refractory B-cell lymphomas with CAR T-cell therapy. *New England Journal of Medicine* 384: 673–74.

Christiano T. 1997. The significance of public deliberation. In *Deliberative Democracy: Essays on Reason and Politics*, edited by J Bohman, W Rehg. Cambridge, MA: MIT Press, 243–78.

Clackson S. 2008. Ronald Dworkin's "prudent insurance" ideal for healthcare: idealisations of circumstance, prudence and self-interest. *Health Care Analysis* 16: 31–38.

Clarke MF. 2019. Clinical and therapeutic implications of cancer stem cells. *New England Journal of Medicine* 380: 2237–45.

Claxton K. 2015. The UKs Cancer Drugs Fund does more harm than good. *New Scientist* (Jan. 13). Accessed 10/10/2020. https://www.newscientist.com/article/dn26785-the-uks-cancer-drugs-fund-does-more-harm-than-good/

Clazton G, Cox C, Damico A, Levitt L, Pollitz K. 2019. Pre-existing condition prevalence for individuals and families. Kaiser Family Foundation (Oct. 4). Accessed 4/28/2022. https://www.kff.org/health-reform/issue-brief/pre-existing-condition-prevalence-for-individuals-and-families/.

Cohen D. 2017. Most drugs paid for by £1.27bn Cancer Drugs Fund had no "meaningful benefit." *BMJ* (April 28). Accessed 7/30/2020. https://www.bmj.com/content/357/bmj.j2097

Cohen J. 1997. Deliberation and democratic legitimacy. In *Deliberative Democracy: Essays on Reason and Politics*, edited by J Bohman, W Rehg. Cambridge, MA: MIT Press, 67–92.

Cohen J. 1993. Moral pluralism and political consensus. In *The Idea of Democracy*, edited by D Copp, J Hampton, J Roemer. Cambridge, UK: Cambridge University Press, 270–91.

Cohen SB, Yu W. 2012. The concentration and persistence in the level of health expenditures over time: estimates for the U.S. population, 2008–2009. Agency for Health Care Research and Quality Statistical Brief #354. Accessed 7/24/2020. https://meps.ahrq.gov/data_files/publications/st354/stat354.shtml

Cohn WE, Timms DL, Frazier OH. 2015. Total artificial hearts: past, present, and future. *Nature Reviews: Cardiology* 12: 609–17.

Cole MB, Ellison JE, Trivedi AN. 2020. Association between high-deductible health plans and disparities in access to care among cancer survivors. *JAMA Network Open* 3(6): e208965. doi: 10/1001/jamanetworkopen.2020.8965

Collins M, Latimer N. 2013. NICE's end of life decision making scheme: impact on population health. *BMJ* 346: f1363.

Columbus G. 2020. NICE cites cost in deciding against atezolizumab for frontline advanced small cell lung cancer. *OncLive*. Accessed 4/30/2022. https://www.onclive.com/view/nice-cites-cost-in-deciding-against-atezolizumab-for-frontline-advanced-small-cell-lung-cancer.

Constine LS, Hudson MM, Seibel NL. 2020. Late effects of treatment for childhood cancer. National Cancer Institute (March 10). Accessed 10/23/2020. https://www.cancer.gov/types/childhood-cancers/late-effects-hp-pdq

Cookson R. 2013. Can the NICE "end-of-life premium" be given a coherent ethical justification? *Journal of Health Politics, Policy, and Law* 38: 1129–48.

Cookson R, Dolan P. 2000. Principles of justice in health care rationing. *Journal of Medical Ethics* 26: 323–29.

Cookson R, McCabe C, Tsuchiya A. 2008. Public healthcare resource allocation and the rule of rescue. *Journal of Medical Ethics* 34: 540–44.

Corless GL, Barnett CM, Heinrich MC. 2011. Gastrointestinal stromal tumors: origin and molecular oncology. *Nature Reviews Cancer* 11: 865–78.

Cortes J, Cescon DW, Rugo HS, Nowecki Z, Im S, Yusof M, et al. 2020. Pemrolizumab plus chemotherapy versus placebo plus chemotherapy for previously untreated locally recurrent inoperable or metastatic triple-negative breast cancer (KEYNOTE-355): a randomized placebo-controlled, double-blind, phase 3 clinical trial. *Lancet* 396 (10265): 1817–28.

Courtney PT, Yip AT, Cherry DR, Salans MA, Kumar A, Murphy JD. 2020. Cost effectiveness of combination ipilimumab–nivolumab in advanced non-small-cell lung cancer. *Journal of Clinical Oncology* 38 (15, Supplement): e19387.

Coyle D, Cheung MC, Evans GA. 2014. Opportunity cost of funding drugs for rare diseases: the cost-effectiveness of eculizumab in paroxysmal nocturnal hemoglobinuria. *Medical Decision Making* 34: 1016–29.

Crisp R. 2003. Equality, priority, and compassion. *Ethics* 113: 745–63.

Cubanski J, Neuman T, True S, Freed M. 2019. What's the latest on Medicare drug price negotiations? *Henry Kaiser Family Foundation Issue Brief* (Oct. 17). Accessed 8/26/2020. https://www.kff.org/medicare/issue-brief/whats-the-latest-on-medicare-drug-price-negotiations/

Cuckler GA, Sisko AM, Poisal JA, Keehan SP, Smith SD, Madison AJ, et al. 2018. National health expenditure projections, 2017–26: despite uncertainty, fundamentals primarily drive spending growth. *Health Affairs* 37: 482–92.

Daily Mail Reporter. 2008. Life-and-death decisions of drugs rationing body are "less fair than tossing a coin" says ethics expert. Accessed 5/6/2016. http://www.dailymail.co.uk/sciencetech/article-1080212/Life-death-decisions-drugs-rationing-body-fair-tossing-coin-says-ethics-expert.html

Daniels N. 1988. *Am I My Parents' Keeper? An Essay on Justice Between the Young and the Old.* New York: Oxford University Press.

Daniels N. 2015. Can there be moral force in favoring an identified over a statistical life? In *Identified Versus Statistical Lives: An Interdisciplinary Perspective,* edited by IG Cohen, N Daniels, N Eyal. New York: Oxford University Press, 110–23.

Daniels N. 1985. *Just Health Care.* Cambridge, UK: Cambridge University Press.

Daniels N. 1986. Why saying no to patients in the United States is so hard: cost containment, justice, and provider autonomy. *New England Journal of Medicine* 314: 1381–83.

Daniels N, Sabin J. 1998a. Last chance therapies and managed care: pluralism, fair procedures and legitimacy. *Hastings Center Report* 28(2): 27–41.

Daniels N, Sabin J. 1997. Limits to health care: fair procedures, democratic deliberation, and the legitimacy problem for insurers. *Philosophy and Public Affairs* 26: 303–50.

Daniels N, Sabin J. 2008. *Setting Limits Fairly: Learning to Share Resources for Health.* New York: Oxford University Press.

Daniels N, Sabin J. 1998b. The ethics of accountability and the reform of managed care organizations. *Health Affairs* 17(5): 50–69.

Davis DM. 2018. *The Beautiful Cure: The Revolution in Immunology and What It Means for Your Health.* Chicago: University of Chicago Press.

DeCamp M, Sulmasy LS. 2021. Ethical and professionalism implications of physician employment and health care business practices: a policy paper from the American College of Physicians. *Annals of Internal Medicine* 174(6): 844–51. doi: 10.7326/M20-7093.DeRosier J. 2019. New indications may accelerate "explosion" in CAR T-cell therapy, but more education still needed. *HemOnc Today* (March 25). Accessed 7/7/2020. https://www.healio.com/news/hematology-oncology/20190312/new-indications-may-accelerate-explosion-in-car-tcell-therapy-but-more-education-still-needed

DiLoreto R, Khush K, Vlaminck ID. 2017. Precision monitoring of immunotherapies in solid organ and hematopoietic stem cell transplantation. *Advanced Drug Delivery Reviews* 114: 272–84.

Drilon A, Laetsch DW, Kummar S, DuBois SG, Steven G, Lassen UN, et al. 2018. Efficacy of larotrectinib in TRK fusion-positive cancers in adults and children. *New England Journal of Medicine* 378: 731–39.

Drilon A, Oxnard GR, Tan DSW, Loong HHF, Johnson M, Gainor J, et al. 2020. Efficacy of selpercaptinib in RET fusion-positive non-small-cell lung cancer. *New England Journal of Medicine* 383: 813–24.

Duckett S. 2022. Challenges of economic evaluation in rare diseases. *Journal of Medical Ethics* 48: 93–4.

Dudley JC, Lin MT, Le DT, Eshleman JR. 2016. Microsatellite instability as a biomarker for PD-1 blockade. *Clinical Cancer Research* 22: 813–20.

Dunbar SB, Khavjou OA, Bakas T, Hunt G, Kirch RA, Leib AR, et al. 2018. Projected costs of informal caregiving for cardiovascular disease: 2015 to 2025: A policy statement from the American Heart Association. *Circulation* 137: e558–e577.

Durkee BY, Qian Y, Pollom EL, King MT, Dudley SA, Shaffer JL, et al. 2015. Cost-effectiveness of perytuzumab in human epidermal growth factor receptor 2—positive metastatic breast cancer. *Journal of Clinical Oncology* 34: 902–09.

Dworkin R. 2000. *Sovereign Virtue: The Theory and Practice of Equality.* Cambridge, MA: Harvard University Press.

Dworkin R. 1981. What is equality? Part 1: equality of welfare. *Philosophy & Public Affairs* 10: 228–40.

Eddy DM. 1996. *Clinical Decision Making: From Theory to Practice.* Boston: Jones and Bartlett.

Eisenstein M. 2020. Taking cancer out of circulation. *Nature* 579 (March 26): S6–S8.

Emanuel E. 2020. *Which Country Has the World's Best Health Care?* New York: Public Affairs Press.

Engelhardt T. 1996. *The Foundations of Bioethics* (2nd ed). New York: Oxford University Press.

Epanomeritakis IK. 2019. Moral ambivalence towards the Cancer Drugs Fund. *Journal of Medical Ethics* 45: 623–26.

Estlund DM. 2008. *Democratic Authority: A Philosophic Framework.* Princeton: Princeton University Press.

Eyal N. 2013. Denial of treatment to obese patients—the wrong policy on personal responsibility for health. *International Journal of Health Policy and Management* 1(2): 107–10.

Feller S. 2015. Study: superlative use by media overhypes medical research. *UPI Health News* (Nov. 2). Accessed 1/4/2019. https://www.upi.com/Health_News/2015/11/02/Study-Superlative-use-by-media-overhypes-medical-research/9381446470460/

Ferkol T, Quinton P. 2015. Precision medicine: at what price? *American Journal of Respiratory and Critical Care Medicine* 192: 658–59.

Ferlay J, Colombet M, Soerjomataram I, Dyba T, Randi G, Bettio M, et al. 2018. Cancer incidence and mortality patterns in Europe: estimates for 40 countries and 25 major cancers in 2018. *European Journal of Cancer* 103: 356–87.

Figueroa JF, Wadhera RK, Jha AK. 2020. Eliminating wasteful health care spending—is the United States simply spinning its wheels? *JAMA Cardiology* 5: 9–10.

Fink S. 2021. The rationing of last-resort COVID treatment. *New York Times* (July 12). https://www.nytimes.com/2021/07/12/us/covid-treatment-ecmo.html

Finkel RS, Mercuri E, Darras BT, Connolly AM, Kuntz NL, Kirschner J, et al. 2017. Nusinersen versus sham control in infantile-onset spinal muscular atrophy. *New England Journal of Medicine* 377: 1723–32.

Fleck LM. 2021. Alzheimer's and aducanumab: unjust profits and false hopes. *Hastings Center Report* 51(4): 7–9.

Fleck LM. 2016a. Choosing wisely: is parsimonious care just rationing? *Cambridge Quarterly of Healthcare Ethics* 25: 366–76.

Fleck, LM. 2016b. Just caring: the insufficiency of the sufficiency principle in health care. In *What is Enough? Sufficiency, Justice, and Health*, edited by C Fourie, A Rid. New York: Oxford University Press, 223–43.

Fleck LM. 1987. DRGs: justice and the invisible rationing of health care resources. *Journal of Medicine and Philosophy* 12: 165–96.

Fleck LM. 2013. Just caring: can we afford the ethical and economic costs of circumventing cancer drug resistance? *Journal of Personalized Medicine* 3(3): 124–43.

Fleck LM. 2009. *Just Caring: Health Care Rationing and Democratic Deliberation*. New York: Oxford University Press.

Fleck LM. 1994. Just caring: Oregon, health care rationing, and informed democratic deliberation. *Journal of Medicine and Philosophy* 19: 367–88.

Fleck LM. 2018. Just caring: precision medicine, cancer biomarkers, and ethical ambiguity. In *Cancer Biomarkers: Ethics, Economics, and Society*, edited by A Blanchard, R Strand. Kokstod, Norway: Megaloceros Press, 73–94.

Fleck LM. 1992. Just health care rationing: a democratic decision making approach. *University of Pennsylvania Law Review* 140(5): 1597–1636.

Fleck LM. 1990. Justice, HMOs, and the invisible rationing of health care resources. *Bioethics* 4: 97–120.

Fleck LM. 2022. Precision medicine and the fragmentation of solidarity (and justice). *Medicine, Health Care, and Philosophy*. 1–16. doi: 10.1007/s11019-022-10067-2

Fleck LM. 2012. Whoopie pies, super-sized fries: "just" snacks? "just" des(s)erts?" *Cambridge Quarterly of Healthcare Ethics* 20: 5–19.

Ford C. 2020. Lansing man celebrates coronavirus recovery after 90 days in the hospital. WILX-TV (June 19). Accessed 6/25/2020. https://www.wilx.com/search?searchK eywords=Lansing+man+celebrates+coronavirus+recovery+after+90+days+in+the+ hospital

Fourie C. 2017. Sufficiency of capabilities, social equality, and two-tiered health care. In *What Is Enough? Sufficiency, Justice, and Health*, edited by C Fourie, A Rid. New York: Oxford University Press, 185–204.

Fousek K, Watanabe J, Joseph SK, George A, An X, Byrd TA, et al. 2021. CAR T-cells that target acute B-lineage leukemia irrespective of CD19 expression. *Leukemia* 35: 75–89. https://doi.org/10.1038/s41375-020-0792-2

Frangoul H, Altschuler D, Cappellini MD, Chen YS, Domm J, Eustace BK, et al. 2021. CRISPR-cas9 gene-editing for sickle cell disease and β-thalassemia. *New England Journal of Medicine* 384(3): 252–60. doi: 10.1056NEJMoa2031054

Frankfurt H. 1987. Equality as a moral ideal. *Ethics* 98: 21–43.

Friesen P. 2018. Personal responsibility within health policy: unethical and ineffective. *Journal of Medical Ethics* 44: 53–58.

Fuerst ML. 2019. TMB predicts immunotherapy success in colorectal cancer. *MedPage Today* (Oct. 11). Accessed 11/8/2020. https://www.medpagetoday.com/reading-room/ asco/immunotherapy/82653

Garon EB, Hellman MD, Rizvi NA, Cercereny E, Leighl NB, Ahn M, et al. 2019. Five-year overall survival for patients with advanced non-small-cell lung cancer treated with pembrolizumab: results from the phase I Keynote-001 study. *Journal of Clinical Oncology* 37: 2518–27.

Garraway LA. 2013. Genomics-driven oncology: framework for an emerging paradigm. *Journal of Clinical Oncology* 31: 1806–14.

Gaus GF. 1997. Reason, justification, and consensus: why democracy cannot have it all. In *Deliberative Democracy: Essays on Reason and Politics*, edited by J Bohman, W Rehg. Cambridge, MA: MIT Press, 205–42.

Gauthier J, Hirayuama AV, Purusche J, Hay KA, Lymp J, Li DH, et al. 2020. Feasibility and efficacy of CD19-targeted CAR T cells with concurrent ibrutinib for CLL after ibrutinib failure. *Blood* 135: 1650–60.

George J. 2021a. Novel Alzheimer's drug appears to slow decline. *MedPage Today* (Jan. 11). Accessed 1/12/2021. https://www.medpagetoday.com/neurology/alzheimersdisease/90636

George J. 2021b. Another Duchenne treatment gets FDA nod. *MedPage Today* (Feb. 25). Accessed 2/28/2021. https://www.medpagetoday.com/neurology/generalneurology/91367

Gerlinger M, Rowan AJ, Horswell S, Larkin J, Endesfelder D, Gronroos E, et al. 2012. Intratumor heterogeneity and branched evolution revealed by multiregion sequencing. *New England Journal of Medicine* 366: 883–92.

Gettinger SN, Horn L, Gandhi L, Spigel GL, Antonia SJ, Rizvi NA, et al. 2015. Overall survival and long term safety of nivolumab (anti-programmed death 1 antibody, BMS-936558, ONO-4538) in patients with previously treated advanced non-small-cell lung cancer. *Journal of Clinical Oncology* 33: 2004012.

Giugliano RP, Pedersen TR, Saver JL, Sever PS, Keech AC, Bohula EA, et al. 2020. Stroke prevention with the PCSK9 (proprotein convertase subtilisin-kexin type 9) inhibitor evolocumab added to statin in high-risk patients with stable atherosclerosis. *Stroke* 51: 1546–54.

Goldstein DA, Den RB. 2019. Patient-centered oncology or population-centered oncology—which do you want, and which tradeoffs are we willing to accept? *The Oncologist* 24: 288–90.

Goodin RE. 2003. *Reflective Democracy*. New York: Oxford University Press.

Grady D. 2016. 1 Patient, 7 Tumors, and 100 Billion Cells Equal 1 Striking Recovery. *New York Times* (Dec. 7). https://www.nytimes.com/2016/12/07/health/cancer-immunotherapy.html

Graeber C. 2018. *The Breakthrough: Immunotherapy and the Race to Cure Cancer.* New York: Twelve Publishing.

Greenhouse L. 1993. Hospital appeals ruling on treating baby born with most of brain gone. *New York Times* (Sept. 24). Accessed 10/5/2020. https://www.nytimes.com/1993/09/24/us/hospital-appeals-ruling-on-treating-baby-born-with-most-of-brain-gone.html

Grens K. 2019. The next frontier of CAR T-cell therapy: solid tumors. *The Scientist* (March 31). https://www.the-scientist.com/features/the-next-frontier-of-car-t-cell-therapy-solid-tumors-65612

Gutmann A, Thompson D. 2003. Deliberative democracy beyond process. In *Debating Deliberative Democracy*, edited by J Fishkin, P Laslett. London: Blackwell, 31–53.

Gutmann A, Thompson D. 1996. *Democracy and Disagreement: Why Moral Conflict Cannot Be Avoided in Politics and What Should Be Done About It.* Cambridge, MA: Harvard University Press.

Gutmann A, Thompson D. 2004. *Why Deliberative Democracy?* Princeton: Princeton University Press.Ham C. 1999. Tragic choices in health care: lessons from the child B case. *BMJ* 319: 1258–61.

Hamid O, Robert C, Daud A, Hodi FS, Hwu WJ, Kefford R, et al. 2019. Five-year survival outcomes for patients with advanced melanoma treated with pembrolizumab in Keynote-001. *Annals of Oncology* 30: 582–88.

Harris J. 1987. QALYfying the value of human life. *Journal of Medical Ethics* 13: 117–23.

Harris J. 1985. *The Value of Life*. Oxford, UK: Routledge and Kegan Paul.

Harris R. 2016. Medicare pays for a kidney transplant, but not the drugs to keep it viable. National Public Radio (Dec. 22). Accessed 3/22/2018. https://www.npr.org/sections/health-shots/2016/12/22/506319553/medicare-pays-for-a-kidney-transplant-but-not-the-drugs-to-keep-it-viable

Harrison C. 2018. RCC treatment costs could negatively affect health. *Renal and Urology News* (Jan. 22). Accessed 11/26/2018. https://www.renalandurologynews.com/kidney-cancer/renal-cell-carcinoma-treatment-costs-barrier/article/738290/

Hassel JC. 2016. Ipilimumab versus nivolumab in advanced melanoma. *Lancet Oncology* 17: 1471–72.

Hausman DM. 2015. *Valuing Health: Well-Being, Freedom, and Suffering*. New York: Oxford University Press.

Hellman MD, Ciuleanu TE, Pluzanski A, Lee JS, Otterson GA, Audigier-Valette C, et al. 2018. Nivolumab plus ipilimumab in lung cancer with a high tumor mutational burden. *New England Journal of Medicine* 378: 2093–2104.

Hellman MD, Paz-Ares L, Caro RB, Zurawski B, Kim SW, Costa EC, et al. 2019. Nivolumab plus ipilimumab in advanced non-small-cell lung cancer. *New England Journal of Medicine* 381: 2020–31.

Herder M. 2017. What is the purpose of the Orphan Drug Act? *PLoS Medicine* 14(1): e1000291. Accessed 3/14/2018. http://journals.plos.org/plosmedicine/article/file?id=10.1371/journal.pmed.1002191&type=printable

Himmelstein D, Campbell T, Woolhandler S. 2020. Health care administrative costs in the United States and Canada, 2017. *Annals of Internal Medicine* 172: 134–42.

Hirsch FR, Suda K, Wiens J, Bunn PA. 2016. New and emerging targeted treatments in advanced non-small-cell lung cancer. *Lancet* 388: 1012–24.

Hlatky MA. 2019. A pound of prevention? Assessing the value of new cholesterol-lowering drugs. *Annals of Internal Medicine* 170(4): 264–65. doi: 10.7326/M18-3632

Hlatky MA, Kazi DS. 2017. PCSK9 inhibitors: economics and policy. *Annals of Internal Medicine* 70: 2677–87.

Hofmann B. 2013. Priority setting in health care: trends and models from Scandinavian Countries. *Medicine, Health Care and Philosophy* 16: 349–56.

Hofmarcher T, Lingren P, Wilking N, Jonsson B. 2020. The cost of cancer care in Europe 2018. *European Journal of Cancer* 129: 41–49.

Holguin F. 2018. Triple CFTR modulator therapy for cystic fibrosis. *New England Journal of Medicine* 379: 1671–72.

Holstein SA, Lunning MA. 2020. CAR T-cell therapy in hematologic malignancies: a voyage in progress. *Clinical Pharmacology & Therapeutics* 107: 112–22.

Holtug N. 2006. Prioritarianism. In *Egalitarianism: New Essays on the Nature and Value of Equality*, edited by N Holtug, K Lippert-Rasmussen. Oxford: Clarendon Press, 125–56.

Honey K. 2017. FDA approves fourth ALK inhibitor for lung cancer. *American Association for Cancer Research blog* (May 5). Accessed 1/14/2018. http://blog.aacr.org/fda-approves-fourth-alk-inhibitor-for-lung-cancer/

Hong DS, Fakih MG, Strickler JH, Desai J, Durm GA, Shapiro GI, et al. 2020. KRAS (F12C) inhibition with sotorasib in advanced solid tumors. *New England Journal of Medicine* 383: 1207–17.

Horgan J. 2020. The cancer industry: hype vs. reality. *Scientific American* (Feb. 12). Accessed 9/20/2020. https://blogs.scientificamerican.com/cross-check/the-cancer-industry-hype-vs-reality/?print=true

Hunt L. 2015. The case for two-tiered health care: a three-pronged defense. Linked in (Oct. 17). Accessed 1/21/2021. https://www.linkedin.com/pulse/case-two-tiered-health-care-three-pronged-defense-liam-hunt/

Ingram I. 2020. Chemo-free combo boosts PFS in first-line CLL. *MedPage* (Dec. 8). https://www.medpagetoday.com/meetingcoverage/ashhematology/90091?xid=nl_mpt_DHE_2020-12-09&eun=g322269d0r&utm_source=Sailthru&utm_medium=email&utm_campaign=Daily%20Headlines%20Top%20Cat%20HeC%20%202020-12-09&utm_term=NL_Daily_DHE_dual-gmail-definition

Institute for Clinical and Economic Review. 2016. A look at treatments for non-small cell lung cancer. (October). Accessed 3/18/2018. https://icer.org/news-insights/press-releases/nsclc-evidence-report/

Institute for Clinical and Economic Review. 2020. Modulator treatments for cystic fibrosis: effectiveness and value. Evidence report (May 3). Accessed 4/24/2022. https://icer.org/wp-content/uploads/2020/08/ICER_CF_Evidence_Report_042720.pdf https://www.sciencedaily.com/releases/2019/02/190221130242.htm

iSpot.tv. 2015. Longer life [TV ad for Opdivo]. Accessed 1/29/2017. https://www.ispot.tv/ad/AL_Z/opdivo-longer-life

iSpot.tv. 2017. A chance to live longer [TV ad for Opdivo]. Accessed 9/20/2020. https://www.ispot.tv/ad/wIsF/opdivo-a-chance-to-live-longer

Jacobson CA, Hunter BD, Redd R, Rodig SJ, Chen PH, Wright K, et al. 2020. Axicabtagene ciloleucel in the non-trial setting: outcomes and correlates of response, resistance, and toxicity. *Journal of Clinical Oncology* 38: 3095–3106.

Jain N, Keating M, Thompson P, Ferrajoli A, Burger J, Borthakur G, et al. 2019. Ibrutinib and venetoclax for first-line treatment of CLL. *New England Journal of Medicine* 380: 2095–2103.

Jamal-Hanjani M, Wilson GA, McGranahan N, Birkbak NJ, Watkins TB, Veeriah S, et al. 2017. Tracking the evolution of non-small-cell lung cancer. *New England Journal of Medicine* 376: 2109–21.

James A, Mannon RB. 2015. The cost of transplant immunosuppressant therapy: is this sustainable? *Current Transplantation Reports* 2(2): 113–21.

Jones S. 2018. Pharma CEO says its "moral" to increase drug price by 400%. *New Republic* (Sept. 11). Accessed 12/11/2018. https://newrepublic.com/minutes/151165/pharma-ceo-says-its-moral-increase-drug-price-400

Joy K. 2019. A $34,000 drug for postpartum depression brings praise, price concerns. *Michigan Health Lab blog* (April 5). Accessed 1/10/2021. https://labblog.uofmhealth.org/rounds/a-34000-drug-for-postpartum-depression-brings-praise-price-concerns

June CH. 2016. Drugging the undruggable Ras—immunotherapy to the rescue? *New England Journal of Medicine* 375: 2286–89.

June CH, Sadelain M. 2018. Chimeric antigen receptor therapy. *New England Journal of Medicine* 379: 64–73.

Kaiser J. 2018. "Liquid biopsy" promises early detection of cancer. *Science* (Jan. 18). Accessed 1/23/2019. http://www.sciencemag.org/news/2018/01/liquid-biopsy-promises-early-detection-cancer

Kaiser J. 2015. The cancer stem cell gamble. *Science* 347(6219): 226–29.

Kamm F. 1993. *Morality, Mortality: Death and Whom to Save From It.* Vol. 1. New York: Oxford University Press.

Kant, Immanuel. 2008. (orig. 1781, first edition; 1787, second edition). *Critique of Pure Reason.* Translate by Ma Muller. New York: Penguin Classics.

Kasakovski D, Xu L, Li Y. 2018. T cell senescence and CAR-T cell exhaustion in hematological malignancies. *Journal of Hematology & Oncology* 11: 91. https://doi.org/10.1186/s13045-018-0629-x

Kaufman S. 2015. *Ordinary Medicine: Extraordinary Treatments, Longer Lives, and Where to Draw the Line.* Durham, NC: Duke University Press.

Kazi DS. 2020. Making tafimidis cost-effective for TTR amyloid cardiomyopathy may require 93% price reduction. *Cardiology Today* (Feb. 19). Accessed 8/2/2020. https://www.healio.com/news/cardiology/20200219/making-tafimidis-costeffective-for-ttr-amyloid-cardiomyopathy-may-require-93-price-reduction

Kazi DS, Bellows BK, Baron SJ, Shen C, Spertus JA, Yeh RW, et al. 2020. Cost-effectiveness of tafamidis therapy foe transthyretin amyloid cardiomyopathy. *Circulation* 141: 1214–24.

Kazi DS, Moran AE, Coxson PG, Penko J, Ollendorf DA, Pearson SD, et al. 2016. Cost-effectiveness of PCSK9 inhibitor therapy in patients with heterozygous familial hypercholesterolemia or atherosclerotic cardiovascular disease. *JAMA* 316: 743–53.

Kazi DS, Penko J, Coxson PG, Guzman D, Wei PC, Bibbens-Domingo K. 2019. Cost-effectiveness of alirocumab: a just-in-time analysis based on the ODYSSEY outcomes trial. *Annals of Internal Medicine* 170(4): 221–29. doi: 10.7326/M18-1776

Keehan SP, Cuckler GA, Poisal JA, Sisko AM, Smith SD, Madison AJ, et al. 2020. National health expenditure projections, 2019–28: expected rebound in prices drives rising spending growth. *Health Affairs* 39: 704–14.

Knight C, Stemplowska Z. (eds). 2011. *Responsibility and Distributive Justice.* New York: Oxford University Press.

Knox R. 2015. Cancer drug mark-ups: year of Gleevec costs $159 to make but sells for $106K. Accessed 4/25/2022 https://www.wbur.org/news/2015/09/25/cancer-drug-cost.

Knox R. 2018. New cancer treatments top $500,000 and raise daunting questions about how to pay [WBUR broadcast transcript]. (Jan. 11). Accessed 2/2/2019. https://www.wbur.org/commonhealth/2018/01/11/cancer-drug-costs

Kolata G. 2022. A cancer treatment makes leukemia vanish, but creates more mysteries. *New York Times* (Feb. 2). Accessed 4/24/2022. https://www.nytimes.com/2022/02/02/health/leukemia-car-t-immunotherapy.html.

Kolata G. 2019. Two new drugs help relieve sickle-cell disease. *New York Times* (Dec. 7). Accessed 7/9/2020. https://www.nytimes.com/2019/12/07/health/sickle-cell-adakveo-oxbryta.html

Komisar H. 2017. Premium support is the wrong direction for Medicare. *AARP Insight on the Issues* (October). Accessed 8/27/2020. https://www.aarp.org/content/dam/aarp/ppi/2017/10/premium-support-is-the-wrong-direction-for-medicare.pdf

Kopetz S, Grothey A, Yaeger R, Van Cutsem E, Desai J, Yoshino T, et al. 2019. Encorafenib, binimetinib, and cetuximab in BRAF V600E–mutated colorectal cancer. *New England Journal of Medicine* 381: 1632–43.

Krohmal BJ, Emanuel EJ. 2007. Access and ability to pay: the ethics of a tiered health care system. *Archives of Internal Medicine* 167: 433–37.

Kuehn BM. 2018. High costs and caution yield slow start to new heart drugs. *Circulation* 137: 197–99.

Kurella M, Covinsky KE, Collins AJ, Chertow GM. 2007. Octogenarians and nonagenarians starting dialysis in the United States. *Archives of Internal Medicine* 146: 177–83.

Lafont K. 2020. *Democracy Without Shortcuts: A Participatory Conception of Deliberative Democracy.* New York: Oxford University Press.

Larkin J, Chiarion-Sileni V, Gonalez R, Grob JJ, Rutkowski P, Lao CD, et al. 2019. Five-year survival with combined nivolumab and ipilimumab in advanced melanoma. *New England Journal of Medicine* 381: 1535–46.

Lathia J, Liu H, Matei D. 2020. The clinical impact of cancer stem cells. *The Oncologist* 25: 123–31.

Lawrence L. 2018. Single-agent ibrutinib active at 5 years in CLL, SLL. *Cancer Network* (Feb. 20). Accessed 2/21/2018. http://www.cancernetwork.com/news/single-agent-ibrutinib-active-5-years-cll-sll

Le QA, Bae YH, Kang JH. 2016. Cost-effectiveness analysis of trastuzumab emtansine (T-DM1) in human epidermal growth factor receptor 2 (HER2): positive advanced breast cancer. *Breast Cancer Research and Treatment* 159: 565–73.

LeMieux J. 2018. Cancer stem cells redefine how we think about cancer. *Cell Science* (March 21). Accessed 12/19/2018. https://www.technologynetworks.com/cell-scie nce/articles/cancer-stem-cells-redefine-how-we-think-about-cancer-298848

Lemonick MD, Park A. 2001. New hope for cancer. *Time* (May 28). Accessed 4/25/2022. http://content.time.com/time/subscriber/article/0,33009,999978,00.html.

Leopold C, Peppercorn JM, Zafar SY, Wagner AK. 2018. Defining value of cancer therapeutics—a health system perspective. *Journal of the National Cancer Institute* 110: 699–703.

Levenson D. 2020. A new era for liquid biopsy. *Clinical Laboratory News* (Nov. 1). Accessed 2/1/2021. https://www.aacc.org/cln/articles/2020/november/a-new-era-for-liquid-biopsy

Levy N. 2019. Taking responsibility for responsibility. *Public Health Ethics* 12(2): 103–13.

Liao JM, Fischer MA. 2017. Restrictions of hepatitis C treatment for substance-using Medicaid patients: cost versus ethics. *American Journal of Public Health* 107: 893–99.

Lim WA, June CH. 2017. The principles of engineering immune cells to treat cancer. *Cell* 168: 724–40.

Lin JK, Muffly LS, Spinner MA, Barnes JI, Owens DK, Goldhaber-Fiebert JD. 2019. Cost effectiveness of chimeric antigen receptor T-cell therapy in multiply relapsed or refractory adult large B-cell lymphoma. *Journal of Clinical Oncology* 37: 2105–19.

Linley WG, Hughes DA. 2013. Societal views on NICE, cancer drugs fund and value based pricing criteria for prioritizing medicines: a cross-sectional survey of 4118 adults in Great Britain. *Health Economics* 22: 948–64.

Liu S, Watcha D, Holodniy M, Goldhaber-Fiebert JD. 2014. Sofosbuvir-based treatment regimens for chronic, genotype 1 hepatitis C virus infection in US incarcerated populations: a cost-effectiveness analysis. *Annals of Internal Medicine* 161(8): 546–53.

Lo JH, U KP, Yiu T, Ong MT, Lee WY. 2020. Sarcopenia: current treatment and new regenerative approaches. *Journal of Orthopedic Translation* 23: 38–52.

Locke, John. 1998 (orig.1689). *An Essay Concerning Human Understanding.* New York: PenguinClassics.

Lomasky L. 1980. Medical progress and national health care. *Philosophy and Public Affairs* 10: 65–88.

Longo DL. 2012. Tumor heterogeneity and personalized medicine. *New England Journal of Medicine* 366: 956–57.

Lunning M, Vose J, NastoupilL, Fowler N, Burger JA, Wierda WG, et al. 2019. Ublituximab and umbralisib in relapsed/reflectory B-cell non-Hodgkin lymphoma and chronic lymphocytic leukemia. *Blood* 134: 1811–20.

Magalhaes M. 2022. Should rare diseases get special treatment? *Journal of Medical Ethics* 48: 86–92.

Mahlangu J, Oldenburg J, Paz-Priel I, Negrier C, Niggli M, Mancuso E, et al. 2018. Emicizumab prophylaxis in patients who have hemophilia A without inhibitors. *New England Journal of Medicine* 379: 811–22.

Maj E, Papiernik D, Wietrzyk J. 2016. Antiangiogenic cancer treatment: the great discovery and greater complexity (review). *International Journal of Oncology* 49: 1773–84.

Majzner RG, Mackall CL. 2019. Clinical lessons learned from the first leg of the CAR T cell journey. *Nature Medicine* 25: 1341–55.

Makena MR, Ranjan A, Thirumala V, Reddy AP. 2020. Cancer stem cells: road to therapeutic resistance and strategies to overcome resistance. *BBA—Molecular Basis of Disease* 1866: 165339.

Mallal S, Phillips E, Carosi G, Molina JM, Workman C, Tomazic J, et al. 2008. HLA-B*5701 screening for hypersensitivity to abacavir. *New England Journal of Medicine* 358: 568–79.

Malone ER, Oliva M, Sabatini PJB, Stockley TL, Siu LL. 2020. Molecular profiling for precision cancer therapies. *Genome Medicine* 12: 8. doi: 10.1186/s13073-019-0703-1

Mandavilli A. 2021. F.D.A. approves monthly shots to treat H.I.V. *New York Times* (Jan. 21). Accessed 1/21/2021. https://www.nytimes.com/2021/01/21/health/hiv-cabenuva.html

Marcus AD. 2020. Gene editing shows promise in sickle-cell disease. *Wall Street Journal* (Dec. 5). https://www.wsj.com/articles/gene-editing-shows-promise-in-sickle-cell-disease-11607189442

Masters GA, Temin S, Azzoli CG, Giaccone G, Baker S, Brahmer JR, et al. 2015. Systemic therapy for stage IV non-small-cell lung cancer: American Society of Clinical Oncology clinical practice guideline update. *Journal of Clinical Oncology* 33: 3488–3516.

McGinley L, Johnson CY. 2017. FDA clears first gene-altering therapy—'a living drug'—for childhood leukemia. *Washington Post* (August 30). Accessed 4/22/2022. https://www.washingtonpost.com/news/to-your-health/wp/2017/08/30/fda-approves-first-of-its-kind-living-drug-for-childhood-leukemia/.

McKerlie D. 1996. Equality. *Ethics* 106: 274–96.

McKie J, Richardson J. 2003. The rule of rescue. *Social Science and Medicine* 56: 2407–19.

McMahon C. 2009. *Reasonable Disagreement: A Theory of Political Morality*. Cambridge, UK: Cambridge University Press.

Mechanic D. 1997. Muddling through elegantly: finding the proper balance in rationing. *Health Affairs* 16(5): 83–92.

Mega JL, Close SL, Wiviott SD, Shen L, Hockett RD, Brandt JT, et al. 2009. Cytochrome P-450 polymorphisms and response to clopidogrel. *New England Journal of Medicine* 360: 354–62.

Mello MM, Brennan TA. 2001. The controversy over high-dose chemotherapy with autologous bone marrow transplant for breast cancer. *Health Affairs* 20: 101–17.

Mendes E. 2017. More than 4 in 10 cancers and cancer deaths linked to modifiable risk factors. American Cancer Society. Accessed 5/22/2020. https://www.cancer.org/latest-news/more-than-4-in-10-cancers-and-cancer-deaths-linked-to-modifiable-risk-factors.html

Menzel PT. 1983. *Medical Costs, Moral Choices*. New Haven: Yale University Press.

Menzel PT. 2012. The variable value of life and fairness to the already ill: two promising but tenuous arguments for treatment's priority. In *Prevention vs. Treatment: What's the Right Balance?*, edited by HS Faust, PT Menzel. New York: Oxford University Press, 194–218.

Mercuri E, Darras BT, Chiriboga CA, Day JW, Campbell C, Connolly AM, et al. 2018. Nusinersen versus sham control in later-onset spinal muscular atrophy. *New England Journal of Medicine* 378: 625–35.

Mickelson D, Ciafaloni E, Ashwal S, Lewis E, Narayanaswami P, Oskoui M, Armstrong MJ. 2018. Evidence in focus: nusinersen use in spinal muscular atrophy. Report of the Guideline Development, Dissemination, and Implementation Subcommittee of the American Academy of Neurology. *Neurology* 91: 923–33.

Miller J. 2018. U.S. FDA expands approval of Roche hemophilia drug. *Reuters* (Oct. 4). Accessed 10/4/2020. https://www.reuters.com/article/us-roche-hldg-hemlibra-appro val/u-s-fda-expands-approval-of-roche-hemophilia-drug-idUSKCN1ME29T

Millman J. 2015. The coming revolution in much cheaper life-saving drugs. *Washington Post* (Jan. 16). Accessed 4/24/2016. https://www.washingtonpost.com/news/wonk/wp/ 2015/01/16/the-coming-revolution-in-much-cheaper-life-saving-drugs/

Minckwitz G, Huang CS, Mano MS, Loibl S, Mamounas EP, Untch M, et al. 2019. Trastuzumab emtansine for residual invasive HER2-positive breast cancer. *New England Journal of Medicine* 380: 617–28.

Mintun MA, Lo AC, Evans CD, Wessels AM, Ardayfio PA, Andersen SW, et al. 2021. Donanemab in early Alzheimer's disease. *New England Journal of Medicine* 384(18): 1691–1704. doi: 10.1056/NEJMoa2100708

Mok TS, Wu WL, Kudaba I, Kowalski DM, Cho BC, Turna HC, et al. 2019. Pembrolizumab versus chemotherapy for previously untreated, PD-L1-expressing, locally advanced or metastatic non-small-cell lung cancer (Keynote-042): a randomized, open-label, con- trolled, phase 3 trial. *Lancet* 393: 1819–30.

Moriates C, Arora V, Shah N. 2015. *Understanding Value-Based Health Care.* New York: McGraw Hill Lange.

Morshuis M, Rojas SV, Hakim-Meibodi K, Rozumov A, Gummert JF, Schramm R. 2020. Heart transplantation after Syncardia total artificial heart implantation. *Annals of Cardiothoracic Surgery* 9(2): 98–103.

Moscoso A, Grothe MJ, Ashton NJ, Karikari TK, Rodriquez JL, Snellman A, et al. 2021. Longitudinal associations of blood phosphorylated tau181 and neurofilament light chain with neurodegeneration in Alzheimer disease. *JAMA Neurology* 78(4): 396–406. doi: 10.1001/jamaneurol.2020.4986

Mukherjee S. 2018. Cancer, our genes, and the anxiety of risk-based medicine. *Health Affairs* 37: 817–20.

Mukherjee S. 2010. *The Emperor of All Maladies.* New York: Simon and Schuster.

Mukherjee S. 2016. The improvisational oncologist. *New York Times Sunday Magazine* (May 15). Accessed 5/15/2016. http://www.nytimes.com/2016/05/15/magazine/onc ologist-improvisation.html?_r=0

Mullin E. 2017. Promising new cancer drugs won't go far unless everyone gets genetic testing. *MIT Technology Review* (June 6). Accessed 4/28/22 https://www.technologyrev iew.com/2017/06/06/151379/promising-new-cancer-drugs-wont-go-far-unless-every one-gets-genetic-testing/.

Murthy RK, Loi S, Okines A, Paplomata E, Hamilton E, Hurviz SA, et al. 2020. Tucatinib, trastuzumab, and capecitabine for HER2-positive metastatic breast cancer. *New England Journal of Medicine* 382: 597–609.

National Cancer Institute. 2022. Car T cells: engineering patients' immune cells to treat their cancers. (March 10). Accessed 4/24/2022. https://www.cancer.gov/about-cancer/ treatment/research/car-t-cells

National Cancer Institute: Surveillance, Epidemiology, and End Results Program. 2020. Cancer stat facts: cancer of any site. Accessed 5/5/2020. https://seer.cancer.gov/statfacts/html/all.html

National Institute for Health Care Management. 2012. The concentration of health care spending: NIHCM Foundation data brief. (July). Accessed 4/28/2022. https://nihcm.org/assets/articles/databrief3final.pdf

National Research Council: Committee on a Framework for Development of a New Taxonomy of Disease. 2011. *Toward Precision Medicine: Building a Knowledge Network for Biomedical Research and a New Taxonomy of Disease*. Washington, D.C.: National Academies Press.

Neelapu SS, Tummala S, Kebriaei P, Wierda W, Gutierrez C, Locke FL, et al. 2018. Chimeric antigen receptor T-cell therapy—assessment and management of toxicities. *Nature Reviews Clinical Oncology* 15: 47–62.

Nogrady B. 2016. Targeted therapies predicted to blow out costs for CLL. *Hematology News* (Nov. 21). Accessed 2/21/2018. https://www.mdedge.com/hematologynews/article/118611/cll/targeted-therapies-predicted-blow-out-costs-cll

Norwegian Ministry of Health and Care Services. 2017. *Principles for Priority Setting in Health Care* [White paper]. Oslo, Norway.

Olson D. 2018. A breakthrough in cancer treatment—a patient's story. *CLL Society Newsletter* (June 28). Accessed 2/3/2019. https://cllsociety.org/2018/06/a-breakthrough-in-cancer-treatment-a-patients-story/

Olson DJ, Eroglu Z, Brockstein B, Peklepovic AS, Bajaj M, Babu N, et al. 2021. Pembrolizumab plus ipilimumab following anti-PD-1/L1 failure in melanoma. *Journal of Clinical Oncology* 39(24): 2647–55. doi: 10.1200/JCO.21.00079Olson S, Robinson S, Giffin R.

O'Riordan M. 2020. "Outrageous" $225,000 per year list price for tafamidis draws outcry. *tctMD/the heart beat.* (Jan. 10). Accessed 6/18/2020. https://www.tctmd.com/news/outrageous-225000-year-list-price-tafamidis-draws-outcry

Ortega J, Vigil CE, Chodkiewicz C. 2010. Current progress in targeted therapy for colorectal cancer. *Cancer Control* 17: 7–15.

Oxnard G. 2019. New blood test capable of detecting multiple types of cancer. *Dana-Farber Cancer Institute News Release* (Sept. 28). https://www.dana-farber.org/newsroom/news-releases/2019/new-blood-test-capable-of-detecting-multiple-types-of-cancer/

Pandya A. 2018. Adding cost-effectiveness to define low-value care. *JAMA* 319: 1977–78.

Papanicolas I, Woskie LR, Jha AK. 2018. Health care spending in the United States and other high income countries. *JAMA* 319: 1024–39.

Parfit D. 2012. Another defense of the priority view. *Utilitas* 24: 399–440.

Parfit D. 1991. *Equality or Priority* (The Lindley Lecture, The University of Kansas). https://www.stafforini.com/docs/Parfit%20-%20Equality%20or%20priority.pdf

Patient Power. 2020. Mike Boston: CLL patient and advocate. https://patientpower.info/bio/mike-boston/

Pazdur R. 2019. FDA approves crizanlizumab-tmca for sickle cell disease. American Society of Clinical Oncology (Nov. 15). Accessed 10/5/20. https://www.asco.org/practice-policy/policy-issues-statements/asco-in-action/fda-approves-crizanlizumab-tmca-sickle-cell

Peacock SJ, Regier DA, Raymakers AJ, Chan KK. 2019. Evidence, values, and funding decisions in Canadian cancer systems. *Healthcare Management Forum* 32(6): 293–98.

Pendleton R. 2018. In health care, it's time to get a second opinion on what "value" stands for. *Stat* (Aug. 15). Accessed 12/2/2018. https://www.statnews.com/sponsor/2018/08/15/health-care-value-u-of-utah/

Peppercorn J. 2017. Financial toxicity and societal costs of cancer care: distinct problems require distinct solutions. *The Oncologist* 22: 123–25.

Persad G. 2015. Priority setting, cost-effectiveness, and the Affordable Care Act. *American Journal of Law and Medicine* 41: 119–66.

Pettitt DA, Raza S, Naughton B, Roscoe A, Ramakrishnan A, All A, et al. 2016. The limitations of QALY: a literature review. *Journal of Stem Cell Research and Therapy* 6: 4. doi: 10.4172/2157-7633.1000334

Pietrantonio F, Loupakis F, Randon G, Raimondo A, Salati M, Trapani D, et al. 2020. Efficacy and safety of immune checkpoint inhibitors in patients with microsatellite instability-high end-stage cancers and poor performance status related to high disease burden. *The Oncologist* 25: 803–09.

Pineda S, Sigdel TK, Chen J, Jackson AM, Sirota M, Sarwal MM. 2017. Novel non-histocompatibility antigen mismatch variants improve the ability to predict antibody-mediated rejection risk in kidney transplant. *Frontiers in Immunology* 8: 1687. doi: 10.3389/fimmu.2017.01687

Poisal JA, Sisko AM, Cuckler GA, Smith SD, Keehan SP, Fiore JA, et al. 2022. National health expenditure projections, 2021–30: growth to moderate as COVID-19 impacts wane. *Health Affairs* 41:474–86.

Pollack A. 2016. F.D.A. approves an immunotherapy drug for bladder cancer. *New York Times* (May 19). Accessed 5/19/2016. http://www.nytimes.com/2016/05/19/business/food-and-drug-administration-immunotherapy-bladder-cancer.html?emc=edit_th_20160519&nl=todaysheadlines&nlid=62793687&_r=0

Porter DL, Hwang WT, Frey NV, Lacey SF, Shaw PA, Loren AW, et al. 2015. Chimeric antigen receptor T cells persist and induce sustained remissions in relapsed refractory chronic lymphocytic leukemia. *Science Translational Medicine* 7(303): 303ra139.

Powers V. 2017. Study finds hyperprogression after immunotherapy in NSCLC subset. *OncLive* (Sept. 14). Accessed 2/9/2018. http://www.onclive.com/conference-coverage/esmo-2017/study-finds-hyperprogression-after-immunotherapy-in-nsclc-subset?p=1

Prakash V. 2017. Spinraza—a rare disease success story. *Gene Therapy* 24: 497.

Prasad V. 2020. Malignant: *How Bad Policy and Bad Evidence Harm People with Cancer*. Baltimore, MD: Johns Hopkins University Press.

Prasad V. 2018. Tisangenlecleucel—the first approved CAR-T-cell therapy: implications for payers and policymakers. *Nature Reviews: Clinical Oncology* 15: 11–12.

Prasad V, Kaestner V, Mailonkody S. 2018. Cancer drugs approved on biomarkers and not tumor type—FDA approval of pembrolizumab for mismatch repair-deficient solid tumors. *JAMA Oncology* 4: 157–58.

Prasad V, Vandross A. 2015. Characteristics of exceptional or super responders to cancer drugs. *Mayo Clinic Proceedings* 90: 1639–49.

Querido J. 2012. Imatinib—the dawn of targeted treatment. *Cancer Research UK* (Oct. 25). Accessed 4/25/2022. https://news.cancerresearchuk.org/2012/10/25/imatinib-the-dawn-of-targeted-treatments/

Raez LE, Santos ES. 2018. Tumor type-agnostic treatment and the future of cancer therapy. *Targeted Oncology* 13: 541–44.

Rahib L, Smith BD, Aizenberg R, Rosenzweig AB, Fleshman JM, Matrisian LM. 2014. Projecting cancer incidence and deaths to 2030: the unexpected burden of thyroid, liver, and pancreas cancers in the United States. *Cancer Research* 74: 2913–21.

Rahman M, Deleyrolle L, Vedam-Mai V, Azari H, Abd-El-Barr M, Reynolds BA. 2011. The cancer stem cell hypothesis: failures and pitfalls. *Neurosurgery* 68: 531–45.

Ramalingam SS, Vansteenkiste J, Planchard D, Cho BC, Gray JE, Ohe Y, et al. 2020. Overall survival with osimertinib in untreated, EGFR-mutated advanced NSCLC. *New England Journal of Medicine* 382: 41–50.

Ramsey BW, Davies J, McElvaney NG, Tullis E, Bell SC, Drevenik P, et al. 2011. A CFTR potentiator in patients with cystic fibrosis and the G551D mutation. New England Journal of Medicine 365: 1663–1672

Ram-Tiktin E. 2017. Basic human functional capabilities as the currency of sufficientarian distribution in health care. In *What Is Enough? Sufficiency, Justice, and Health*, edited by C Fourie, A Rid. New York: Oxford University Press, 144–63.

Raspe E, Decraene C, Berx G. 2012. Gene expression profiling to dissect the complexity of cancer biology: pitfalls and promise. *Seminars in Cancer Biology* 22: 250–60.

Rawls J. 1971. *A Theory of Justice.* Cambridge, MA: Harvard University Press.

Rawls J. 1996. *Political Liberalism.* New York: Columbia University Press.

Raza A. 2019. *The First Cell: And the Human Costs of Pursuing Cancer to the Last.* New York: Basic Books.

Reck M, Rodriguez-Abreu D, Robinson AG, Hui R, Csoszi T, Fulop A, et al. 2016. Pembrolizumab versus chemotherapy for PD-L1-positive non-small-cell cancer. *New England Journal of Medicine* 375: 1823–33.

Reckers-Droog VT, Exel NJA, Brouwer WBF. 2018. Looking back and moving forward: on the application of proportional shortfall in healthcare priority setting in the Netherlands. *Health Policy* 122: 621–29.

Regalado A. 2016. Should we sequence the DNA of every cancer patient? *MIT Technology Review* (June 14). Accessed 11/26/2018. https://www.technologyreview.com/s/601 611/should-we-sequence-the-dna-of-every-cancer-patient/

Rein DB, Wittenborn JS, Smith BD, Liffman DK, Ward JW. 2015. The cost-effectiveness, health benefits, and financial costs of new antiviral treatments for hepatitis C virus. *Clinics in Infectious Disease* 61(2): 157–68.

Reindl JC. 2018. Heart transplant patient told to fundraise gets $30,000. *Detroit Free Press* (Nov. 30). Accessed 4/22/2022 https://www.freep.com/story/news/health/2018/11/30/ hedda-martin-spectrum-health-transplant/2162187002/.

Reinhardt U. 1982. Table manners at the health care feast. In *Financing Health Care: Competition versus Regulation*, edited by D. Yaggy and W.G. Anylan. Cambridge, MA: Ballinger, 13–34.

Reiter-Brennan C, Osei AD, Uddin SM, Orimoloye OA, Obisesan OH, Mirbolouk M, et al. 2020. ACC/AHA lipid guidelines: personalized care to prevent cardiovascular disease. *Cleveland Clinic Journal of Medicine* 87: 231–39.

Remon J, Lopes G. 2020. Upfront osimertinib—winner takes it all? *Nature Reviews Clinical Oncology* 17: 202–03.

Remon J, Steuer CE, Ramalingam SS, Felip E. 2018. Osimertinib and other third-generation EGFR TKJI in EGFR-mutant NSCLC patients. *Annals of Oncology* 29 (Supplement 1): i20–i127.

Richardson HS. 2002. *Democratic Autonomy: Public Reasoning About the Ends of Policy.* New York: Oxford University Press.

Rittel H, Webber M. 1973. Dilemmas in a general theory of planning. *Policy Science* 4: 155–69.

Robert C, Ribas A, Hamid O, Daud A, Wolchok JD, Joshua AM, et al. 2017. Durable complete response after discontinuation of pembrolizumab in patients with metastatic melanoma. *Journal of Clinical Oncology* 36: 1668–74.

Robert C, Ribas A, Hamid O, Daud A, Wolchok JD, Joshua AM, et al. 2016. Three-year overall survival for patients with advanced melanoma treated with pembrolizumab in KEYNOTE-001. Abstract presented at 2016 annual ASCO meeting. Accessed 4/28/ 2022. https://ascopubs.org/doi/abs/10.1200/JCO.2016.34.15_suppl.9503

Robert C, Ribas A, Schachter J, Arance A, Grob J, Mortier L, et al. 2019. Pembrolizumab versus ipilimumab in advanced melanoma (Keynote-006): post-hoc 5-year results from an open-label, multicentre, randomized, controlled phase 3 study. *Lancet Oncology* 20: 1239–51.

Rockoff JD. 2018. The million-dollar cancer treatment: who will pay? *Wall Street Journal* (April 27). Accessed 4/27/2018. https://www.wsj.com/articles/the-million-dollar-cancer-treatment-no-one-knows-how-to-pay-for-1524740401

Rosenbaum L. 2017. Tragedy, perseverance, and chance—the story of CAR-T therapy. *New England Journal of Medicine* 377: 1313–15.

Rosenthal E. 2017. *An American Sickness: How Healthcare Became Big Business and How You Can Take It Back.* New York: Penguin Press.

Rosoff P. 2017. *Drawing the Line: Healthcare Rationing and the Cutoff Problem.* New York: Oxford University Press.

Ross C. 2018. A new cancer care dilemma: patients want immunotherapy even when evidence is lacking. *Statnews* (June 4). Accessed 1/25/2019. https://www.statnews.com/ 2018/06/04/cancer-care-dilemma-immunotherapy/

Rumbold B, Weale A, Rid A, Wilson J, Littlejohns P. 2017. Public reasoning and health care priority: the case of NICE. *Kennedy Institute of Ethics Journal* 27: 107–34.

Russell L. 2010. *Is Prevention Better Than Cure?* Washington, D.C.: Brookings Institution Press.

Ruzzo A, Graziano F, Canestrari E, Magnani M. 2010. Molecular predictors of efficacy to anti-EGFR agents in colorectal cancer patients. *Current Cancer Drug Targets* 10: 68–79.

Sabatine MS, Giugliano RP, Keech AC, Honarpour N, Wiviott SD, Murphy SA, et al. 2017. Evolucumab and clinical outcomes in patients with cardiovascular disease. *New England Journal of Medicine* 376: 1713–22.

Salas-Vega S, Iliopoulos O, Mossialos E. 2017. Assessment of overall survival, quality of life, and safety benefits associated with new cancer medicines. *JAMA Oncology* 3: 382–90.

Salcher-Konrad M, Naci H, Davis C. 2020. Approval of cancer drugs with uncertain therapeutic value: a comparison of regulatory decisions in Europe and the United States. *Milbank Quarterly* 98: 1219–56. doi: 10.1111/1468-0009.12476

Scanlon T. 1976. Nozick on rights, liberty, and property. *Philosophy and Public Affairs* 6: 3–25.

Schauer F. 1995. Giving reasons. *Stanford Law Review* 47: 635–59.

Schmidt AF, Career JL, Pearce LS, Wilkins JT, Overington JP, Hingorani AD, Casas JP. 2020. PCSK9 monoclonal antibodies for the primary and secondary prevention of cardiovascular disease. *Cochrane Database Systematic Reviews* 10: CD011748. doi: 10.1002/146518858.CD011748.pub3

Schnipper LE, Bastian A. 2016. New frameworks to assess value of cancer care: strengths and Limitations. *The Oncologist* 21: 654–58.

Schoenberger SP, Cohen E. 2017. Neoantigens enable personalized cancer immuno-therapy. *The Scientist Magazine* (April). Accessed 1/12/2018. https://www.the-scient ist.com/?articles.view/articleNo/49000/title/Neoantigens-Enable-Personalized-Can cer-Immunotherapy/

Schrag D, Basch E. 2018. Oncology in transition: changes, challenges and opportunities. *JAMA* 320: 2203–04. doi: 10.1001/jama.2018.17057

Schuster SJ, Bishop MR, Tam CS, Waller EK, Borchmann P, McGuirk JP et al. 2019. Tisagenlecleucel in adult relapsed or refractory diffuse large B-cell lymphoma. *New England Journal of Medicine* 380: 45–56.

Search Collaborative Group, Link E, Parish S, Armitage J, Bowman L, Heath S, Matsuda F, et al. 2008. SLCO1B1 variants and statin-induced myopathy—a genomewide study. *New England Journal of Medicine* 359: 789–99.

Segall S. 2010. *Health, Luck, and Justice*. Princeton: Princeton University Press.

Serrano MJ, Garrido-Navas MC, Mochon JJ, Cristofanilli M, Gil-Bazo G, Pauwels P, et al. 2020. Precision prevention and cancer interception: the new challenges of liquid bi-opsy. *Cancer Discovery* 10: 1635–44.

Shah KK, Tsuchiya A, Wailoo AJ. 2015. Valuing health at the end of life: a stated prefer-ence discrete choice experiment. *Social Science & Medicine* 124: 48–56.

Shanafelt TD, Borah BJ, Finnes HD, Chafee KG, Ding W, Leis JF, et al. 2015. Impact of ibrutinib and idelalisib on the pharmaceutical cost of treating chronic lymphocytic leukemia at the individual and societal levels. *Journal of Oncology Practice* 11: 252–58.

Sharma P, Hu-Lieskovan S, Wargo JA, Ribas A. 2017. Primary, adaptive, and acquired re-sistance to cancer immunotherapy. *Cell* 168: 707–23.

Shaw AT, Felip E, Bauer TM, Besse B, Navarro A, Postel-Vinay S, et al. 2017. Lorlatinib in non-small-cell lung cancer with ALK or ROS1 rearrangement: an international, multi-center, open-label, single-arm, first-in-man phase 1 trial. *Lancet Oncology* 18: 1590–99.

Shitara K, Yatabe Y, Matsuo K, Sugano M, Kondo C, Takahari D, et al. 2013. Prognosis of patients with advanced gastric cancer by HER2 status and trastuzumab treatment. *Gastric Cancer* 16: 261–67.

Shohdy KS, West H. 2020. Circulating tumor DNA testing—liquid biopsy of a cancer. *JAMA Oncology* 6: 792.

Shrank WH, Rogstad TL, Parekh N. 2019. Waste in the US health care system: estimated costs and potential savings. *JAMA* 322: 1501–09.

Siegal RL, Miller KD, Fuchs HE, Jemal A. 2021. Cancer statistics, 2021. *CA: Cancer Journal for Clinicians* 712: 7–33.

Silverman E. 2016. FDA designated a record number of orphan drugs last year. *StatNews* (Feb. 11). Accessed 3/14/2018. https://www.statnews.com/pharmalot/2016/02/11/fda-designates-record-number-of-orphan-drugs/

http://blogs.wsj.com/pharmalot/2015/05/05/how-much-global-spending-on-cancer-medicines-hit-100b-last-year/

Simon S. 2019. Population of US cancer survivors grows to nearly 17 million. American Cancer Society. Accessed 5/19/2020. https://www.cancer.org/latest-news/population-of-us-cancer-survivors-grows-to-nearly-17-million.html

Sisko AM, Keehan SP, Poisal JA, Cuckler GA, Smith SD, Madison AJ, et al. 2019. National health expenditure projections, 2018–27: economic and demographic trends drive spending and enrollment growth. *Health Affairs* 38: 491–501.

Skarzynski J. 2019. Mosunetuzumab produces complete remissions in patients with non-Hodgkin lymphoma. *Cure* (Dec. 8). https://www.curetoday.com/view/mosunetuzu mab-produces-complete-remissions-in-patients-with-nonhodgkin-lymphoma

Slater H. 2021. FDA grants breakthrough therapy designation to trigolumab combo for PD-L1-high NSCLC. *Cancer Network* (Jan. 5). Accessed 1/18/2021. https://www.cancer network.com/view/fda-grants-breakthrough-therapy-designation-to-tiragolumab-combo-for-pd-l1-high-nsclc?utm_source=sfmc&utm_medium=email&utm_campa ign=1.15.21_CN_NSCLC%20TRC-AMG-21-OND0353-Amgen%20510&eKey=Zmx lY2tAbXN1LmVkdQ

Sleijfer S, Verweij J. 2016. Affordability of drugs used in oncology health care. *Nature Reviews: Clinical Oncology* 13: 331–32. doi: 10.1038/nrclinonc.2016.77

Smit EF, deLangen AJ. 2019. Pembrolizumab for all PD-L1-positive NSCLC. *Lancet* 393: 1776–78.

Soloman JP, Hechtman JF. 2019. Detection of NTRK fusions: merits and limitations of current diagnostic platforms. *Cancer Research* 79: 3163–68.

Sorenson C. 2012. Valuing end-of-life care in the United States: the case of new cancer drugs. *Health Economics, Policy and Law* 7: 411–30.

Sorin M, Franco EL, Quesnell-Vallee A. 2019. Inter- and intraprovincial inequities in public coverage of cancer drug programs across Canada: a plea for the establishment of a pan-Canadian pharmacare program. *Current Oncology* 26: 266–69.

Sparano JA, Gray RJ, Makower DF, Pritchard KI, Albain KS, Hayes DF, et al. 2015. Prospective validation of a 21-gene expression assay in breast cancer. *New England Journal of Medicine* 373: 2005–14.

Sprangers B, Nair V, Launay-Vacher V, Riella LV, Jhaveri KD. 2018. Risk factors associated with post-kidney transplant malignancies: an article from the Cancer-Kidney International Network. *Clinical Kidney Journal* 11: 315–29. doi: 10.1093/ckj/sfx122

Sprung A. 2016. Paul Ryan wants to Trump Medicare as we know it. *The Medicare Resource Center blog* (Nov. 19). Accessed 10/10/2020. https://www.medicareresources.org/blog/ 2016/11/19/paul-ryan-wants-to-trump-medicare-as-we-know-it/

Stadtmauer EA, O'Neill A, Goldstein LJ, Crilley PA, Mangan KF, Ingle JN, et al. 2000. Conventional-dose chemotherapy compared with high-dose chemotherapy plus autologous hematopoietic stem-cell transplantation for metastatic breast cancer. Philadelphia Bone Marrow Transplant Group . *New England Journal of Medicine* 342: 1069–76.

Steenhuysen J, Burger L. 2019. Inside drugmakers' strategy to boost cancer medicines "Lazarus effect." *London South East Finance News* (Sept. 6). Accessed 11/11/2020. https://www.lse.co.uk/news/insight-inside-drugmakers-strategy-to-boost-cancer-medicines-with-lazarus-effect-xidlsjwp7zpxknq.html

Stein MS. 2012. A utilitarian approach to justice in health care. In *Medicine and Social Justice: Essays on the Distribution of Health Care* (2nd ed), edited by R Rhodes, M Battin, A Silvers. New York: Oxford University Press, 47–57.

Stein R. 2020a. A year in, 1st patient to get gene editing for sickle cell disease is thriving. NPR (June 23). https://www.npr.org/sections/health-shots/2020/12/15/944184405/ 1st-patients-to-get-crispr-gene-editing-treatment-continue-to-thrive

Stein R. 2020b. Gene therapy shows promise for hemophilia, but could be most expensive U.S. drug ever. *Shots: Health News from NPR* (July 20). Accessed 7/28/2020. https:// www.npr.org/sections/health-shots/2020/07/20/800556057/gene-therapy-shows-promise-for-hemophilia-but-could-be-most-expensive-u-s-drug-e

Szabo L. 2018. Are we being misled about precision medicine? *The New York Times* (Sept. 11). Accessed 11/11/2018. https://www.nytimes.com/2018/09/11/opinion/cancer-genetic-testing-precision-medicine.html

Szabo L. 2017. Cancer treatment hype gives false hope to many cancer patients. *USA Today* (April 27). https://www.usatoday.com/story/news/2017/04/27/cancer-treatment-hype-gives-false-hope-many-patients/100972794/

Tarhini A, McDermott D, Ambavane A, Gupte-Singh K, Aponte-Ribero V, Ritchings C, et al. 2019. Clinical and economic outcomes associated with treatment sequences in patients with BRAF-mutant advanced melanoma. *Immunotherapy* 11(4): 283–95.

Taylor NP. 2020. Illumina inks $8B Grail buyout for liquid biopsy market. Investors are not sold. *MedTech Drive* (Sept. 21). Accessed 2/3/2021. https://www.medtechdive.com/news/illumina-inks-8b-grail-buyout-for-liquid-biopsy-market-investors-are-not/585584/

Taylor P. 2018. Novartis says $4m price is reasonable for SMA gene therapy. *Pharmaphorum* (Nov. 6). Accessed 11/19/2018. https://pharmaphorum.com/news/novartis-says-4m-price-is-reasonable-for-sma-gene-therapy/

Temel JS, Gainor JF, Sullivan RJ, Greer JA. 2018. Keeping expectations in check with immune checkpoint inhibitors. *Journal of Clinical Oncology* 36: 1654–57.

Temel JS, Greer JA, Muzikansky A, Gallagher ER, Admane S, Jackson VA, et al. 2010. Early palliative care for patients with non-small-cell lung cancer. *New England Journal of Medicine* 363: 733–42.

Temkin L. 1993. *Inequality*. Oxford, UK: Oxford University Press.

Temkin L. 2003. Inequality defended. *Ethics* 113: 764–82.

Thomasma DC, Muraskas J, Marshall PA, Myers T, Tomich P, O'Neill JA. 1996. The ethics of caring for conjoined twins: the Lakeberg twins. *Hastings Center Report* 26(4): 4–12.

Thompson A. 2019. A targeted agent for sickle cell disease—changing the protein but not the gene. *New England Journal of Medicine* 381: 579–80.

Thompson PA, Kantarjian HM, Cortes JE. 2015. Diagnosis and treatment of chronic myeloid leukemia in 2015. *Mayo Clinic Proceedings* 90: 1440–54.

Thorsteinsdottir B, Swetz KM, Albright RC. 2015. The ethics of chronic dialysis for the older patient: time to reevaluate the norms. *Clinical Journal of the American Society of Nephrology* 10: 2094–99.

Tilburt JC, Cassel CK. 2013. Why the ethics of parsimonious medicine is not the ethics of rationing. *JAMA* 309: 773–74.

Titov A, Valiullina A, Zmievskaya E, Zaikova E, Petukhov A, Miftakhova R, et al. 2020. Advancing CAR T-cell therapy for solid tumors: lessons learned from lymphoma treatment. *Cancers* 12(1): 125. doi: 10.3390/cancers12010125

Topalian SL, Hodi FS, Brahmer JR, Gettinger SN, Smith DC, McDermott DF, et al. 2019. Five-year survival and correlates among patients with advanced melanoma, renal cell carcinoma, or non-small-cell lung cancer treated with nivolumab. *JAMA Oncology* 5: 1411–20.

Tran E, Robbins PF, Yong-Chen L, Prickett TD, Gartner JJ, Jia L, et al. 2016. T-cell transfer therapy targeting mutant KRAS in cancer. *New England Journal of Medicine* 375: 2255–62.

Tranvag E, Norheim OF. 2018. How can biomarkers influence priority setting for cancer drugs? In *Cancer Biomarkers: Ethics, Economics, and Society*, edited by A Blanchard, R Strand. Kokstod, Norway: Megaloceros Press, 55–72.

Tu SM. 2010. *Origin of Cancers: Clinical Perspectives and Implications of a Stem-Cell Theory of Cancer*. New York: Springer.

Tumber MB. 2017. Restricted access: state Medicaid coverage of sofosbuvir hepatitis C treatment. *Journal of Legal Medicine* 37(1–2): 21–64.

Turtle CJ, Hay KA, Hanafi LA, Li D, Cherian S, Chen X, et al. 2017. Durable molecular remissions in chronic lymphocytic leukemia treated with CD19-specific chimeric antigen receptor-modified T-cells after failure of ibrutinib. *Journal of Clinical Oncology* 35: 3010–20.

Ubel PA. 2000. *Pricing Life: Why It's Time for Health Care Rationing.* Cambridge, MA: MIT Press.

Ugurel S, Schadendorf D, Horny K, Sucker A, Schramm S, Utikal J, et al. 2020. Elevated baseline serum PD-1 or PD L-1 predicts poor outcome of PD-1 inhibition therapy in metastatic melanoma. *Annals of Oncology* 31: 144–52.

United States Renal Data System. 2020. *2020 Annual Data Report.* Accessed 4/22/2022. https://adr.usrds.org/2020/

University of Chicago Medical Center. 2018. Supercharging your blood cells to defeat cancer. Accessed 1/31/2019. https://www.uchicagomedicine.org/conditions-services/cancer/car-t-cell-therapy?_vsrefdom=cartcelltherapy_google&gclid=EAIaIQobChM IxPe62uSY4AIVybXACh2UAw-xEAAYASAAEgKCZPD_BwE

Van Allen EM, Wagle N, Sucker A, Treacy DJ, Johannessen CM, Goetz EM, et al. 2014. The genetic landscape of clinical resistance to RAF inhibition in metastatic melanoma. *Cancer Discovery* 4: 94–109.

Van Cutsem E, Dicato M, Arber N, Berlin J, Cervantes A, Ciardiello F, et al. 2010. Molecular markers and biological targeted therapies in metastatic colorectal cancer: expert opinion and recommendations derived from the 11th ESMO/World Congress on Gastrointestinal Cancer, Barcelona, 2009. *Annals of Oncology* 21(Supplement 6): vi1–10.

Van Dussen L, Biegstraaten M, Hollak CEM, Dijkgraaf MGW. 2014. Cost-effectiveness of enzyme replacement therapy for type 1 Gaucher disease. *Orphanet Journal of Rare Diseases* 9: 51. Accessed 3/15/2018. http://www.ojrd.com/content/9/1/51

Vichinsky E, Hoppe CC, Ataga KI, Ware RE, Nduba V, El-Beshlawy A, et al. 2019. A phase 3 randomized trial of voxelotor in sickle cell disease. *New England Journal of Medicine* 381: 509–19.

Vokinger KN, Hwang TJ, Grischott T, Reichert S, Tibau A, Rosemann T, Ksselheim AS. 2020. Prices and clinical benefit of cancer drugs in the USA and Europe: a cost–benefit analysis. *Lancet Oncology* 21: 664–70.

Wagner J, Wickman E, DeRenzo C, Gottschalk S. 2020. CAR T-cell therapy for solid tumors: bright future or dark reality? *Molecular Therapy* 28: 2320–39.

Wainwright CE, Elborn JS, Ramsey BW, Marigowda G, Huang X, Cipolli M, et al. 2015. Lumacaftor–ivacaftor in patients with cystic fibrosis homozygous for Phe508del CFTR. *New England Journal of Medicine* 373: 220–31.

Walker T. 2018. Is precision medicine worth the hype? Oncologists weigh in. *Managed Health Care Executive* (June 27). Accessed 1/6/2019. http://www.managedhealthca reexecutive.com/leukemia-and-lymphoma/precision-medicine-worth-hype-oncologi sts-weigh

Wang S, Cang S, Liu D. 2016. Third-generation inhibitors targeting *EGFR* T790M mutation in advanced non-small cell lung cancer. *Journal of Hematology & Oncology* 9: 34. Accessed 2/4/2018. https://jhoonline.biomedcentral.com/articles/10.1186/s13 045-016-0268-z

Watanabe K, Kuramitsu S, Posey AD, June CH. 2018. Expanding the therapeutic window for CAR T-cell therapy in solid tumors: the knowns and unknowns of CAR T-cell biology. *Frontiers in Immunology* 9: 2486. doi: 10.3389/fimmu.2018.02486

Weissmann J. 2012. 5% of Americans made up 50% of U.S. health care spending. *The Atlantic* (Jan. 13). Accessed 7/24/2020. https://www.theatlantic.com/business/archive/2012/01/5-of-americans-made-up-50-of-us-health-care-spending/251402/

Wharam JF, Zhang F, Lu CY, Wagner AK, Nekhlyudov L, Earle CC, et al. 2018. Breast cancer diagnosis and treatment after high-deductible insurance enrollment. *Journal of Clinical Oncology* 36: 1121–27.

Wiebe C, Ho J, Gibson IW, Rush DN, Nickerson PW. 2018. Carpe diem—time to transition from empiric to precision medicine in kidney transplantation. *American Journal of Transplantation* 18: 1615–25. doi: 10.1111/ajt.14746

Wildavsky A. 1977. Doing better and feeling worse: the political pathology of healthcare policy. In *Doing Better and Feeling Worse: Health Care in the United States*, edited by JH Knowles. New York: W.W. Norton, 105–23.

Wilking N, Lopes G, Meier K, Simoens S, van Harten W, Vulto A. 2017. Can we continue to afford access to cancer treatment? *European Oncology & Haematology* 13(2): 114–19.

Wilper AP, Woolhandler S, Lasser KE, McCormick D, Bor DH, Himmelstein DU. 2009. Health insurance and mortality in US adults. *American Journal of Public Health* 99: 2289–95.

Winger BA, Shah NP. 2015. PPARγ: welcoming the new kid on the CML stem cell block. *Cancer Cell* 28: 409–11.

Winslow R. 2016. Cancer treatment's new direction: genetic testing helps oncologists target tumors and tailor treatments. *Wall Street Journal* (March 28). Accessed 4/22/22 https://www.wsj.com/articles/cancer-treatments-new-direction-1459193085.

Winslow R. 2014. Cancer's super-survivors: how the promise of immunotherapy is transforming oncology. *Wall Street Journal* (Dec. 4). Accessed 5/15/2016. http://www.wsj.com/articles/cancers-super-survivors-how-immunotherapy-is-transforming-oncology-1417714379

Winslow R. 2013. Gene breakthroughs spark a revolution in cancer treatment. *Wall Street Journal* (Aug. 13). Accessed 5/7/2016. http://www.wsj.com/articles/SB10001424127887323300004578557473861805376

Wolchok JD, Chiarion-Sileni V, Gonzalez R, Rutkowski P, Grob JJ, Cowey CL, et al. 2017. Overall survival with combined nivolumab and ipilimumab in advanced melanoma. *New England Journal of Medicine* 377: 1345–56.

Woolhandler S, Himmelstein D. 2017. The relationship of health insurance and mortality: is lack of insurance deadly? *Annals of Internal Medicine* 167: 424–31.

Workman P, Draetta GF, Schellens JH, Bernards R. 2017. How much longer will we put up with $100,000 cancer drugs? *Cell* 168: 579–83.

Wouters S, van Exel J, Baker R, Brouwer W. 2017. Priority to end of life treatments? Views of the public in the Netherlands. *Value in Health* 20: 107–17.

Woyach JA, Ruppert AS, Heerema NA, Zhao W, Booth AM, Ding W, et al. 2018. Ibrutinib regimens versus chemoimmunotherapy in older patients with untreated CLL. *New England journal of Medicine* 379: 2517–28.

Wu Q, Liao W, Zhang M, Huang J, Zhang P, Li Q. 2020. Cost-effectiveness of tucatinib in human epidermal growth factor receptor 2—positive metastatic breast cancer from the US and Chinese perspectives. *Frontiers in Oncology* 10: 1336. doi: 10.3389/fonc.2020.01336

Yabroff KR, Gansler T, Wender RC, Cullen KJ, Brawley OW. 2019. Minimizing the burden of cancer care in the United States: goals for a high-performing health care system. *CA: A Cancer Journal for Clinicians* 69: 166–83.

Yancy CW. 2020. COVID-19 and African Americans. *JAMA* 323: 1891–92.

Yap TA, Omlin A, de Bono JS. 2013. Development of therapeutic combinations targeting major cancer signaling pathways. *Journal of Clinical Oncology* 31: 1592–1605.

Yeo CJ, Simmons Z, Vivo DC, Darras BT. 2022. Ethical perspectives on treatment options with spinal muscular atrophy patients. *Annals of Neurology* 91: 305–16.

Yi M, Jiao D, Xu H, Liu Q, Zhao W, Han X, Wu K. 2018. Biomarkers for predicting efficacy of PD-1/PD L-1 inhibitors. *Molecular Cancer* 17: 129–43.

Young IM. 2003. Activist challenges to deliberative democracy. In *Debating Deliberative Democracy*, edited by J Fishkin, P Laslett. London: Blackwell, 102–20.

Younossi Z, Gordon SC, Ahmed A, Dieterich D, Saab S, Beckerman R. 2017. Treating Medicaid patients with hepatitis C: clinical and economic impact. *American Journal of Managed Care* 23(2): 107–24.

Yu HA, Tian SK, Drilon AE, Borsu L, Riely GJ, Arcila M, Ladanyi M. 2015. Acquired resistance of EGFR-mutant lung cancer to a T790M-specific EGFR inhibitor: emergence of a third mutation (C797S) in the EGFR tyrosine kinase domain. *JAMA Oncology* 1: 982–83.

Zafar SY. 2016. Financial toxicity of cancer care: it's time to intervene. *Journal of the National Cancer Institute* 108(5): djv 370.

Zaretsky JM, Garcia-Diaz A, Shin DS, Escuin-Ordinas H, Hugo W, Hu-Lieskovan S, et al. 2016. Mutations associated with acquired resistance to PD-1 blockade in melanoma. *New England Journal of Medicine* 375: 819–29.

Zimmerman S, Peters S. 2019. Appraising the tail of the survival curve in the era of PD-1/PD-L1 checkpoint blockade. *JAMA Oncology* 5: 1403–05.

Index